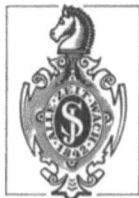

CAPD
in Children

Edited by
R. N. Fine K. Schärer O. Mehls

With 61 Figures

Springer-Verlag
Berlin Heidelberg New York Tokyo

RICHARD N. FINE, M.D., Professor of Pediatrics, UCLA School of
Medicine, Head, Division of Pediatric Nephrology, UCLA Center for the
Health Sciences, 10833 Le Conte Avenue, Los Angeles, California 90024,
USA

KARL SCHÄRER, M.D., Professor, Head, Division of Pediatric Nephrology,
University Children's Hospital, Im Neuenheimer Feld 150,
D-6900 Heidelberg, FRG

OTTO MEHLS, M.D., Professor, Head, Pediatric Dialysis Unit,
University Children's Hospital, Im Neuenheimer Feld 150,
D-6900 Heidelberg, FRG

ISBN-13: 978-3-642-70215-0   e-ISBN-13: 978-3-642-70213-6
DOI: 10.1007/978-3-642-70213-6

Library of Congress Cataloging in Publication Data. Main entry under title: CAPD in children.
Papers presented at the First International Symposium on CAPD in Children held May 14–15,
1984 at Heidelberg, Germany. Bibliography: p. 1. Peritoneal dialysis, Continuous ambulatory,
in children–Congresses. I. Fine, Richard N. II. Schärer, K. (Karl), 1929–   . III. Mehls, O.
(Otto), 1939–   . IV. International Symposium on CAPD in Children (1st : 1984 : Heidelberg,
Germany) RJ470.5.P47C37 1985 617'.461059 85-2704

2125/3130-543210

Preface

The renewal of interest in peritoneal dialysis as a treatment modality for patients with end-stage renal disease was stimulated by the report of Popovich and his colleagues in 1976 on the technique of CAPD. With the introduction of commercial dialysate-containing plastic bags, which markedly reduced the incidence of peritonitis, the use of CAPD as a primary treatment modality has increased significantly. At the present time, more than 12% of the patients undergoing dialysis in the United States are utilizing CAPD; however, the use of CAPD among pediatric patients is considerably greater.

The First International Symposium on CAPD in Children was organized in order to gather together experts with experience in treating children undergoing CAPD in an attempt to exchange current information on the utilization of this emerging technique in children. Since pediatric patients comprise a small percentage of the CAPD population and since limited data were available concerning specific methodology and complications of CAPD in children, it was hoped that an international symposium would provide a forum for an exchange of experience that would ultimately lead to better adaptation and increased utilization of this technique.

In this volume, the symposium participants present their experience with various aspects of the use of CAPD in children. The authors hope that the information will be helpful in the management of children with end-stage renal disease who require CAPD and that it will improve understanding of the use of peritoneal dialysis in general.

The Editors

Acknowledgments

The First International Symposium on CAPD in Children was supported by Stiftung Volkswagenwerk, Hannover, and by a number of firms listed in the printed program. Substantial financial contributions to this publication were received from both Fresenius AG, Bad Homburg, Fed. Rep. of Germany and Travenol Laboratories, Deerfield, Illinois, USA. We wish to extend our thanks to all authors and participants of the Symposium and to Dr. T. Thiekötter from Springer-Verlag who made it possible to produce this monograph within a reasonable time after the meeting. Mrs. Cornelia Meye and Mrs. Barbara Korn kindly assisted in preparing the workshop and the manuscripts.

Contents

List of Contributors

F. C. B. ABBAD, M.D., Department of Pediatric Nephrology, Kindergenees-kunde, Academisch Ziekenhuis, University of Amsterdam, Meiberg-dreef 9, NL 1105 AZ Amsterdam, The Netherlands

S. R. ALEXANDER, M.D., Department of Pediatrics, Oregon Health Sciences University, 3181 S.W. Sam Jackson Park Road, Portland, Oregon 97201, USA

G. AMATO, M.D., Nefrologia pediatrica, First Faculty of Medicine, University of Naples, Padiglioni 17, via Pansini, I-80131 Naples, Italy

W. ARNOLD, M.D., Southwest Pediatric Nehrology Study Group, Department of Pediatrics, University of Arkansas, Little Rock, Arkansas, USA

U. ASSOGBA, M.D., Department of Nephrology, Hôpital de la Pitié, 83, boulevard de l'Hôpital, F-75013 Paris 13, France

J. AUGUSTIN, M.D., Department of Internal Medicine, University of Heidelberg, Bergheimerstraße 56, D-6900 Heidelberg, FRG

A. BALAS, M.D., Research Assistant, EDTA Registration Committee, St. Thomas' Hospital, London SE1 7EH, United Kingdom

J. W. BALFE, M.D., F.R.C.P. (C), Division of Nephrology, The Hospital for Sick Children, 555 University Avenue, Toronto, Ontario M5G 1X8, Canada

G. BASILE, M.D., Department of Nephrology and Dialysis, G. Gaslini Institute, via V Maggio 39, I-16148 Genova, Italy

D. BESSARIONE, M.D., Endocrinology Chair, University of Genova, I-16148 Genova, Italy

K. E. BONZEL, M.D., Division of Pediatric Nephrology, University Children's Hospital, Im Neuenheimer Feld 150, D-6900 Heidelberg, FRG

A. BOUDJEMAA, M.D., Department of Nephrology, Hôpital de la Pitié, 83, boulevard de l'Hôpital, F-75013 Paris 13, France

M. BROYER, M.D., Professor of Pediatrics, Director, Department of Pediatric Nephrology, Hôpital Necker – Enfants Malades, 149, rue de Sèvres, F-75730 Paris Cédex 15, France

F. BRUNNER, M.D., Member, EDTA Registration Committee, Department of Internal Medicine, University of Basel, CH-4000 Basel, Switzerland

H. BRYNGER, M.D., Member, EDTA Registration Committee, Department of Surgery I, Sahlgrenska Sjukhuset, Göteborg, Sweden

B. BUSCH, M.D., Dialysis Unit, University Children's Hospital, Joseph-Stelzmann-Straße 9, D-5000 Köln 41, FRG

G. CAPASSO, M.D., Faculty of Medicine, University of Naples, Padiglioni 17, via Pansini, I-80131 Naples, Italy

G. CAPODICASA, M.D., Institute of Internal Medicine and Nephrology, University of Naples, Padiglioni 17, via Pansini, I-80131 Naples, Italy

C. CARELLA, M.D., Nefrologia pediatrica, First Faculty of Medicine, University of Naples, Padiglioni 17, via Pansini, I-80131 Naples, Italy

A. CARREA, M.D., Department of Nephrology and Dialysis, G. Gaslini Institute, via V Maggio 39, I-16148 Genova, Italy

C. CHANTLER, M.A., M.D., M.R.C.P., Professor of Paediatric Nephrology, Evelina Department of Pediatrics, Guy's Hospital, St. Thomas' Street, London SE1 9RT, United Kingdom

J.W. COBURN, M.D., Medical and Research Service, VA Wadsworth Medical Center, Department of Medicine, UCLA School of Medicine, Los Angeles, California 90024, USA

A.T. CORNEIL, R.N., Pediatric CAPD/CCPD Program, Doernbecher Memorial Hospital for Children, 3181 SW Sam Jackson Park Road, Portland, Oregon 97201, USA

P.Y. COSSETTE, M.D., Department of Nephrology, Hôpital de la Pitié, 83, boulevard de l'Hôpital, F-75013 Paris 13, France

A.-M. DARTOIS, Dietician, Unité de Recherches de Néphrologie Pédiatrique, Hôpital Necker – Enfants Malades, 149, rue de Sèvres, F-75730 Paris Cédex 15, France

D. DAVIDSON, R.N., BSN., Division of Pediatric Nephrology, UCLA Center for the Health Sciences, 10833 Le Conte Avenue, Los Angeles, California 90024

N. G. DE SANTO, M.D., Professor of Pediatrics, Nefrologia pediatrica, First Faculty of Medicine, University of Naples, Padiglioni 17, via Pansini, I-80131 Naples, Italy

V. DE SIMONE, M.D., Nefrologia pediatrica, First Faculty of Medicine, University of Naples, Padiglioni 17, via Pansini, I-80131 Naples, Italy

R. DONCKERWOLCKE, M.D., Professor of Pediatrics, Wilhelmina Kinderziekenhuis, University of Utrecht, Nieuwe Gracht 137, NL 3512 LK Utrecht, The Netherlands

R. DRACHMAN, M.D., Department of Pediatric Nephrology, Hôpital Nekker – Enfants Malades, 149, rue de Sèvres, F-75730 Paris Cédex 15, France

S. DUTTA, M.D., Department of Pediatrics, University of Oklahoma, 618 Northeast 15th Street, Oklahoma City, Oklahoma 73190, USA

R. N. FINE, M.D., Professor of Pediatrics, UCLA School of Medicine, Head, Division of Pediatric Nephrology, UCLA Center for the Health Sciences, 10833 Le Conte Avenue, Los Angeles, California 90024, USA

S. E. FINE, R.N., Clinical Nurse Specialist, Division of Pediatric Nephrology, UCLA Center for the Health Sciences, 10833 Le Conte Avenue, Los Angeles, California 90024, USA

J. FOLEY, R.N., M.S., Division of Pediatric Nephrology, UCLA Center for the Health Sciences, 10833 Le Conte Avenue, Los Angeles, California 90024, USA

G. M. GAHL, M.D., Department of Nephrology, Hôpital de la Pitié, 83, boulevard de l'Hôpital, F-75013 Paris 13, France

F. GINEVRI, M.D., Department of Nephrology and Dialysis, G. Gaslini Institute, via V Maggio 39, I-16148 Genova, Italy

C. GIORDANO, Professor, Istituto di Medicina interna e nefrologia, Università degli studi di Napoli, Policlinico Cappella Cangiani, Padiglione 17, via Pansini, I-80131 Naples, Italy

M. GIUSTI, M.D., Endocrinology chair, University of Genova, I-16148 Genova, Italy

A. GNASSO, M.D., Department of Internal Medicine, University of Heidelberg, Bergheimerstraße 56, D-6900 Heidelberg, FRG

M. GRÄNING, cand. med., Division of Pediatric Nephrology, University Children's Hospital, Im Neuenheimer Feld 150, D-6900 Heidelberg, FRG

M. C. GUBLER, M.D., Unité de Recherches de Néphrologie pédiatrique, Hôpital Necker – Enfants Malades, 149, rue de Sèvres, F-75730 Paris Cédex 15, France

R. GUSMANO, M.D., Professor of Pediatrics, Department of Nephrology and Dialysis, G. Gaslini Institute, via V Maggio 39, I-16148 Genova, Italy

W. HABERBOSCH, M.D., Department of Internal Medicine, University of Heidelberg, Bergheimerstraße 56, D-6900 Heidelberg, FRG

T. HALL, R.N., M.S., Division of Pediatric Nephrology, UCLA Center for the Health Sciences, 10833 Le Conte Avenue, Los Angeles, California 90024, USA

R. M. HANNING, M.D., Division of Nephrology, The Hospital for Sick Children, 555 University Avenue, Toronto, Ontario M5G 1X8, Canada

C. C. HEUCK, M.D., Head, Division of Laboratory Medicine, University Children's Hospital, Im Neuenheimer Feld 150, D-6900 Heidelberg, FRG

R. J. HOGG, M.D., Director, Southwest Pediatric Nephrology Study Group, Department of Pediatrics, University of Texas Health Science Center at Dallas, 5323 Harry Hines Boulevard, Dallas, Texas 75235, USA

B. ISSAD, M.D., Department of Nephrology, Hôpital de la Pitié, 83, boulevard de l'Hôpital, F-75013 Paris 13, France

C. JACOBS, M.D., EDTA Registration Committee, Centre Pasteur – Vallery – Radot, 26, rue des Peupliers, F-75013 Paris, France

H. KANGARLOO, M.D., UCLA Center for the Health Sciences, 10833 Le Conte Avenue, Los Angeles, California 90024, USA

E. C. KOHAUT, M.D. Professor of Pediatrics, Director of Pediatric Nephrology, Department of Pediatrics, University of Alabama, 1601 Sixth Avenue South, Birmingham, Alabama 35233, USA

P. KRAMER, M.D., Member, EDTA Registration Committee, Department of Internal Medicine, University of Göttingen, D-3400 Göttingen, FRG (deceased)

G. LAMA, M.D., Nefrologia pediatrica, First Faculty of Medicine, University of Naples, Padiglioni 17, via Pansini, I-80131 Naples, Italy

P. LANGLOIS, M.D., Department of Nephrology, Hôpital de la Pitié, 83, boulevard de l'Hôpital, F-75013 Paris, France

H. E. LEICHTER, M.D., Division of Pediatric Nephrology, UCLA Center for the Health Sciences, 10833 Le Conte Avenue, Los Angeles, California 90024

E. LEUMANN, M.D., University Children's Hospital, Steinwiesstraße 75, CH-8032 Zürich, Switzerland

G. M. LUM, M.D., Department of Pediatrics, University of Colorado Health Sciences Center, Denver, Colorado 80262

R. H. K. MAK, M.D., Lecturer in Paediatrics and Metabolic Medicine, Evelina Department of Paediatrics, Guy's Hospital, St. Thomas Street, London SE1 9RT, United Kingdom

B. MATTER, M.D., Department of Pediatrics, University of Oklahoma, 618 Northeast 15th Street, Oklahoma City, Oklahoma 73190, USA

H. MEHAMHA, M.D., Department of Nephrology, Hôpital de la Pitié, 83, boulevard de l'Hôpital, F-75013 Paris 13, France

O. MEHLS, M.D., Head, Pediatric Dialysis Unit, University Children's Hospital, Im Neuenheimer Feld 150, D-6900 Heidelberg, FRG

J. METCOFF, M.D., P.M.D., George Lynn Cross Research Professor, Departments of Pediatrics, Biochemistry and Molecular Biology, University of Oklahoma, 618 Northeast 15th Street, Oklahoma City, Oklahoma 73190, USA

D. E. MÜLLER-WIEFEL, M. D., Division of Pediatric Nephrology, University Children's Hospital, Im Neuenheimer Feld 150, D-6900 Heidelberg, FRG

J. NEMETH, M.D., Division of Pediatric Nephrology, University Children's Hospital, Steinwiesstraße 75, CH-8032 Zürich, Schwitzerland

P. NIAUDET, M.D., Department of Pediatric Nephrology, Hôpital Necker – Enfants Malades, 149, rue de Sèvres, F-75730 Paris Cédex 15, France

F. NUZZI, M.D., Nefrologia pediatrica, First Faculty of Medicine, University of Naples, Padiglioni, 17, via Pansini, I-80131 Naples, Italy

R. OLEGGINI, M.D., Department of Nephrology and Dialysis, G. Gaslini Institute, via V Maggio 39, I-16148 Genova, Italy

L. PAUNIER, M.D., Professor of Pediatrics, University Children's Hospital, 30, boulevard de la Cluse, CH-1211 Genève 4, Switzerland

J. PEDERSON, Department of Medicine, The Veterans Administration Hospital, Oklahoma City, Oklahoma 73190, USA

F. PERFUMO, M.D., Department of Nephrology and Dialysis, G. Gaslini Institute, via V Maggio 39, I-16148 Genova, Italy

S. L. B. PLOOS VAN AMSTEL, M.D., Department of Pediatric Nephrology, Kindergeneeskunde, Academisch Ziekenhuis, University of Amsterdam, Meibergdreef 9, NL-1105 AZ Amsterdam, The Netherlands

U. QUERFELD, M.D., Division of Pediatric Nephrology, University Children's Hospital, Im Neuenheimer Feld 150, D-6900 Heidelberg, FRG

G. RIZZONI, M.D., Head Dialysis Unit, Istituto Clinica Pediatrica, Universita degli Studi di Padova, via Giustiniani 3, I-35100 Padova, Italy

B. ROTH, M.D., University Children's Hospital, Joseph-Stelzmann-Straße 9, D-5000 Köln 41, FRG

J. ROTTEMBOURG, M.D., Department of Nephrology, Hôpital de la Pitié, 83, boulevard de l'Hôpital, F-75013 Paris, France

I. B. SALUSKY, M.D., Assistant Professor of Pediatrics, Director, Dialysis Program, Division of Pediatric Nephrology, UCLA Center for the Health Sciences, 10833 Le Conte Avenue, Los Angeles, California 90024, USA

K. SCHÄRER, M.D. Head, Division of Pediatric Nephrology, University Children's Hospital, Im Neuenheimer Feld 150, D-6900 Heidelberg, FRG

N. H. SELWOOD, M.D., Member, EDTA Registration Committee, United Kingdom Transplant, Bristol, United Kingdom

E. SLATOPOLSKY, M.D., Department of Medicine, Washington University School of Medicine, St. Louis, Missouri, USA

F. SCOPPA, M.D., Nefrologia pediatrica, First Faculty of Medicine, University of Naples, Padiglioni 17, via Pansini, I-80131 Naples, Italy

E.S. TANK, M.D., Division of Pediatric Urology, Oregon Health Sciences University, 3181 SW Sam Jackson Park Road, Portland, Oregon 97201, USA

A. VIGNEUX, M.D., Division of Nephrology, The Hospital for Sick Children, 555 University Avenue, Toronto, Ontario M5G 1X8, Canada

R. WARTHA, M.D., Division of Pediatric Nephrology, University Children's Hospital, Im Neuenheimer Feld 150, D-6900 Heidelberg, FRG

A.R. WATSON, M.D., Division of Nephrology, The Hospital for Sick Children, 555 University Avenue, Toronto, Ontario M5G 1X8, Canada

M. WILSON, R.N., Division of Pediatric Nephrology, UCLA Center for the Health Sciences, 10833 Le Conte Avenue, Los Angeles, California 90024, USA

A. WING, M.D., Chairman, EDTA Registration Committee, St. Thomas' Hospital, London SE1 7EH, United Kingdom

S.H. ZLOTKIN, M.D., Division of Nephrology, The Hospital for Sick Children, 555 University Avenue, Toronto, Ontario M5G 1X8, Canada

Cellular Abnormalities in Uremia *

J. Metcoff, J. Pederson, B. Matter, and S. Dutta, with the technical assistance of G. Burns, J. Stow, and J. Gable

Introduction

Numerous metabolic abnormalities have been documented in patients with chronic renal failure and uremia. Among these, abnormal energy, amino acid, and protein metabolism are prominent [1–4]. Abnormalities in these major metabolic pathways may be related in part to uremic toxins. Most of these are dialyzable and should therefore be removed by maintenance dialysis therapy. However, some of the abnormalities in energy and protein metabolism may reflect a subtle form of chronic malnutrition at the cellular level. This type of malnutrition would affect substrate availability and the activity of enzymes related to energy metabolism and protein synthesis, as found in protein-calorie malnutrition of children [5]. To evaluate this possibility, a cell model is required. Classically, muscle biopsies have been used as a cell source. The studies of Fürst, Bergström, Alvestrand, and their co-workers [1, 2, 6] have provided important information concerning amino acid pools in tissues, using muscle as a model. Circulating polymorphonuclear leukocytes (granulocytes) are commonly used to study the mechanism of phagocytosis but also may be used to quantify enzyme activities [7], metabolic functions such as glucose utilization [8–10], cell amino acid pools [11], energy levels [12–15], and protein synthesis (7, 16–18). This tissue has the advantage of being easily accessible through relatively nontraumatic procedures. We have used the granulocyte to examine several major metabolic parameters at the cellular level in normal subjects, in nondialyzed chronic uremics, in uremics with hemodialytic maintenance therapy, in some of the hemodialyzed patients supplemented by amino acid infusions for a period of 3 months, and in a few patients being treated with continuous ambulatory peritoneal dialysis (CAPD).

Methods

Subjects

In this study, approved by the Human Experimentation Committee, all subjects gave written informed consent to participate.

---

* The studies of the CAPD patients were supported by a research award from Travenol Laboratories, Inc., Deerfield, Illinois. The studies on the nondialyzed uremics, hemodialyzed patients and control subjects was supported by a grant from NIH, NIAMDD, AM 19503.

Controls: 32 healthy, volunteer donors (21–42 years of age) provided blood for normal reference data.

Uremics: Nine patients were studied before any dialysis procedures were started. A group of 40 uremics with end stage renal disease (ESRD) undergoing maintenance hemodialysis three times weekly were studied after they had been stabilized for at least 2 months on dialysis. Blood samples were obtained prior to a dialysis session. Of these patients, 18 subsequently received a course of commercially available amino acid infusions (10% Aminosyn, Abbott Laboratories) after each dialysis session, dialyzer disconnected, for a 3month period. Observations were made before the infusions were begun and at monthly intervals during the infusion periods. Ten patients stabilized on CAPD for at least 3 months were studied in the morning after completion of the previous night's exchange, with the abdominal cavity drained, and before the next dialysate was introduced. All subjects and patients were asked to fast for at least 8 hours prior to the study.

Laboratory Methods

Leukocytes were isolated by heparin-dextran sedimentation, followed by Ficoll-Hypaque isolation in the cold (approximately 4 °C), and the isolated granulocytes were then suspended in 0.16 M KCl [19]. The suspension contains 95%–98% granulocytes, and approximately 97% are viable, based on trypan-blue exclusion. Enzyme activities (pyruvate kinase, phosphofructokinase, glucose-6-phosphate dehydrogenase, adenylate kinase) were assayed spectrophotometrically; protein synthesis was determined by incorporation of ^{3}H-Leucine, in vitro. Nucleotides were assayed following perchloric acid precipitation of the KCl suspension of granulocytes and neutralization. All determinations were performed by standardized methods [20]. The utilization of glucose at the cellular level was measured by incubation of leukocytes in a medium containing 5-mM glucose for 30 min at 37 °C. Approximately $2–4 \times 10^7$ cells were used. The reaction was stopped with 6 M perchloric acid and the metabolites assayed fluorometrically. Amino acids were determined from a trichloracetic acid extract of the isolated granulocytes suspension, adjusted to a pH 2.0 with sodium citrate, using a high-pressure liquid chromatography system with automatic sample injection and fluorometric detection following column elution with sodium citrate buffers at two temperatures and three or five pH's [21]. All leukocyte data for each subject were obtained from the same blood sample and use DNA as a reference. DNA was determined by a modification of the method of Giles [22].

Data Analyses

All data were recorded on previously prepared special forms. They were entered into a computerized data base, verified, screened for outliers, with appropriate transformations made, and subsequently analyzed using statistical analytical systems (SAS) procedures with appropriate interface programs.

Results

Glycolysis

Glycolytic Enzyme and Adenylate Kinase Activities (Table 1)

Leukocytes may be considered experimental animals reflecting human cell metabolism. Their energy is derived from glycolysis. Phosphofructokinase is the major rate-controlling enzyme in the glycolytic pathway, but from a biological point of view, pyruvate kinase, at the end of the glycolytic stream, is also rate-limiting. It is a unidirectional enzyme which catalyzes the transfer of a high-energy bond from phosphoenolpyruvate to ADP in order to form ATP and the substrate product pyruvate.

Among three major enzymes in the glycolytic stream, glucose-6-phosphate dehydrogenase, phosphofructokinase, and pyruvate kinase, only the latter was significantly reduced in nondialyzed and hemodialyzed uremics compared to controls. In these preliminary studies of the CAPD patients, pyruvate kinase activity was elevated and significantly greater than found in the other two groups of uremics or in normal controls.

Although not a glycolytic enzyme, adenylate kinase catalyzes the reaction $ATP + AMP = 2\,ADP$ and thereby regulates the balance of nucleotides contributing to the energy level. Adenylate kinase activities also were significantly reduced in the uremics compared to controls.

Energy Charge (Fig. 1)

Energy charge is a concept proposed by Atkinson [23]. It relates the balance of nucleotides with respect to their potential for generating or utilizing ATP sequences. An equilibrium energy charge ratio is 0.82–0.84. An energy charge level signifi-

Table 1. Glycolytic enzymes (n mol/min/mg DNA)

Enzymes		Nondialyzed	HEMO	CAPD	Controls
Pyruvate Kinase	m	n, 9	n, 40	n, 9	n, 32
		13 278[a]	12 385[a]	16 598[a, b]	14 520
	SE	851	525	701	488
Adenylate Kinase		1 047[a]	1 016[a]	721[a, b]	1 206
		58	52	55	43
Phosphofructokinase		322	315	287[a]	333
		16	13	15	14
Glucose-6-PO₄-dehydrogenase		2 372	2 317	2 621	2 552
		191	121	171	82

[a] $P < 0.05$ vs controls.
[b] $P < 0.05$ vs hemodialyzed.

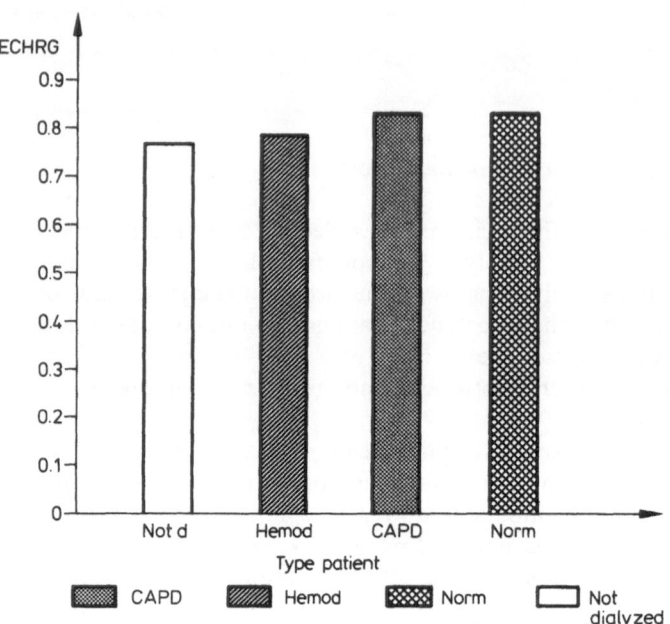

Fig. 1. Cell energy charge. (ECHRG = ATP + 0.5) (ADP)/(ATP + ADP + AMP). Normals: $n = 32$; non-dialyzed uremics: $n = 9$; hemodialysis: $n = 40$; CAPD: $n = 10$

cantly lower than this is consistent with inhibition of ATP-utilizing sequences. Energy charge in the "resting" leukocytes was significantly reduced in nondialyzed uremics and in those undergoing hemodialysis compared to control subjects ($P < 0.05$). Although our data for CAPD-treated patients is very limited, the preliminary results suggest that the energy charge levels were not significantly different from control subjects.

Glucose Utilization (Fig. 2)

Preliminary studies showed that lactate formation was very active starting from glucose-6-phosphate, while the formation of other metabolites was negligible. Glucose-6-phosphatase activity was minimal as well, suggesting the absence of a futile cycle. Thus the metabolites of glycolytic flux derived from the utilization of the exogenous glucose could be inferred to reflect glucose utilization by the cells. The results indicate that there is an abnormal metabolite generation pattern at the level of the triose phosphates. No significant difference was detected either in the formation of glucose-6-phosphate or in lactate formation. Thus, glycolysis did not appear to be significantly reduced in the uremics. However, activities of enzymes which participate in the interconversion of the triose phosphate metabolites were not analyzed. The large accumulation of glucose-6-phosphate and relatively low levels of fructose 1-6-diphosphate observed in the incubated uremic leukocytes suggests a defect in regulation of glycolytic flux at the level of phosphofructokinase. Curiously, however, activity of this enzyme in the hemodialyzed uremic patients was not significantly decreased. Also unexplainable at the present time, the formation of pyruvate from phosphoenolpyruvate was not reduced in these uremic leukocytes, although the ac-

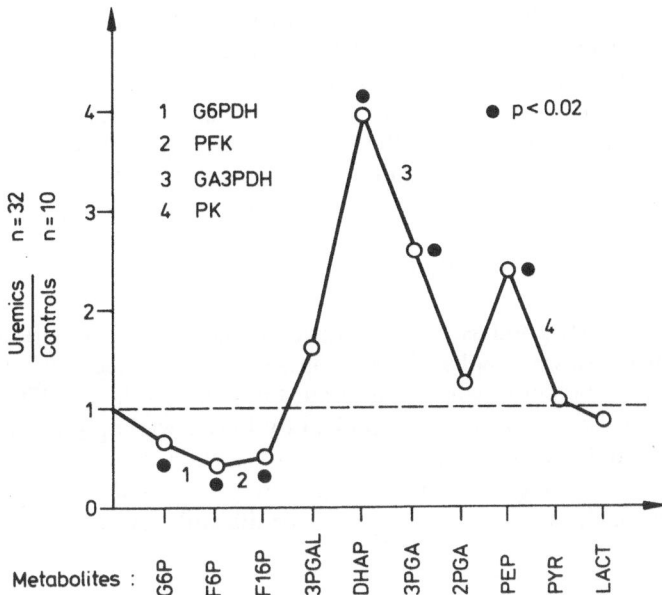

Fig. 2. Use of glucose by uremic vs normal cells (cells incubated with 5 m*M* glucose for 30 min at 37 °C)

tivity of the catalyzing enzyme, pyruvate kinase, was significantly reduced. It is conceivable that isoenzyme patterns for phosphofructokinase and pyruvate kinase are different in uremic cells compared with control cells. It is also possible that the enzyme activity does not reflect content of the active enzyme or that a statistically significant reduction of enzyme activity may not have equivalent biological significance.

Adenine Nucleotides in Incubated Uremic Leukocytes

Nucleotide production by the leukocytes incubated with 5-m*M* glucose was abnormal with respect to ADP and AMP, both of which were significantly reduced compared with controls. ATP production was normal, thus suggesting that ATP generation was not suppressed in the presence of glucose utilization. However, the total nucleotide pool in uremics was lower than in controls. Nonetheless, the energy charge in these incubated leukocytes metabolizing glucose achieved normal levels [24].

Protein Metabolism

Plasma Essential Amino Acids

In the stable, hemodialyzed patients, the plasma levels of the essential amino acids were similar to those found in controls. Only histidine and arginine differed, both exhibiting higher levels than in controls [20]. Among the CAPD patients, plasma methionine, isoleucine, and phenylalanine levels were higher than those found in either controls or hemodialysis patients. Tyrosine levels were equivalent to those in the controls, but higher than those in hemodialysis patients. These preliminary studies suggest that the CAPD treatment is associated with normal or slightly elevated levels for the essential amino acids.

Plasma Nonessential Amino Acids

Among the nonessential amino acids, plasma levels in virtually all the hemodialyzed patients, were higher than in controls with the exception of taurine, which was lower, and alanine, which was about the same. In the CAPD patients, levels of taurine and aspartic acid were significantly lower, while glycine was increased, relative to control subjects. The remaining nonessential amino acids were within the normal range for control subjects. Compared to hemodialyzed patients, taurine, aspartic acid, glycine, and ornithine were significantly lower.

Leukocyte Essential Amino Acids

In hemodialyzed patients, we found a significant reduction of the cellular levels of the branched-chain amino acids and methionine [20]. The levels of the other intracellular essential amino acids were similar to those in normal subjects. The relative intracellular concentrations of the branched-chain amino acids and methionine are illustrated in Fig. 3. The cellular level of leucine in the CAPD patients was not significantly different from normal. However, with the exception of leucine, levels of virtually all of the other essential intracellular amino acids were significantly reduced compared with both controls and hemodialyzed patients ($P < 0.05$).

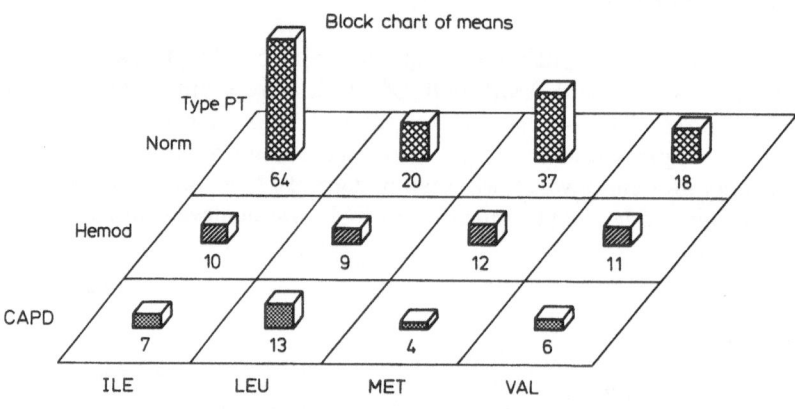

Fig. 3. Some cell amino acid levels in dialysis patients vs normals (numbers in *squares,* mean cell amino acid values). Normals: $n = 10$; hemodialysis: $n = 37$; CAPD: $n = 10$. See text.

Leukocyte Nonessential Amino Acids

Among the nonessential amino acids, cell levels of taurine and glutamic acid were significantly elevated, while that of ornithine was reduced in hemodialyzed uremics [20]. For the CAPD patients, only aspartic, glutamic, and ornithine levels were significantly lower than control subjects. Levels of these amino acids also were lower than those noted in the hemodialyzed patients.

These preliminary comparisons of the amino acid pools among CAPD, hemodialyzed, and control subjects suggests that the CAPD treatment may be associated with normal or high plasma essential amino acid levels, compared with control subjects. On the other hand, uremia is characterized by significant deficits of the intracellular branched-chain amino acids and methionine. With the exception of leucine, this situation appears to persist in the first ten CAPD patients we have studied. Cell levels of threonine, histidine, and lysine also were reduced in the CAPD patients.

Protein Synthesis (Fig. 4)

Protein synthesis was significantly reduced in the nondialyzed and stabilized hemodialysis patients compared with control subjects ($P < 0.05$). In contrast, preliminary data from CAPD patients suggest that the rate of protein synthesis is higher and does not differ significantly from control subjects. Since the incorporation of the labelled leucine into protein may be modified both by transport of the amino acid across the cell membrane and by the intracellular amino acid pool size, and since

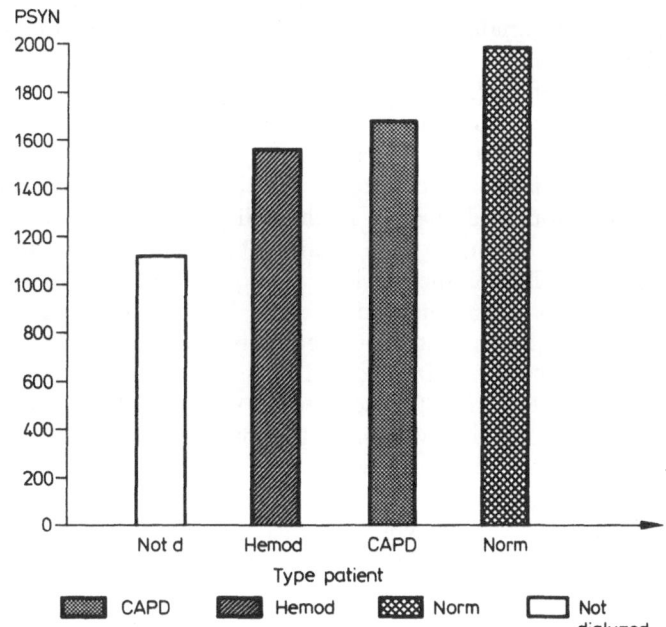

Fig. 4. Cell protein synthesis in uremics vs controls (3H-Leu incorporation in pmol/h/mg DNA). Normals: $n = 32$; nondialyzed uremics: $n = 9$; hemodialysis: $n = 40$; CAPD: $n = 10$.

membrane transport could be different in uremics compared with controls, we contrasted the apparent incorporations of label for protein synthesis in leukocytes of three uremics and three controls, measuring the total intracellular concentration of leucine to determine specific activity. The differences between the two groups remained essentially the same after adjusting for pool size. Thus, we believe it is reasonable to assume that the observed differences between uremics and controls are valid.

Attempts To Improve Protein Synthesis and Energy Levels in Uremics

We know from the studies of Harper's group that amino acid imbalance, that is, disproportionate amounts of one or more amino acids with respect to the others, will impair intracellular transport of some essential amino acids and limit protein synthesis and energy metabolism in experimental animals [25]. Thus, we reasoned that to improve protein synthesis and energy levels in uremics would require reestablishing appropriate proportions by correcting imbalance among the intracellular amino acids. Presumably, the critical amino acids whose relative concentrations require adjustment are those most closely related to the bioactivities. However, there were virtually no significant product : moment self-correlations between extracellular and intracellular amino acids among the 37 stabilized uremics on hemodialysis, with the exception of ornithine, which had a simple correlation coefficient ($r = 0.37$) between its intracellular and extracellular levels.

Multiple regression analysis makes it possible to determine which combinations of a series of independent variables best explain the variance, i.e., predicts the values, of a dependent variable. Taking intracellular energy charge or protein synthesis as dependent variables and the intracellular levels of the amino acids as independent variables, it was possible to identify sets of intracellular amino acids which accounted for a significant proportion of the variance in energy charge and protein synthesis [20].

Using a commercially available concentrated (10%) amino acid mixture, 500 ml was infused in each of 22 patients for a 3-month period following each dialysis session, with dialyzer disconnected. Baseline values were obtained prior to the amino acid infusions and changes in the cell parameters were examined at monthly intervals. Blood samples were obtained before the dialysis session. This usually was 2 or 3 days following the previous amino acid infusion. In all, these patients received 1.6–1.8 kg of free amino acids over the 3-month treatment interval.

Table 2 [20] indicates the predictors of energy charge and their coefficients observed in the 40 stabilized hemodialysis patients. Also shown are the baseline values for the subset of 18 of these uremics who completed 3 months of amino acid infusions, as compared with the values of control subjects. All nucleotide values were available at all points in only 16 of the 18 patients.

Among the set of five predictors selected by the model, only aspartic acid made significant ($P < 0.05$) contributions to the prediction. However, the other four amino acids, especially ornithine, contributed more than 1.5% to the regression.

Combinations of six cell amino acid levels accounted for a significant proportion of the variance in protein synthesis (Table 3) [20]. The baseline values for these

Table 2. Combination of cell-amino acid levels as predictors of energy level in uremics [20]

Predictors[a]	B Value	P	Baseline values[b]	
			Uremics	Controls
Intercept	0.766		n mol/mg DNA	
ASP	−0.00075	0.007	115***	81
GLU	0.00018	0.225	251	209
GLY	0.00059	0.209	118***	82
ORN	0.00053	0.052	84**	121
ARG	−0.00325	0.159	13**	7
			Energy charge[c]	
$R^2 = 0.333$; Df = 35; $P = 0.036$			0.77*	0.84

*, $P < 0.01$; **, $P < 0.05$; ***, $P < 0.08$ vs controls.
[a] Derived by multiple regression best subset analysis from data of 27 uremics.
[b] Values from 16 uremics completing 3 months of amino acid infusions and 10 control subjects.
[c] Data from 18 uremics and 32 controls.

Table 3. Combination of plasma amino acid levels as predictors of level of protein synthesis in uremics [20]

Predictors[a]	B Value	P	Baseline values[b]	
			Uremics	Controls
Intercept	11.153		n mol/mg DNA	
GLY	−0.027	0.002	372***	219
ALA	0.010	0.176	320	331
VAL	−0.059	0.011	149	174
MET	0.254	0.081	26	19
TYR	0.102	0.164	39	44
ORN	0.084	0.012	76*	41
ARG	0.048	0.076	116**	73
			Protein synthesis[c] (pmol/h/mg DNA)	
$R^2 = 0.433$; Df = 37; $P = 0.006$			1483*	1998

*, $P < 0.01$; **, $P < 0.05$; ***, $P < 0.08$ vs controls.
[a] Derived by multiple regression best subset analysis from data of 37 uremics.
[b] Values from 16 uremics completing 3 months of amino acid infusions and 21 control subjects.
[c] Data from 18 uremics and 32 controls.

amino acids in the uremic subjects are also compared with values in controls. Isoleucine was the only statistically significant predictor in this set, but each of the other amino acids contributed more than a 1.5% increment to the prediction and were therefore selected by the model.

We could not detect improvement in the level of energy charge or in the activity of the enzymes pyruvate kinase and adenlyate kinase following 3 months of the amino acid infusions [20]. Levels of ATP appeared to be reduced, particularly at the 2-month study interval.

After 3 months of amino acid infusions, there was a slight, but not statistically significant, increase in protein synthesis for 17 of the 18 patients for whom data were complete. However, while the level of protein synthesis was still below the mean value for the normal subjects, the difference between the means of the uremic and control subjects after 3 months of infusions was not statistically significant, suggesting that the gap may have been narrowed [20].

Our inability to detect a significant increment in the level of energy charge or of protein synthesis following 3 months of amino acid infusions was accompanied by failure to improve the imbalance among the intracellular amino acid predictors.

For those amino acids predictive of protein synthesis, all declined further from baseline values by at least 25%. The already low values for the branched-chain amino acids valine and isoleucine were reduced by 50% from their starting value. These reductions were significant for valine, isoleucine, lysine, and ornithine.

For the amino acid predictors of energy charge, the level of ornithine was significantly reduced by 43%, while the other amino acids, with the exception of glutamate, showed less reduction from their baseline values. Glutamate levels increased, but the increment was not statistically significant (Table 4) [20].

Summary of Results

The circulating granulocyte was used as a model to study cellular abnormalities in uremia in three groups of uremic patients: 9 non-dialyzed, 40 hemodialyzed and 10 on CAPD. These were compared to 32 normal subjects. Glucose utilization, energy levels (ATP, ADP, AMP), energy charge (Ech = ATP + 0.5 ADP/[ATP + ADP + AMP]), protein synthesis (^{3}H-LEU incorporation), glycolytic enzyme activities, and amino acid pools were studied. Significant reductions in energy charge, protein synthesis and pyruvate kinase activities were found in the undialyzed and hemodialyzed uremics, compared to normals. Protein synthesis, energy charge and pyruvate kinase activity in CAPD did not differ significantly from controls. The intracellular amino acid pools, particularly branched chain amino acids, were significantly reduced in the uremics. Multiple regression analysis identified a set of intracellular amino acids related to protein synthesis and energy charge in hemodialyzed

Table 4. Effect of amino acid infusions on combinations of cell amino acids [20][a]

Predictors of protein synthesis	% Change	Predictors of energy charge	% Change
Aspartic	− 24	Aspartic	− 24
Valine	− 48[b]	Glutamic	+ 39
Isoleucine	− 54[b]	Glycine	− 6
Ornithine	− 43[b]	Ornithine	− 43[b]
Lysine	− 36[b]	Arginine	− 24
Tryptophan	− 76		

[a] Using paired values only, $n = 11$ patients. % change is $\dfrac{\text{Baseline value} - 3 \text{ months value}}{\text{Baseline value}} \times 100$.

[b] $P < 0.05$ vs baseline.

uremics. Infusions of a 10% amino acid solution for 3 months in these hemodialyzed patients did not correct either the cellular amino acid imbalance, protein synthesis, or energy charge. We conclude that intracellular malnutrition occurs in uremia and requires correction to improve protein synthesis and energy levels. CAPD seems to improve some cell bioactivities and may be a corrective step toward improvement of cellular malnutrition in uremics.

Discussion

The observations in this report confirm the concept originally derived from muscle analysis, as described by Fürst, Alvestrand, Bergström, and their colleagues [1, 2, 6], that intracellular amino acid imbalance and energy level are related and may modulate protein synthesis. The circulating granulocyte is a readily available, viable cell model. It is increasingly being used in place of muscle biopsies. Multiple regression analysis, as a statistical tool, extends the conceptual model. The data presented here indicate that extensive cellular abnormalities persist in apparently adequately nourished, stabilized adult uremics undergoing various types of dialytic procedures.

The reductions in cellular protein synthesis, energy levels, and glycolytic enzyme activities are similar to those found in muscle in protein-calorie malnutrition (PCM) of children [5]. The reductions of pyruvate kinase and adenylate kinase activities and of nucleotide levels in leukocytes were also similar to those reported for PCM [14, 15]. The deviations of the intracellular amino acid levels in the leukocytes of the uremics were similar to the patterns found in muscle of some patients of Alvestrand et al. [26] and/or those of Broyer et al. [27]. We have not encountered values for intracellular amino acids in either muscle or leukocytes of PCM patients. Wells and Smits indicated that leukocyte amino acid concentrations seemed to resemble more closely those in muscle than in plasma; however, they did not study muscle [11].

Infusions of a commonly used, commercially available amino acid solution administered for as long as 3 months in uremic patients stabilized by hemodialysis did not seem to improve the intracellular environment sufficiently to correct the abnormalities of cellular amino acid imbalance, reduced energy level, or protein synthesis [20]. The data from the ten CAPD patients reported here is too preliminary to be conclusive. However, the changes in cellular bioactivities appear to be in the right direction. For these patients who had been on CAPD management for at least 3 months, plasma amino acid levels were within the normal range. Protein synthesis and energy charge levels appeared to be more nearly normal and did not differ significantly from controls. However, the intracellular amino acid pools were still abnormal.

Conclusions

1. The circulating granulocyte appears to be a useful cell model to detect and monitor cellular abnormalities in uremia.

2. Uremic patients with ESRD, including those stabilized by maintenance hemodialysis, are characterized by cellular abnormalities in glycolytic enzyme activities, energy metabolism, and protein synthesis, all being decreased relative to controls. These abnormalities were similar to those reported for children with severe PCM.

3. The levels of cell energy and protein synthesis in uremics were largely accounted for by particular combinations of intracellular amino acid levels, as determined by a multiple regression model.

4. Supplementary amino acid infusions for 3 months in patients undergoing hemodialysis did not significantly improve intracellular levels of those amino acids which were predictive of the energy levels or protein synthesis. Neither energy charge nor protein synthesis were significantly improved by the intravenous amino acid supplements.

5. Preliminary data from a few CAPD patients suggests that the cellular abnormalities were similar to those found in hemodialyzed patients but that energy level and protein synthesis were nearly normal. However, further data are required before these preliminary, though encouraging, observations can be considered conclusive.

Acknowledgments We appreciate the technical support provided by Gayle Burns, James Gable, Marie Smith, R. N., and Mitzi Klarich, R. N. We are indebted to Paul Costiloe, Ph. D., for guidance in experimental design and data analyses, to Don Wood, systems analyst, for assistance in programming, and to Edith Alyce for preparation of the manuscript.

References

1. Fürst P, Bergström J, Josephson B, Noree LO (1970) The effect of dialysis and administration of essential amino acids on plasma and muscle protein synthesis studied with ^{15}N in uremic patients. Proc Eur Dial Transpl Assoc 7:175–180
2. Bergström J, Fürst P, Noree LO, Vinnars E (1975) Intracellular free amino acids in uremic patients as influenced by amino acid supply. Kidney Int 7:S345–348
3. Mitch WE, Clark AS (1983) Muscle protein turnover in uremia. Kidney Int 24, Suppl 16:S2–S8
4. Rubenfeld S, Garber AJ (1978) Abnormal carbohydrate metabolism in chronic renal failure. J Clin Invest 62:20–28
5. Metcoff J (1975) Cellular energy metabolism in protein-calorie malnutrition. In: Olson R (ed) Protein-calorie malnutrition. Academic, New York pp 65–91
6. Alvestrand A, Fürst P, Bergström J (1983) Intracellular amino acids in muscle. Kidney Int 24 Suppl 16:S9–S16
7. Metcoff J, Lindeman R, Baxter D, Pederson J (1978) Cell metabolism in uremia. Am J Clin Nutr 31:1627–1634
8. Beck WS (1958) The control of leukocyte glycolysis. J Biol Chem 232:251–270
9. Baehner RL, Gilman N, Karnovsky (1970) Repiration and glucose oxidation in human and guinea pig leukocytes: comparative studies. J Clin Invest 49:692–700
10. Stjernholm RL, Burns CP, Hohnadel JH (1972) Carbohydrate metabolism by leukocytes. Enzyme 13:7
11. Wells FE, Smits BJ (1980) Leukocyte amino acid concentrations and their relationship to changes in plasma amino acids. J Parent Enteral Nutr 4:264–267

12. Foster M, Terry L (1967) Studies on the energy metabolism of human leukocytes I. Oxidative phosphorylation by human leukocyte mitochondria. Blood 30:168–175
13. Jemelin M, Frei J (1970) Leukocyte energy metabolism: anaerobic and aerobic ATP production and related enzymes. Enzym Biol Clin 2:289
14. Yoshida T, Metcoff J, Frenk S, de la Pena C (1967) Intermediary metabolites and adenine nucleotides in leukocytes of children with protein-calorie malnutrition. Nature 214:525–526
15. Yoshida T, Metcoff J, Frenk S (1968) Reduced pyruvic kinase activity, altered growth patterns of ATP in leukocytes and protein-calorie malnutrition. Am J Clin Nutr 21:162
16. Winkler K, Heller-Shoch G, Neth R (1972) Protein synthesis in human leukocytes. IV. Mutual inhibition of amino acids in cell suspensions and cell-free systems. Hoppe Seylers Z Physiol Chem 353:787–792
17. Winkler K (1972) Protein synthesis in human leukocytes II. Kinetics of the flow of amino acids from the extracellular space and the intracellular pools resulting in protein synthesis. Hoppe Seylers Z Physiol Chem 353:782–786
18. Metcoff J, Wikman-Coffelt J, Yoshida T et al. (1973) Energy metabolism and protein synthesis in human leukocytes during pregnancy and in placenta related to fetal growth. Pediatrics 51:866–877
19. Boyum A (1968) Isolation of mononuclear cells and granulocytes from human blood. Scand J Clin Lab Invest 21 [Suppl 97]:77–83
20. Metcoff J, Dutta S, Burns G, Pederson J, Matter B, Rennert O (1983) Effects of amino acid infusions on cell metabolism in hemodialyzed patients with uremia. Kidney Int 24 Suppl 16:S87–S92
21. Benson JR (1976) Single column analysis of amino acids. In: Simmons IL, Ewing GW (eds) Applications of the newer techniques of analysis. Plenum, New York, p 233
22. Giles KW, Myers H (1965) An improved diphenylamine method for the estimation of deoxyribonucleic acid. Nature 105:93
23. Atkinson DE (1968) The energy charge of the adenylate pool as a regulatory parameter. Interaction with feedback modifiers. Biochemistry 7:4030
24. Dutta S, Metcoff J, Pederson J, Matter B, Costiloe P (1981) Glycolytic flux and protein synthesis in circulating leukocytes of chronic uremic patients. Fed Proc 40:753
25. Tews JK, Young-Woo LK, Harper AE (1979) Induction of threonine imbalance by dispensable amino acids: Relation to competition for amino acid transport into brain. J Nutr 109:304–315
26. Alvestrand A, Bergström J, Fürst P, Germans G, Widstom V (1978) Effect of essential amino acid supplementation on muscle and plasma free amino acids in chronic uremia. Kidney Int 14:323–329
27. Broyer M, Jean G, Dartois H, Kleinknecht C (1980) Plasma and muscle free amino acids in children at the early stages of renal failure. Am J Clin Nutr 33:1396–1401

A Comparison of Peritoneal Water and Solute Movement in Young and Older Children on CAPD

J. W. Balfe, R. M. Hanning, A. Vigneux, and A. R. Watson

Introduction

Continuous Ambulatory Pertioneal Dialysis (CAPD) has encouraged nephrologists around the world to reassess peritoneal dialysis as an acceptable replacement of renal function. Since CAPD is so applicable to children, especially infants, there is an added incentive for pediatric nephrologists to assess the dialytic characteristics of the child's peritoneal membrane. Anecdotally, pediatric nephrologists have found peritoneal dialysis difficult to perform on very young infants. The most apparent and troublesome difficulty is a perceived reduction in ultrafiltration characteristics. One of the reasons for this impression is that infants, after cardiac surgery, may develop acute renal failure, and acute peritoneal dialysis is often the type of dialysis used. The reasons for the difficulty in removing fluid by ultrafiltration are multiple. Often, SVCH children have very reduced left ventricular function and therefore, a sluggish mesenteric circulation. Therefore, this impression concerning peritoneal dialysis in infants and young children may be incorrect and in fact may be the results of a number of other causes which do not necessarily involve the peritoneal membrane. We have previously reported that the glucose and protein concentration in "spent" or "used" dialysate from CAPD patients is different with respect to age [1]. Using 6 years of age as the dividing age, younger patients have a lower glucose and higher protein concentration in the dialysate compared to older children. Therefore, it would appear that with the loss of the glucose osmotic concentration gradient in the dialysate, there would be a decreased ultrafiltration capacity in younger children. There have been no reports comparing the effect of a child's age on peritoneal membrane morphology. Esperanca et al. [2] reported that the infant's peritoneal membrane is relatively larger than the adult's: 383 cm² as compared with 177 cm²/kg body weight.

In order to examine the differences in some dialysis characteristics related to age, we have studied 19 patients who newly entered our CAPD program. The patients' characteristics are depicted in Table 1. In the younger group, there were

Table 1. Study group

	Young patients	Older patients
Number	7	12
Age (years)	1.2	13.7
Standard deviation	0.6	3.5
Range (years)	0.6 – 2.0	9.3 – 20.16

seven infants with a mean age of 1.2 years, whereas the mean age of the 12 children in the older group was 13.7 years. The solutions used were commercially available dialysate (Dianeal, Baxter Travenol, Canada) with the standard concentration of electrolytes and two osmotic strengths of dextrose, 2.5 g% and 4.25 g%. The mean dialysate volume was 32 ± 2.3 (SE) ml/kg body weight. The children were fasted from midnight and during the study. The antecedent dialysate used prior to the study was 2.5 g% dextrose-dialysate. The dextrose-dialysate to be tested was infused at 07:00 hours and dialysate samples were obtained at 0, 0.5, 1.0, 1.5 and 5 hours. Blood samples were obtained for glucose, urea and creatinine levels at the start and end of the exchange. The final drained volume was used to measure ultrafiltration.

Results

Glucose Concentration in Dialysate

The glucose concentrations in the dialysate after a 5-hour dwell time, using the 2.5 g% dextrose-dialysate, are depicted in Table 2. The glucose concentration in the dialysate at 5 hours is lower in the younger patients; 407 mg/dl versus 677 mg/dl. The same observation is made when the 4.25 g% dextrose-dialysate is studied (Table 2); 384 mg/dl in the younger patients versus 846 mg/dl in the older children. It is of interest that the final dialysate glucose concentration in the young infant is the same for the 2.5 g% dialysate as it is for the 4.25 g% dextrose solution.

Kohaut and Alexander [3] made a similar observation in children and then compared their results with those reported by Nolph et al. for adult CAPD patients [4, 5]. Young children absorb glucose faster than older children, and older children absorb glucose more rapidly than adults.

Peritoneal Creatinine and Urea Clearance

The clearance of urea and creatinine was used to measure solute movement. The formula for clearance is:

$$C_{ml/min} = \frac{D}{P} \times \frac{V_D}{t}.$$

Explanation of symbols: C, clearance ml/min; D, dialysate concentration; P, plasma concentration; V_D, dialysate volume; t, time.

The peritoneal clearance of creatinine was greater in the young patients as compared with older children when expressed as ml/min, ml/min/kg body weight, or ml/min/70 kg body weight (Table 3). However, when expressed on the basis of surface area, they were similar. Peritoneal clearance of urea was greater in the younger patients for every scale used (Table 3). Esperanca et al. [2] reported that peritoneal urea clearance was higher in one neonate as compared to adults and made a similar observation in puppies and mature dogs. Elzouki et al. [6, 7] confirmed this ob-

Table 2. Dialysate glucose content at 5 hours

	Young patients	Older patients
2.5% Dialysate		
Number	6	12
Glucose (mean ± SD) mg/dl	407 ± 170	677 ± 192 [a]
4.25 Dialysate		
Number	2	11
Glucose (mean ± SD) mg/dl	384 ± 8	846 ± 145 [b]

[a] P, 0.01.
[b] P, 0.001; SD, standard deviation.

Table 3. Relationship of peritoneal clearance of creatinine and urea to age (mean ± standard deviation)

	Weight (kg)	ml/min	ml/min/kg	ml/min/70 kg	ml/min/1.73 m^2
Peritoneal creatinine clearance					
Young patients	8.25 ± 1.8	1.13 ± 0.33	0.14 ± 0.02	9.52 ± 1.36	5.06 ± 0.87
Older patients	41.5 ± 12.9	3.68 ± 0.66	0.10 ± 0.03	6.74 ± 2.14	5.18 ± 1.24
P		< 0.0005	0.007	0.007	NS
Peritoneal urea clearance					
Young patients		1.17 ± 0.34	0.14 ± 0.02	9.85 ± 1.43	5.23 ± 0.91
Older patients		2.89 ± 0.54	0.08 ± 0.03	5.36 ± 1.92	4.10 ± 1.11
P		< 0.0005	< 0.0005	< 0.0005	0.035

NS, not significant.

servation in studies where the dialysis mechanics were controlled. However, Gruskin et al. [8] reported that the age at which transperitoneal movement of solute approached values observed in adults was between 1 and 2 years. The corrected peritoneal clearance of urea, creatinine, phosphate, and uric acid expressed in ml/min/kg or ml/min/70 kg were similar in children of all ages [9]. It may be that our results differ from Gruskin et al. [8] in that four of the seven infants we studied were less than 1 year of age. Also, strict control of the peritoneal volume was not possible since the Tenckhoff catheter had been recently implanted.

Ultrafiltration

In peritoneal dialysis, hypertonic dextrose dialysate solution is used to remove excess fluids from the patient. Because of the substantial difference in osmolality between blood and dialysate, fluid will move by osmosis between the two compartments. The rate of fluid transport is called the ultrafiltration rate (UFR). In order to measure the UFR accurately, we added a known amount of a nonabsorbable substance to the dialysate (radioiodinated serum albumin [R^{133}ISA]) and measured

Table 4. Relationship of ultrafiltration with respect to age and dextrose concentration (mean ± standard deviation)

	Young patients	Older patients	
2.5% Dialysate			
Number	6	11	
ml/kg	6.5± 1.4	6.0± 1.0	NS
ml/70 kg	455 ±97	422 ± 67	NS
ml/1.73 m²	240 ±50	324 ± 49	NS
4.25% Dialysate			
Number	2	9	
ml/kg	11.4± 0.65	15.4± 1.8	NS
ml/70 kg	795 ±46	522 ±126	NS
ml/1.73 m²	420 ±13	859 ± 98	NS

NS, not significant.

its rate of dilution by water moving into the peritoneal cavity. Other markers such as dextran-70 (molecular weight 70 000) and inulin have been suggested. The RISA method has been useful in animal studies where it is possible to obtain timed dialysate samples directly from the peritoneal catheter. In the case of human studies, sterile precautions are mandatory. Plastic connecting tubes are necessary and, unfortunately, the RISA sticks to the plastic, thus producing erroneous results.

We present our gravimetric data, even though the interpretation must be guarded because of numerous pitfalls. One assumes that the peritoneal cavity is completely drained, and this is not always true. The percent error in incomplete drainage may be more serious in children.

The ultrafiltration data is presented in Table 4. The results, using the 2.5 g% dialysate, did not differ significantly between the two groups. When expressed as per kg body weight or per 70 kg body weight, the mean values were similar; however, when expressed per 1.73 m², there was a trend toward better ultrafiltration in the older group of children. The 4.25 g% dialysate studies also did not demonstrate a statistically significant difference. However, there was stronger trend to demonstrate better ultrafiltration for the older children when the results were normalized for surface area. It should be noted that the number of children in the younger group was small when we tested the 4.25 g% dialysate.

Dialysate Protein

In order to assess the transperitoneal movement of large molecules, the total protein concentration was measured in the dialysate at the end of the 5-h dwell time. When 2.5 g% dialysate was assessed, the total protein concentration in young infants (< 2 years) was 250 ± 60 mg/dl (n, 4) compared with 130 ± 30 mg/dl (n, 11) in the older children (> 6 years). This is in agreement with our original observation that the younger CAPD patient loses more protein in the dialysate [1].

Summary of Results

We have demonstrated that dextrose is absorbed from the dialysate faster in younger children. At the same time, large molecules such as total protein are excreted in greater amounts in the young patients. This protein loss could be critical for the infant with anorexia. Small molecules such as creatinine and urea were cleared by the peritoneum more efficiently in the younger patients. Finally, there was a trend (though not statistically significant) for better ultrafiltration of water in the older patients.

Conclusion

It would appear that there is still considerable controversy about peritoneal function in young patients receiving peritoneal dialysis. Clearly, more accurate and controlled studies are necessary. We know the peritoneal surface area of the infant [2] is proportionately larger than the adult's, and thus the dialysate volume is critical [10]. Mathematical modelling is currently being used to study peritoneal kinetics in adult CAPD patients. Pyle et al. [11] has demonstrated that diffusive transport can be measured by the mass transfer area coefficient (MTAC) and convective transport by the reflection coefficient (RC). Similar preliminary studies have been done on children [12]. Such studies require a fair degree of mathematical and computer sophistication. Even though such studies should be encouraged, we need to develop simple techniques to measure the kinetics of peritoneal transport so that many academic centers can easily test new dialysis solutions as to their suitability for children of varying age and size.

References

1. Balfe JW, Vigneux A, Willumsen J, Hardy BE (1981) The use of CAPD in the treatment of children with end stage renal disease. Perit Dial Bull 1:35–38
2. Esperanca MJ, Collins DJ (1966) Peritoneal dialysis efficiency in relation to body weight. J Pediatr Surg 1:162
3. Kohaut EC, Alexander SR (1981) Ultrafiltration in the young patient on CAPD. In: Moncrief JW, Popovich JW (eds) CAPD update: continuous ambulatory peritoneal dialysis. Masson, New York, pp 221–226
4. Nolph KD, Twardowski ZJ, Popovich RP (1979) Equilibration of peritoneal dialysis solutions during long dwell exchanges. J Lab clin Med 93246–256
5. Nolph KD, Rosenfield PS, Powell JT (1970) Peritoneal glucose transport and hyperglycemia during peritoneal dialysis. Am J Med Sci 259:272–280
6. Elzouki AY, Gruskin AB, Baluarte HJ et al. (1981) Developmental changes in peritoneal dialysis kinetics in dogs. Pediatr Res 15:853
7. Elzouki AY, Gruskin AB, Baluarte HJ et al. (1981) Developmental aspects of peritoneal dialysis. In: Gruskin AB, Norman ME (eds) Developments in nephrology, vol 3. Proceedings fifth international pediatric nephrology symposium. Nijhoff, The Hague, p 517
8. Gruskin AB, Cote ML, Baluarte HJ (1982) Peritoneal diffusion curves, peritoneal clearances and scaling factors in children of differing age. Int J Pediatr Nephrol 3:271

9. Gruskin AB, Morgenstern BZ, Perlman SA (1984) Kinetics of peritoneal dialysis in children. In: Fine RN, Gruskin AB (eds) End stage renal disease in children. Saunders, Philadelphia, pp 95–117
10. Kohaut EC (1983) Effect of dialysate volume on ultrafiltration in young children (Abstract). Eur J Pediatr 140:179
11. Pyle WK, Moncrief JW, Popovich RP (1981) Peritoneal transport evaluation in CAPD. In: Moncrief JW, Popovich RP (eds) CAPD update: Continuous ambulatory peritoneal dialysis. Masson, New York, pp 35–52
12. Popovich RP, Pyle WK, Rosenthal DA, Alexander SR, Balfe JW, Moncrief JW (1981) Kinetics of peritoneal dialysis in children. In: Moncrief JW, Popovich RP (eds) CAPD update: continuous ambulatory peritoneal dialysis. Masson, New York, pp 227–241

Transperitoneal Movements of Solutes of Different Molecular Size in Children on CAPD

K. E. Bonzel, O. Mehls, M. Gräning, R. Wartha, and D. E. Müller-Wiefel

Introduction

Since the first description of a "novel portable/wearable equilibrium peritoneal dialysis technique" by Popovich et al. [1], continuous ambulatory peritoneal dialysis (CAPD) has assumed increasing importance as a therapeutic modality for adults and children with end-stage renal disease (ESRD) [2–12].

An understanding of the transperitoneal movement of solutes and water is fundamental to adapting CAPD and other forms of chronic peritoneal dialysis to infants and young children. Whereas many systematic studies of the peritoneal membrane have been performed in adults [13–21], only a few involving children have been reported [22–27]. Most studies have involved the transperitoneal movement of small molecular weight solutes like electrolytes and urea [22, 25, 26]. Studies of middle and large molecular weight solutes are rare [27].

The aim of this study is to investigate the influence of body weight, dialysate volume, dwell time, duration of CAPD treatment, and peritonitis rate on peritoneal diffusion of exogeneous and endogeneous substances of small and middle molecular weight.

Patients and Methods

Eight children (six boys, two girls) with a median age of 10.5 years (range 2.4–15.5 years) were investigated (Table 1). CAPD had been initiated 1–19 months prior to the study. Dialysis was routinely performed with commercially available dialysate (Fresenius Co.), using four exchanges a day. Whereas the glucose content of the dialysate varied, the exchange volume was approximately 35 ml/kg body weight. None of the children had an appreciable urine output at the time of the investigation. None of the children had had an episode of peritonitis for at least 3 months prior to the study, except for those patients who were studied 7 days after the onset of peritonitis.

Peritoneal mass transfer studies were performed, in the fasting state using a standardized protocol (Fig. 1). In the early morning, 12 h after the last exchange, an intravenous injection of 15 mg/kg inulin (IN) and 40 mg/kg para-aminohuppurate (PAH) was given. The IN (Inutest, Laevosan Co.) contained sinistrin (β-D-fructan of inulin type) with a molecular weight of approximately 4000 dalton [28]. A dialysis exchange with a volume of 35 ml/kg of body weight and a glucose content of 2.3%

Table 1. Clinical data of patients on CAPD with IN and PAH clearances

Patient	Sex	Age years	Weight kg	Body surface area m²	Filling volume ml/kg	Number of studies	Time on CAPD		Diagnosis
							1st study (months)	last study (months)	
1	m	2.4	7.5	0.4	65	2[a]	8	16	renal hypoplasia
2	f	7.0	14.6	0.6	35	2[c]	17	18	nephronophthisis
3	m	4.2	15.0	0.6	35	2[a]	6	11	nephronophthisis
4	m	9.9	24.2	0.9	35	2[b]	7	15	obstructive uropathy
5	m	9.0	26.4	1.0	35	2[a]	1	4	obstructive uropathy
6	f	15.5	27.4	1.0	35	2[b]	3	7	cystinosis
7	m	12.3	30.0	1.1	35	4[b]	9	19	renal hypoplasia
8	m	11.0	43.3	1.4	35	2[a]	1	4	Schönlein-Henoch nephropathy

[a] period free of peritonitis.
[b] one clearance 1 week after peritonitis.
[c] both clearances after peritonitis.

IN/PAH

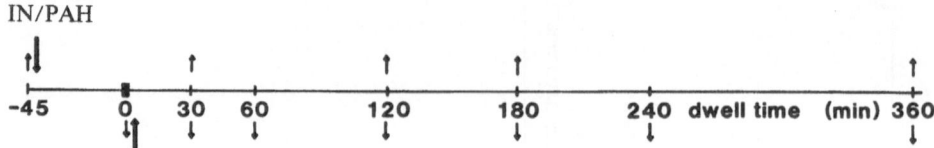

Fig. 1. Protocol of peritoneal transport studies. ↓, IV injection of IN (150 mg/kg body weight) and PAH (40 mg/kg body weight); ↑, filling of the abdomen with dialysis fluid (35 ml/kg body weight); ↑, time at which blood samples were taken; ↓, time at which dialysis fluid samples were taken

was performed 45 min after the intravenous injection. Blood and dialysate samples were then taken at regular intervals up to 360 min as indicated in Fig. 1. For each dialysate sampling, the total volume of dialysate fluid was drained. After the dialysate had been weighed and 10 ml of it removed, the fluid was returned to the peritoneal cavity. For determination of dwell time, 50% of the time required for drainage and reinfusion was subtracted from the overall dwell time.

Urea, creatinine, uric acid, total protein, and electrolyte determinations were performed using standard methods; IN was measured by an anthrone method [29] and PAH using diazo-color reaction method [30]. Both methods were adapted to autoanalyzer measurements [31, 32]. Dialysate IN analysis was performed after the samples had been dialyzed against a glucose-free fluid in order to reduce the high glucose content and to avoid cross reaction.

The ratio of substrate concentration in the dialysate to substrate concentration in the blood (SD/SB) [25, 33] was calculated for all substances up to 720 min of dwell time. Clearances of urea, creatinine, IN, and PAH were calculated using the following formula according to Finkelstein et al. [14]:

$$C = \frac{S_{Dt} \times V_D \times 100 \times 2 \times 1.73}{(S_{B30} + S_{Bt}) \times t \times BSA}$$

(C, Clearance; S_{Dt}, Substrate concentration in dialysate at time t; V_D, Volume of dialysate; S_{B30}, Substrate concentration in blood at time 30'; S_{Bt}, Substrate concentration in blood at time t; t, dwell time in minutes; BSA, body surface area in m^2).

Since we did not continuously infuse IN following the intravenous injection, 24-h IN clearance values could not be measured. The clearance for IN after 24-h was extrapolated from the 4- and 6-h determinations, assuming a constant linear increase of mass transfer with increasing dwell time. Statistical analysis was performed by Wilcoxon tests for paired differences and for random samples.

Results

SD/SB ratios and diffusion curves (Fig. 2) show that the diffusion process for urea, creatinine, and potassium was nearly completed after 240 min. At the same time, the SD/SB ratio for phosphate and PAH was only 0.55 and for IN 0.13. The diffusion curves for IN and for protein are nearly linear presumably because of the slow diffusion of these substances.

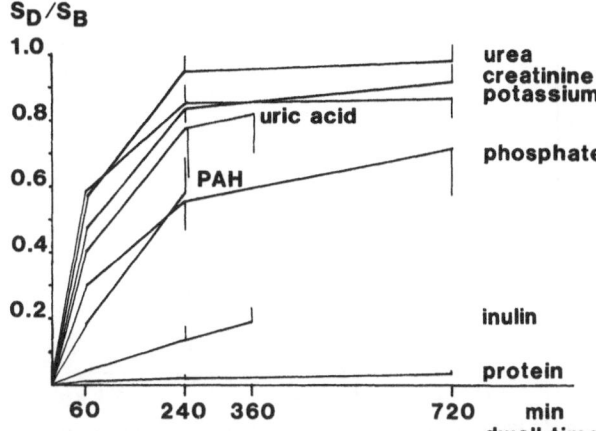

Fig. 2. Peritoneal diffusion curves. Changes of substrate concentration in the dialysate (*SD*) to substrate concentration in the blood (*SB*) with increasing dwell time (mean ± SD)

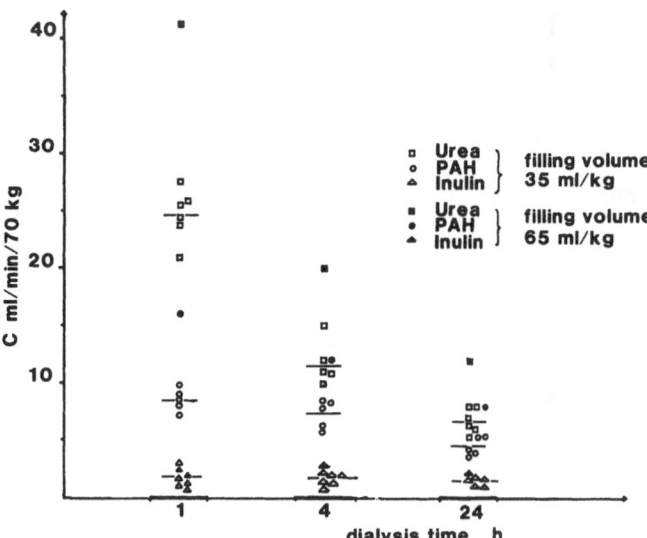

Fig. 3. Influences of dwell time and filling volume on peritoneal clearances of urea, PAH, and IN. C, clearance. The 1- and 4-h values were calculated for dwell times of 1 and 4 h without bag exchanges. The 24-h value was calculated using four bags with dwell times of 4 h for three bags and 12 h for one bag

The clearance of urea expressed in ml/min/70 kg was dependent on both the dwell (dialysis) time and on the filling volume (Fig. 3). The dwell time had a much higher influence on the clearances of low molecule solute (urea) than of middle molecule solute (IN) with an intermediate effect on the clearance of PAH. The influence of the filling volume was suggested by studying patient No. 1 with a filling volume of 65 ml/kg which yielded higher values compared to those obtained by 35 ml/kg.

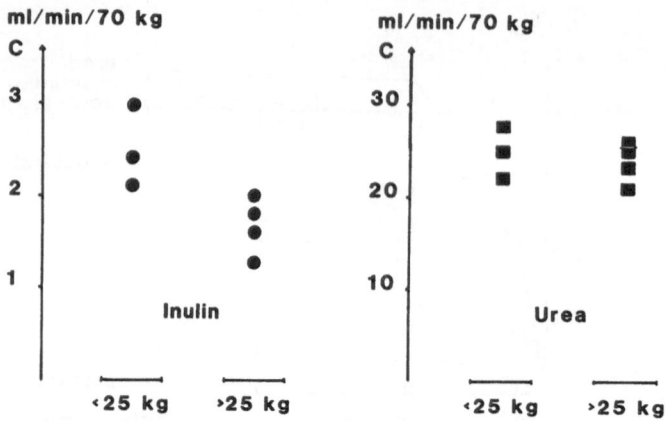

Fig. 4. Peritoneal clearances in relation to body weight. The clearances were calculated for dwell times of 1 h

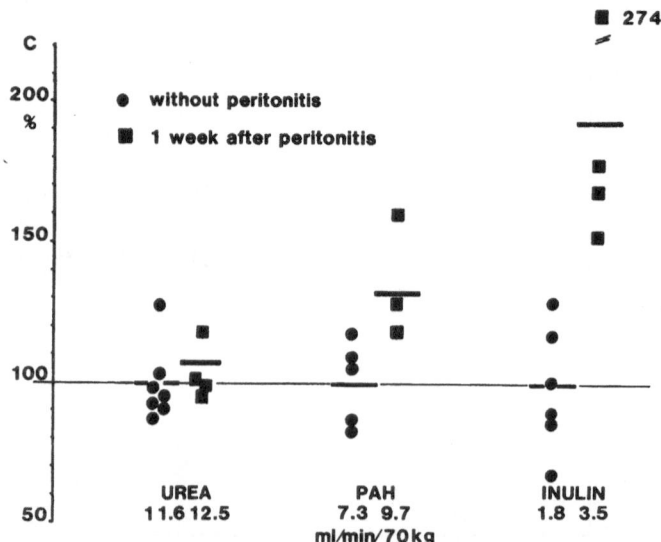

Fig. 5. Changes in peritoneal clearances accompanying peritonitis. The clearances after peritonitis are expressed as the percentage of mean clearance values found under basal conditions. The mean absolute values are indicated at the bottom. All clearances were calculated for dwell times of 4 h

The clearance of IN was higher in three children with a body weight below 25 kg than in four children with a greater body weight (Fig. 4). During the short dwell time of 1 h, there was no relationship between body size and urea clearance.

Peritonitis had a significant influence on the diffusion and clearance of both IN and PAH (Fig. 5). The mean clearances of both substances increased to 195% and to 130% respectively, whereas no significant change in urea clearance was noted.

Repeated clearance studies for urea in six children and for PAH and IN in four children were performed in the absence of peritonitis after 4–8 months (Fig. 6). A significant increase in the clearance of PAH and an even greater increase in the

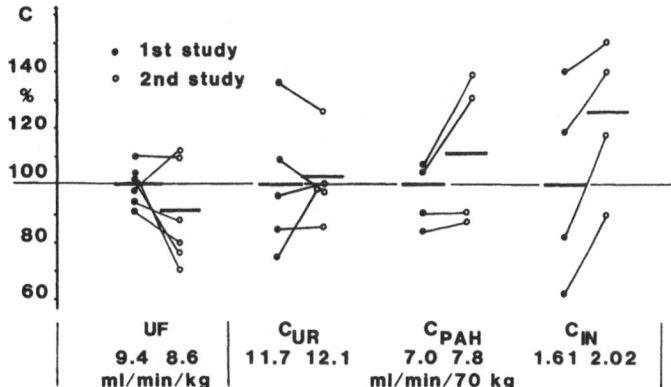

Fig. 6. Changes in peritoneal function apparent 4–8 months of regular CAPD in the absence of peritonitis. The values for clearances in the second study are given as the percentage of the mean clearance values of the first study. The mean absolute values are indicated at the bottom. All clearances were calculated for dwell times of 4 h

clearance of IN was noted, whereas the clearance of urea remained unchanged. At the same time, a small loss of ultrafiltration was noted in four of six children.

Discussion

General Considerations

Of fundamental importance to the long-term use of chronic peritoneal dialysis in children is an understanding of the transperitoneal movement of solute and water. Uniform standards are needed to compare the results of dialysis in children with different body weights and heights. Solute concentration ratios (SD/SB), diffusion curves, and peritoneal clearances are the common standards. It has been shown that comparisons of these tests in different age groups beyond infancy are possible when the dialysis mechanics are constant, the solute concentration ratios remain constant, and the infused dialysate volume is adjusted for the body weight of the patient [23, 25, 27, 34, 35]. Changes in SD/SB reflect differences either in permeability or surface area of the peritoneum. Since neonates have a relative large functional peritoneal surface area [36, 37] and/or a more permeable peritoneal membrane, they have a higher SD/SB ratio than older children [24, 34, 37]. In children beyond the 1st year of life, the SD/SB is constant for each substance at any given duration of dwell time [25].

Clearance values can theoretically be affected by differences of body size, and it remains a question whether clearances should be scaled for body weight or for body surface area. It is not known which is of more physiological relevance. The peritoneal clearance scaled for weight seems to be similar at all ages when the filling volume is scaled for weight [27]. Values scaled for body surface area differ because the surface area is not linearly related to weight alone [25]. With these considerations in mind and for purposes of making comparisons with adult values, we have scaled our clearance data to a body weight of 70 kg.

Movement of Solutes with Low Molecular Size

Our results demonstrate that the diffusion process for urea, creatinine, and potassium is nearly complete after a dwell time of 240 min (Fig. 2). If more effective removal of these substances is needed, the frequency of dialysis has to be changed, using dwell times under 4 h.

Mainly the clearance for low molecular substances (represented by urea in our studies) increased distinctly when a larger filling volume was used (Fig. 3). This is in agreement with the observation of Gruskin et al. [25, 27] and of others [23, 38]. Peritonitis did not significantly increase urea clearance measured for a dwell time of 4 h. This is in contrast to our findings for substances of higher molecular weight (Fig. 5), presumably because the clearance of lower molecular weight substances is already maximal under basal conditions.

No decrease of urea clearance with time was noted after 4–8 months of CAPD. After the same period of time, however, a decrease of ultrafiltration capacity was observed in four of six children studied (Fig. 6). No significant change of urea clearance with time on IPD/CAPD was reported in children [27], whereas both a decrease [14, 39] and no change [19–21, 40] were noted in adults. The loss of ultrafiltration with time on CAPD in some patients has been observed by many groups [41–44]. The reason for this phenomenon is not well understood. Isolated loss of ultrafiltration must be separated from functional loss of peritoneal surface area following progressive sclerosing peritonitis [45–48] (Drachman et al., this volume). The continuous use of the peritoneum [13, 14, 41, 44] and/or the high osmolality of the dialysate [13, 20] have been implicated; however, prospective studies are required before it will be possible to provide a definitive answer.

Movement of Middle and High Molecule Solutes

The IN used in our study has a molecular weight of 4000 dalton and therefore represents a middle molecule. Albumin which represents the majority of proteins in dialysate has a higher molecular weight of about 66 000 daltons.

The increase in the dialysate concentration of IN is nearly linear with dwell time. This relationship is more pronounced for protein (Fig. 2). As a consequence, the daily loss of protein and middle molecular substances is linearly related to the exposure time of the dialysate to the peritoneum. CCPD reduces the exposure time to about 50% of that of CAPD. In agreement with this fact is the reported reduction in protein loss of about 50% by CCPD (see Niaudet et al., this volume).

Whereas the IN clearance was higher in children who weighed < 25 kg than in those weighing > 25 kg, a comparable difference was not noted for urea clearance (Fig. 4). This finding is in accord with previous reports of protein losses that were higher for younger children than for older children [49].

The absolute values of IN clearance in the present report were lower than those obtained in children [25, 27, 34] and adults [23] by other authors. Technical and analytical problems are most likely responsible for the differences.

IN is an ill-defined mixture of polyfructoside molecules with varying molecular weights around 4000 daltons. Furthermore, all preparations of IN contain varying amounts of fructose [28, 50]. Most authors [19, 27, 34] have used a modified method [51] after Walser et al. [50] for analysis of IN. This method is based on hydrolysis of fructan into fructose and a color reaction between fructose and diphenylamine. The analysis is complicated by serious reproduction difficulties caused by several "heating" and "cooling" steps. For our analysis we used the anthrone method [29] modified for the autoanalyzer technique [31]. Both the Walser and the anthrone method show cross-reactions between glucose and fructose which are of minor importance for serum determinations when the glucose content is approximately 100 mg%. However, the glucose content of dialysate is many times higher, and the influence of these high glucose levels on dialysate IN determinations has not been evaluated to date. To avoid these problems, we reduced the glucose content of the dialysate by dialysis against a glucose-free solution prior to the analysis (M. Gräning, unpublished). In our opinion these analytical problems have not been taken into consideration in earlier studies. However, although the absolute values vary in different studies, changes of IN clearance during different conditions are comparable.

IN and PAH clearance increased significantly following episodes of peritonitis (Fig. 5). This is parallel to the well-known increase in protein loss during peritonitis [49]. However, 1 week after peritonitis abated, the protein loss was increased by only 1.25 [49] whereas the IN clearance was increased by 1.9.

The most remarkable result in our study was the increase of IN clearance after 4–8 months of CAPD. In contrast, Gruskin et al. [27] noted a marginally lower IN clearance in four children dialyzed longer than 6 months, as compared with four different children dialyzed less than 1 month. The increase noted in our study cannot be a consequence of peritonitis, since all children with peritonitis were excluded from the study. One possible explanation could be enlargement of pore size and/or the development of a greater active peritoneal area with increasing time of CAPD. The changes could also be the result of a subclinical, chronic (nonbacterial) inflammatory process which leads to the opening of preexisting capillaries or the proliferation of new ones. Further extended studies are necessary to verify these results and to determine if IN clearance is a feasible parameter for evaluation of functional changes in the peritoneum following long-term peritoneal dialysis.

References

1. Popovich RP, Moncrief JW, Decherd JB, Bomar, JB, Pyle WK (1976) The definition of a novel portable/ wearable equilibrium peritoneal dialysis technique. Am Soc Artif Intern Organs 5:64
2. Oreopoulos DG, Robson M, Izatt S, et al. (1978) A simple and safe technique for continuous ambulatory peritoneal dialysis (CAPD). Trans Am Soc Artif Intern Organs 24:484–489
3. Popovich RP, Moncrief JW, Nolph KD (1978) Continuous ambulatory peritoneal dialysis. Ann Intern Med 88:449–456
4. Alexander SR, Clevert AT, Maksym KA, Campbell RA, Talwalkar YB (1980) Clinical parameters in continuous ambulatory peritoneal dialysis for infants and children. In: Moncrief JW, Popovich RP (eds) CAPD update Masson, New York, pp 195–209
5. Balfe JW, Vigneux AB, Willumsen J, Hardy BE (1981) The use of CAPD in the treatment of children with end-stage renal disease. Perit Dial Bull 1:35–37
6. Bonzel KE, Diekmann L, Koch H, Lütkenhaus C (1981) Erfahrungen mit der chronischen Peritonealdialyse (IPD and CAPD) beim Kind. Nieren Hochdruckkr 10:61–67

7. DeSanto NG, Capodicasa G, De Simone V (1981) Experience of CAPD in children – a pilot study. Nephrology, Urology, Andrology 1:62–65
8. Guillot M, Clermont MJ, Gagnadoux MF, Broyer M (1981) Nineteen months' experience with continuous ambulatory peritoneal dialysis (CAPD) in children: Main clinic and biological results. In: Gahl GM, Nolph KD, Kessel M (eds) Advances in peritoneal dialysis. Excerpta Medica, Amsterdam, pp 203–207
9. Kohaut EC (1981) Continuous ambulatory peritoneal dialysis, a preliminary pediatric experience. Am J Dis Child 13:270–273
10. Potter DE, McDaid TK, McHenry K, Mar H (1981) Continuous ambulatory peritoneal dialysis (CAPD) in children. Trans Am Soc Artif Intern Organs 27:64–67
11. Heller-Ackeret C, Ertelt W, Leumann ED (1982) Kontinuierliche ambulante Peritonealdialyse beim Kind; zwei Jahre Erfahrung. Schweiz Med Wochenschr 112:859–864
12. Salusky IP, Lucullo L, Nelson P, Fine RN (1982) Continuous ambulatory peritoneal dialysis in children. Pediatr Clin North Am 29:1005–1012
13. Henderson LW (1969) Altered permeability of peritoneal membrane after using hypertonic peritoneal dialysis fluid. J Clin Invest 48:992–1001
14. Finkelstein FO, Kliger AS, Bastl C, Yap P (1977) Sequential clearance and dialysance measurements of chronic peritoneal dialysis patients. Nephron 18:342–347
15. Villaroel E (1977) Kinetics of intermittent and continuous peritoneal dialysis. J Dialysis 4:333–347
16. Popovich RP, Moncrief JW, Nolph MD (1978) Physiological transport parameters in patients on peritoneal and hemodialysis. In: Mackey BB (ed) Proceedings of 11th annual contractor's conference of the artificial kidney program of the National Institute of Arthritis, Metabolism and Digestive Diseases. Bethesda, Maryland, pp 36–42
17. Nolph KD (1979) Peritoneal clearances. J Lab Clin Med 94:519–525
18. Popovich RP, Moncrief JW (1979) Kinetic modeling of peritoneal transport. Contrib Nephrol 17:59–72
19. Rubin J, Nolph KD, Arfania D, Brown P, Prowant D (1979) Follow-up of peritoneal clearances in patients undergoing continuous ambulatory peritoneal dialysis. Kidney Int 16:619–623
20. Randerson DH, Farrell PC (1981) Long-term clearances in CAPD. In: Atkins RC, Thomson NM, Farrell PC (eds) Peritoneal dialysis. Churchill-Livingstone, Edinburgh, pp 22–29
21. Diaz-Buxo JA, Chandler JT, Farmer CD, Walker PJ, Holt KL, Burgess WP, Orr SL (1983) Long-term observations of peritoneal clearances in patients-undergoing peritoneal dialysis. Trans Am Soc Artif Intern Organs 6:21–25
22. Kohaut EC, Alexander S (1981) Ultrafiltration in the young patient on CAPD. In: Moncrief JW, Popovich RP (eds) CAPD update. Masson, New York, pp 221–226
23. Popovich RP, Pyle WK, Rosenthal DA, Alexander S, Balfe JW, Moncrief JW (1981) Kinetics of peritoneal dialysis in children. In: Moncrief JW, Popovich RP (eds) CAPD update. Masson, New York, pp 227–241
24. Gruskin AB, Elzouki AY, Baluarte HJ, Prebis JW, Polinsky MS (1982) The peritoneal membrane – developmental considerations. In: Spitzer A (ed) The kidney during development. Morphology and function. Masson, New York, pp 315–318
25. Gruskin AB, Cote ML, Baluarte HJ (1982) Peritoneal diffusion curves, peritoneal clearances and scaling factors in children of differing age. Int J Pediatr Nephrol 3:271–278
26. DeSanto NG, Capodicasa G, Gilli G, Giordano G (1982) CAPD in infants and children. In: LaGreca G, Biasioli S, Ronco C (eds) Proceedings of the 1st international course on peritoneal dialysis, Vicenza, Italy, 1982. Wichtig, Milan, pp 263–273
27. Gruskin AB, Rosenbaum H, Baluarte HJ, Morgenstern BZ, Polinsky MS, Perlman SA (1983) Transperitoneal solute movement in children. Kidney Int 24, Suppl 15:S95–S100
28. Nitsch E (1979) Molecular characterization of sinistrin. Carbohydr Res 72:1–12
29. White RP, Samson FE (1954) Determination of inulin in plasma and urine by use of anthrone. J Lab Clin Med 43:475–478
30. Harvey RB, Brothers AJ (1964) Renal extraction of para-amino-hippurate and creatinine measured by continuous in vivo sampling of arterial and renal vein blood. Ann NY Acad Sci 102:46

31. Wright HK, Gann DS (1966) An automatic anthrone method for determination of inulin in plasma and urine. J Lab Clin Med 67:689–696

32. Ardaillou R (1964) Dosage de l'acide para-amino-hippurique par l'autoanalyzer. (Symposium Volume) Compagnie Téchnicon, France

33. Nolph KD, Twardowski ZJ, Popovich RP, Rubin J (1979) Equilibration of peritoneal dialysis solutions during long-dwell exchanges. J Lab Clin Med 93:246–256

34. Elzouki AY, Gruskin AB, Baluarte HJ, Polinsky MS, Prebis JW (1981) Developmental changes in peritoneal dialysis kinetics in dogs. Pediatr Res 15:853–858

35. Esperanca MJ, Collins DL (1966) Peritoneal dialysis efficiency in reaction to body weight. J Pediatr Surg 1:162–169

36. Putiloff PV (1886) Materials for the study of the laws of growth of the human body in relation to the surface areas of different systems; the trial on russian subjects of planigraphic anatomy as a means for exact anthropometry – one of the problems of anthropology. Meeting of the Siberian Branch of the Russian Geographic Society, Oct 29, 1884, Omsk

37. Elzouki AY, Gruskin AB, Baluarte HJ, Prebis JW, Polinsky MS (1981) Developmental aspects of peritoneal dialysis. In: Gruskin AB, Norman ME (eds) Pediatric nephrology. M Nijhoff, The Hague, pp 194–198

38. Twardowski ZJ, Prowant BF, Nolph KD, Martinez AJ, Lampton LM (1983) High volume, low frequency continuous ambulatory peritoneal dialysis. Kidney Int 23:64–70

39. Rubin J, McFarland S, Hellems EW, Brower JD (1981) Peritoneal dialysis during peritonitis. Kidney Int 19:460–464

40. Rubin J, Ray R, Barnes T, Bower J (1981) Peritoneal abnormalities during infectious episodes of continuous ambulatory peritoneal dialysis. Nephron 29:124–127

41. Farrell PC, Randerson DH (1980) Membrane permeability changes in long-term CAPD. Trans Am Soc Artif Intern Organs 26:197–200

42. Oreopoulos DG, Khanna R, Wu G (1983) Sclerosing obstructive peritonitis after CAPD. Lancet 2:409

43. Rottembourg J, Gahl G, Poignet JC, Mertani E, Strippol P, Langlois JP, Legrain M (1983) Severe abdominal complications in patients undergoing continuous ambulatory peritoneal dialysis. Proc Eur Dial Transplant Assoc 20:19–22

44. Nolph KD, Ryan L, Moore H, Legrain M, Mion C, Oreopoulus DG (1984) Factors affecting ultrafiltration in continuous ambulatory peritoneal dialysis. Perit Dial Bull 4:14–19

45. Ghandi VC, Hymayun HM, Ing TS, Daugirdas JT, Jablokow VR, Iwatsuki S, Geis WP, Hano JE (1980) Sclerotic thickening of the peritoneal membrane in maintainance peritoneal dialysis patients. Arch Intern Med 140:1201–1203

46. Bradley JA, McWhinnie DL, Hamilton DNH, Starnes F, MacPherson SG, Seywright M, Briggs JD, Junor BJ (1983) Sclerosing obstructive peritonitis after continuous ambulatory peritoneal dialysis. Lancet 2:113–114

47. Slingeneyer A, Canaud B, Mion C (1983) Permanent loss of ultrafiltration capacity of the peritoneum in long-term peritoneal dialysis: An epidemiological study. Nephron 33:133–138

48. Faller B, Marichal JF (1981) Loss of ultrafiltration in continuous ambulatory peritoneal dialysis: Clinical data. In: Gahl GM, Kessel M, Nolph KD (eds) Advances in peritoneal dialysis. Excerpta Medica, Amsterdam, pp 227–232

49. Bonzel KE, Bonatz K, Senghaas C, Mehls O, Müller-Wiefel DE, Wartha R, Gretz N, Müller E (1985) Nutritional aspects in children on CAPD. In: Maher JF, Winchester JF (eds) Proceedings of the 3rd international symposium on CAPD, Washington 1984. (In press)

50. Walser M, Davidson DG, Orloff J (1955) The renal clearance of alkali-stable inulin. J Clin Invest 34:1520–1523

51. Brown B, Nolph KD (1977) Chemical measurements of inulin concentrations in peritoneal dialysis solution. Clin Chim Acta 76:103–112

CAPD in Children: Data from the European Dialysis and Transplant Association (EDTA) Registry

M. Broyer, G. Rizzoni, R. Donckerwolcke, A. Balas, F. Brunner, H. Brynger, C. Jacobs, P. Kramer, N. Selwood, and A. Wing

The registry of the European Dialysis and Transplant Association (EDTA) collects data from 32 European countries. At the close of 1982, there were more than 2300 pediatric patients alive on dialysis or with a functioning transplant on the registry computer files, and 5.6% of these were being treated by CAPD [4]. This paper reports a study gathering data on CAPD in the pediatric part of the registry. Some of these data have already been published in the last combined reports of the EDTA [1–3].

Patients and Methods

Information used for this study was collected from patient questionnaires which noted sex, date of birth, diagnosis of primary renal disease, and the treatment sequence, recorded by means of a number code designating each method of therapy and entered alongside the date of commencement of that therpay. Special questions on CAPD were also included: 1. reasons for choice of CAPD answered by a number code (1980 and 1981 reports); 2. number of episodes of peritonitis (1981 and 1982 reports); 3. days of hospitalization while treated by CAPD for peritonitis or for other causes (1981 and 1982 reports); 4. reason for abandonment of CAPD (1981 and 1982 reports); 5. number of catheter insertions (1982 report).

The population used in this study was defined as all ED patients included in the pediatric registry starting dialysis before age 15.0 years. We have used data collected by the registration committee from 1979 to 1982. Unfortunately, the 1983 data were not yet available at the time of this study.

Patient survival was calculated using actuarial methodology. Any change in mode of treatment was considered as lost to observation in calculating patient survival. Similarly, if changes are also considered as failure in calculating technique survival, it might have been more appropriate to consider graft as an observation loss, but at the time of this work the program for that purpose was not available. Data for the study on growth were based on information available from the 1982 patient questionnaires and a special pediatric questionnaire of the EDTA Registry.

This growth analysis is restricted to data of prepubertal children whose mode of treatment was not altered during 1982. The prepubertal age group was restricted to boys under 11 years and girls under 10 years in December 1982. Children with a bone age of more than 10 years were excluded. Patients with cystinosis and oxalosis were also excluded.

Growth in children undergoing CAPD was compared to growth in children on hemodialysis. Only linear growth between December 1981 and December 1982 was considered. Growth velocity was evaluated by comparing the linear growth of each patient to the mean normal for chronological age. In this manner, the ratio of observed to expected growth was calculated. Growth retardation was assessed by calculating the standard deviation score (SDS) for height related to the chronological age at the start of treatment. Also, the difference in SDS between the beginning and the end of the study period for those children was recorded.

To compare the nutritional status of patients treated with CAPD with those on hemodialysis weight for height in December 1982 in these prepubertal children was recorded. Also, the difference in SDS for weight between the beginning and the end of 1982 in these patients was calculated.

Results

CAPD in Children in Different Countries

Since 1980, CAPD has contributed significantly to the treatment of ESRD in children in Europe, increasing from 9 patients recorded on December 31, 1979 to 156 on December 31, 1982.

The numbers of pediatric patients treated by CAPD and by other modes of dialytic treatment in European countries on December 31 of 1980, 1981, and 1982 is given in Table 1. The mean percentage of pediatric patients on dialysis treated by CAPD in Europe was 10.3% by the close of 1982, but this percentage varied considerably from one country to another. Among countries with the highest number of patients in the pediatric registry, France, the Federal Republic of Germany, and Spain had a percentage of pediatric patients on CAPD below the European average; the UK was largely above the average with 30% of the pediatric patients on CAPD, while Italy and the Netherlands were around the European average. Taking countries with a small pediatric population to account, little CAPD was done in the eastern European countries, but almost all the others had a percentage of pediatric patients on CAPD above the European mean. This was especially true for Switzerland and the Scandinavian countries.

Age Distribution

Age distribution of 227 pediatric patients treated by CAPD in the year 1982 is shown in Fig. 1. The percentage of patients treated by CAPD has been much higher in the younger age groups, ranging from 2% over 15 years of age to 45% under 1 year of age, according to an analysis of the data for the year 1981 (Table 2). The percentage of pediatric patients on CAPD was higher when only those patients who were less than 15 years of age at the end of the year were taken into account, since CAPD was almost never used in "pediatric patients" over 15 years of age. With this method of calculation, by the close of 1982, the percentage of children treated by CAPD in Europe as a whole was 15%, 50% in the UK and in Sweden, 21% in the Netherlands, 17% in Italy, 14% in the Federal Republic of Germany, 10% in Spain, and 9% in France.

Table 1. Number of pediatric patients on dialysis treated by CAPD and other modes of treatment in the EDTA registry

Year of report	1980		1981		1982	
	CAPD	Other mode of dialysis	CAPD	Other mode of dialysis	CAPD	Other mode of dialysis
Austria	0	19	0	14	0	21
Belgium	1	18	3	17	2	35
Bulgaria	0	8	0	6	0	10
Czechoslovakia	0	9	0	14	1	12
Denmark	1	15	4	18	2	22
GDR	0	22	0	26	0	37
Finland	1	6	0	8	1	8
France	15	238	17	264	22	320
FRG	2	153	3	162	10	193
Greece	0	14	0	13	1	17
Hungary	0	3	0	2	0	1
Ireland	1	1	1	3	1	7
Israel	2	20	1	22	7	24
Italy	1	153	10	141	25	196
Luxemburg	1	4	1	2	0	2
Netherlands	2	30	5	39	6	35
Norway	0	1	1	1	0	5
Poland	0	15	0	14	0	21
Portugal	0	1	1	6	0	22
Spain	0	114	4	146	13	172
Sweden	0	9	2	8	6	13
Switzerland	1	15	4	11	8	11
UK	22	122	32	112	50	114
Yugoslavia	0	12	0	24	0	39
Total	51	1005	89	1077	156	1357

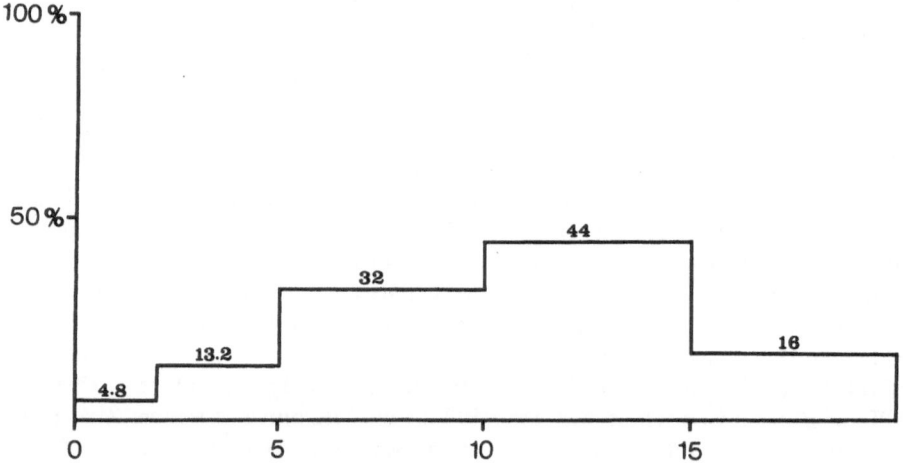

Fig. 1. Age distribution at start of CAPD in the pediatric registry of the EDTA

Table 2. Percentage of pediatric patients on dialysis treated by CAPD according to age (1981 data)

Age	On dialysis number	On CAPD number	On CAPD (%)
< 1	11	5	45
1 – 2	12	3	25
2 – 3	12	5	38
3 – 4	16	8	50
4 – 5	18	5	27
5 – 6	28	7	25
6 – 7	33	2	6
7 – 8	39	6	15
8 – 9	49	7	14
9 – 10	51	5	10
10 – 11	68	6	9
11 – 12	66	3	4.5
12 – 13	96	4	4
13 – 14	130	8	6
14 – 15	114	7	6
> 15	413	8	2

Reasons for CAPD

Analysis of the reasons for choice of CAPD showed that it was considered the first choice in 61% of the pediatric cases versus 53% in adults and was more likely to be used as a temporary therapy while awaiting hemodialysis or transplantation (13%) than in adult patients (9%). The proportion of patients for whom CAPD was dictated by the nonavailability of other modes of therapy was similar in children (16%) and in adult patients (18%).

The method of treatment which preceded CAPD was analyzed for 227 pediatric patients according to age (Table 3): 61% received CAPD as the initial treatment, 19% after intermittent peritoneal dialysis, 14% after hospital hemodialysis, 3% after graft failure, and only 1% after home hemodialysis. There was a definite decrease in the proportion of pediatric patients over 15 years for whom CAPD was the first treatment.

Patient Survival

Patient survival on CAPD was calculated for 36 patients starting CAPD in 1979 and 1980 and for 129 patients who started in 1981 and 1982 (Table 4). There was a clear improvement in the survival rates of both groups. Survival rates on hospital hemodialysis for pediatric patients starting treatment from 1978 to 1982 gave survival rates similar to those of CAPD patients starting treatment in 1981 and 1982. Causes of death on CAPD were recorded in 9 cases: 2 hypertensive cardiac failure, 1 fluid overload, 1 cerebrovascular accident, 2 infections, 1 cachexia, and 2 other causes [4].

Table 3. Previous mode of treatment in pediatric patients treated by CAPD according to age

Age (years)	Hospital hemo-dialysis (n)	Home hemo-dialysis (n)	Intermittent peritoneal dialysis (n)	graft (n)	first treatment with CAPD (n)	total (n)
< 5	2	–	11	–	28	41
5 – 10	10	–	10	1	52	73
10 – 15	13	2	14	2	45	76
> 15	9	1	9	4	14	37
Total	34	3	44	7	139	227
(%)	(15.0)	(1.3)	(19.0)	(3.0)	(61.0)	(100)

Table 4. Pediatric patient survival after starting CAPD. $n =$ number of patients at risk

Duration of treatment (months)		0	3	6	12	18	24
Starting CAPD 1979 – 1980	n	36.5	30	22	17	12	7.5
	%	100	96.6	92.2	77.9	71.4	61.9
Starting CAPD 1981 – 1982	n	129	107	74	37.5	14.5	
	%	100	98.1	95.4	95.4	91.7	
Combined data	n	165.5	137.5	96	54.5	26.5	9
	%	100	97.8	94.7	90.4	84.8	75.4
Starting hospital hemodialysis 1978 – 1981	n	1585	1533	1403	1266		1000
	%	100	97.7	95.7	92.2		87.3

Table 5. Reasons for abandonment of CAPD in pediatric patients

	1981		1982	
	n	%	n	%
Peritonitis	15	(55)	10	(55)
Other abdominal complications	2	(7)	1	(5)
Inadequate dialysis	5	(18)	2	(12)
Patient or family request	2	(7)	2	(12)
Other	3	(13)	3	(16)
Total	27	(100)	18	(100)

Technique Survival

Technique survival was assessed in patients on CAPD including death as technique failure. The mean technique survival was around 50% at 1 year and 30% after 2 years (Fig. 3). Here again, a clear improvement was noted over the years, exceeding 15% at any time interval for patients starting on CAPD in 1981 and 1982 (Fig. 2).

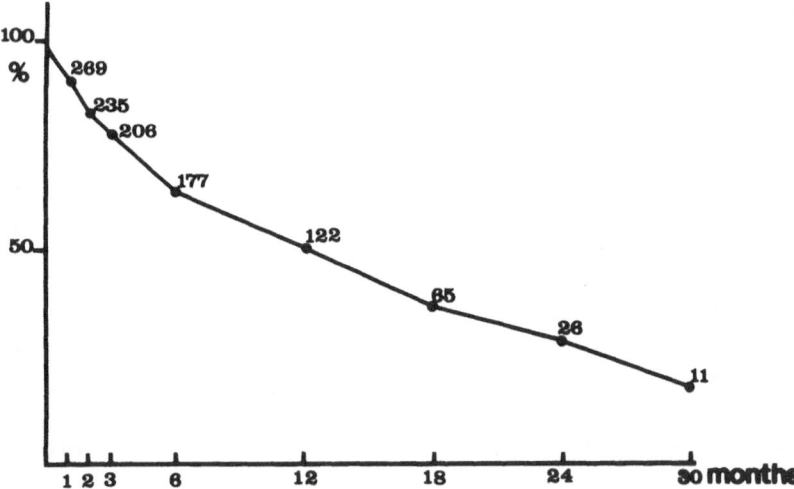

Fig. 2. Technique survival in pediatric patients treated by CAPD

Reasons for abandonment were studied in 1981 and 1982. Peritonitis and abdominal problems were the main causes; the changes observed in 1982 were not significant (Table 5). It should be noted that this information was provided for only a few patients after abandonment of CAPD.

Catheter replacement was studied in one-fifth of the pediatric patients starting CAPD in 1982. Of these, 71% of the patients needed only one catheter insertion, 22% had an additional catheter replacement, 5% had two, and 1% had three replacements.

Peritonitis and Hospitalization

Peritonitis rates were analyzed according to length of time on CAPD for the patients treated in 1981 and 1982: 62 of the patients remained peritonitis-free after 3 months, 30% after 6 months, and 36% after 12 months on CAPD. The number of peritonitis episodes for individual patients was compared with the duration of CAPD treatment. This analysis included all the CAPD treatments recorded in the registry at the close of 1982 (Fig. 3). Patients with three or more episodes represented 10% of the population during the first year of CAPD. This percentage increased to 30% between 12 and 18 months, but decreased again to 15% between 18 and 24 months. The latter was probably due to the dropout of those patients with recurrent peritonitis. The proportion did not change significantly for patients starting in 1981 or 1982 when compared with those starting in 1979 or 1980.

The incidence of peritonitis episodes was calculated for patients starting CAPD in 1981 and 1982. We found an incidence of 0.24 episodes per patient month in 1981 and 0.18 episodes per patient month in 1982 [4].

Data on hospitalization rates were analyzed for 1982 in 146 pediatric patients on CAPD. Out of a total of 2274 hospitalization days, 41% were related to peritonitis and 59% to other causes. A total of 48% of the patients had no hospitalization or fewer than 8 days, while 25% of the patients accounted for two-thirds of the total days of hospitalization.

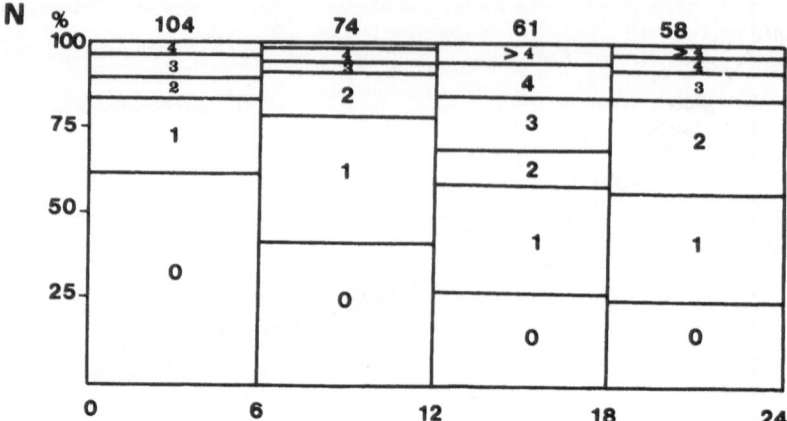

Fig. 3. Number of peritonitis episodes versus time of treatment for children on CAPD

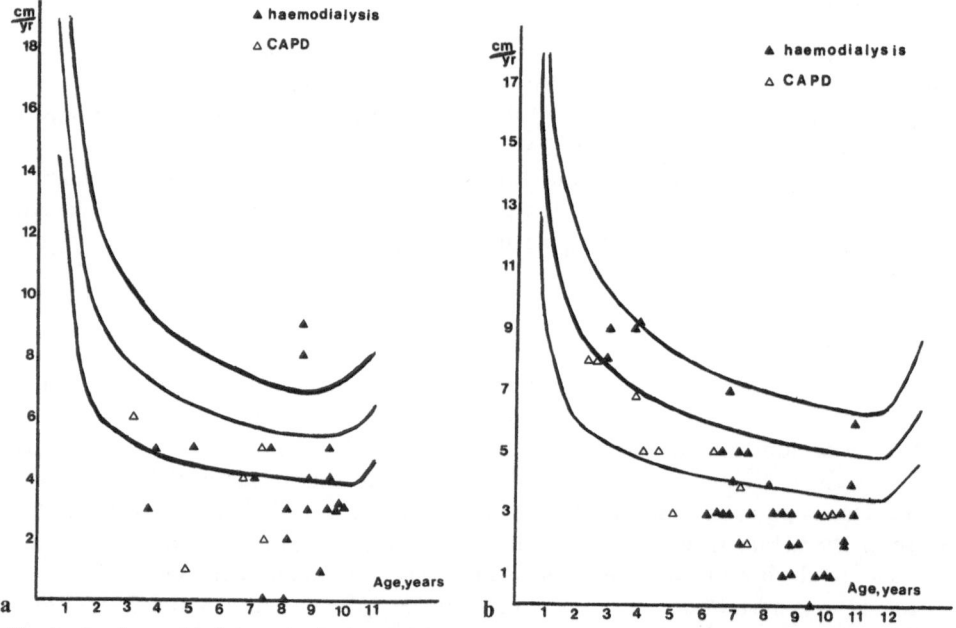

Fig. 4a, b. Annual height gain during 1982 in prepubertal children treated by CAPD and by hemodialysis for girls (*left*) and boys (*right*)

Growth on CAPD

Height Velocity

Growth of prepubertal children on dialysis in 1982 was better in children under 5 years of age, especially in boys. The better growth of the younger children was found with both modes of treatment (Fig. 4).

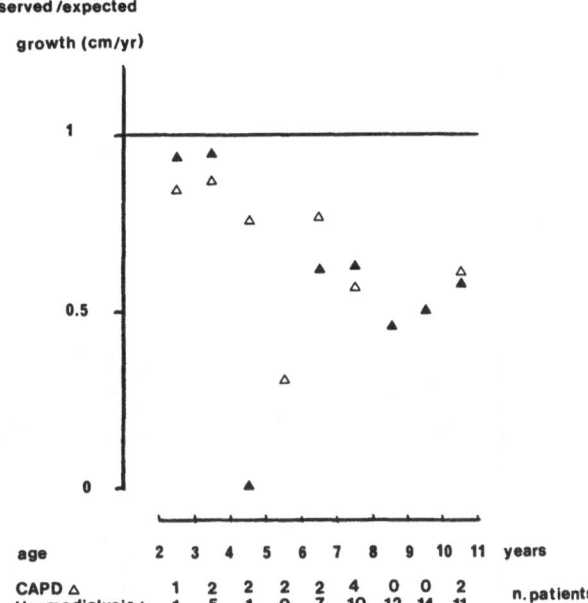

Fig. 5. Linear growth in 1982 for children treated by CAPD and by hemodialysis, according to age

age	2	3	4	5	6	7	8	9	10	11	years
CAPD △		1	2	2	2	2	4	0	0	2	n.patients
Haemodialysis▲		1	5	1	0	7	10	12	14	11	

Growth on CAPD is difficult to compare with growth on hemodialysis, since the number of patients treated for a full year with CAPD is small. The ratio of mean observed growth to expected growth in the children on CAPD (0.63) was higher than the figure observed in children on hemodialysis (0.57). However, because the age distribution was not similar for both groups and great individual variation is present in such a small group of patients, comparison of growth remains difficult (Fig. 5).

Growth Retardation

The height of the majority of the patients treated with either CAPD or hemodialysis was below the 5th percentile for chronological age in January 1982. The average SDS for height in the patients treated with CAPD was −3.18 and for those treated with hemodialysis −3.39 in January 1982. In both groups, height retardation increased, with the difference in SDS during the year being greater in patients treated with CAPD than in those treated with hemodialysis (Fig. 6).

Nutritional Status

Weight for height in prepubertal children dialyzed for more than 1 year is shown in Fig. 7.

Except for patients under 6 years, weight for height was equally distributed around the mean, and patients on CAPD did not behave differently from those on hemodialysis.

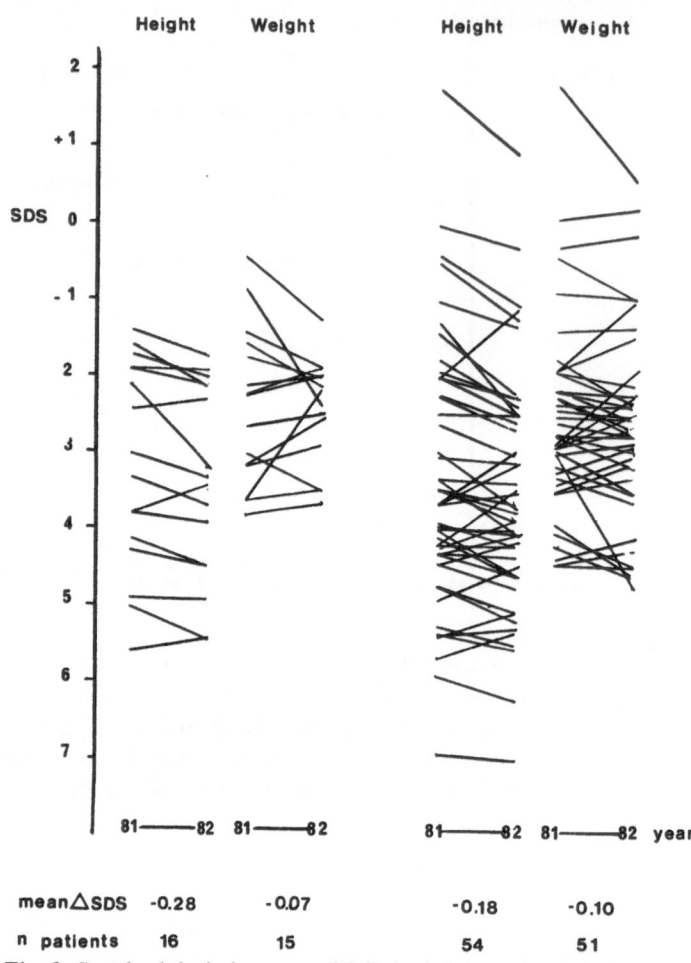

Fig. 6. Standard deviation score (SDS) for height and weight in children treated by CAPD and by hemodialysis in the year 1982

When the difference in SDS for weight during treatment was calculated, no deterioration of weight was noted, and boys on CAPD showed an increase in SDS for weight (Fig. 6).

Results of Transplantation in Children Treated by CAPD.

Results of cadaver transplantation performed in 1980 and thereafter were analyzed according to the mode of dialytic treatment in use at the time of grafting. Both patient and graft survival rates were lower for patients on CAPD when compared with other modes of dialysis, but the difference was not significant.

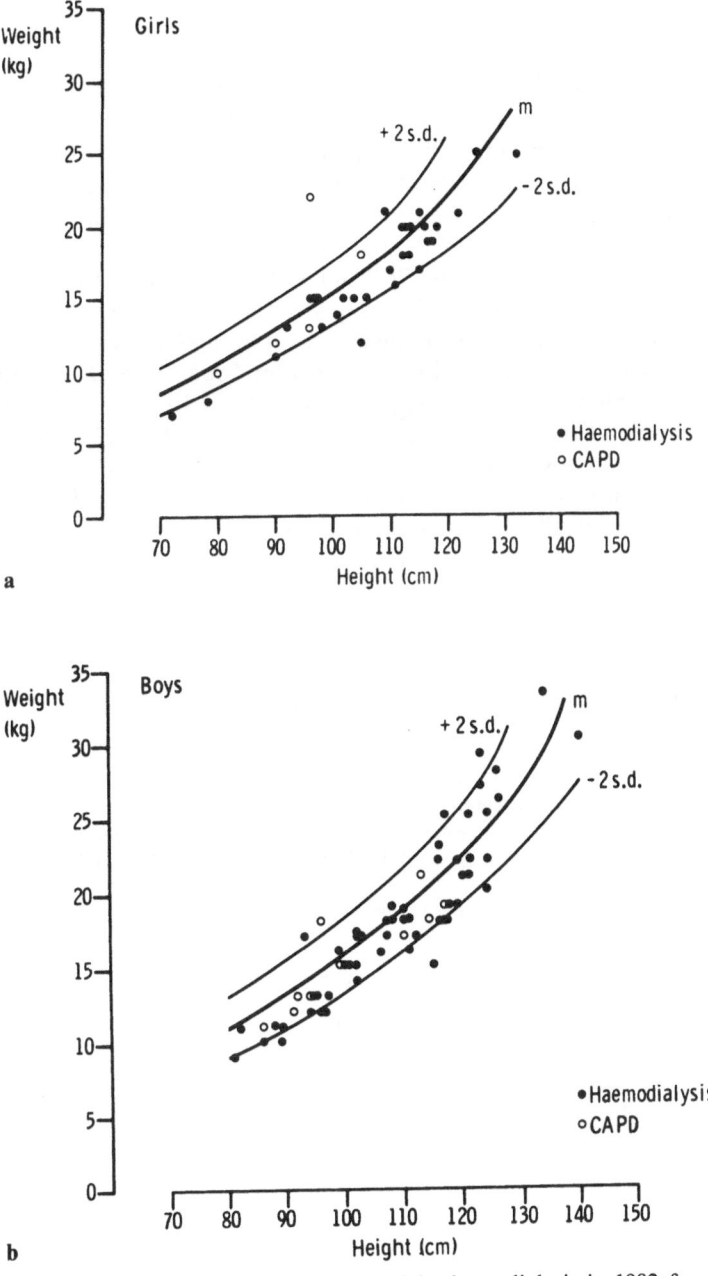

Fig. 7a, b. Weight for height in children treated by CAPD and by hemodialysis in 1982 for girls and boys

Conclusions

Pediatric CAPD developed rapidly in Europe from 1979 to 1982, with 15% of children under 15 years of age treated with this method of dialysis by the close of 1982. The proportion of pediatric patients on CAPD nevertheless differed considerably from one country to another: 50% in the UK and Sweden, 21% in the Netherlands, 17% in Italy, 14% in the FRG, 10% in Spain, and 9% in France. CAPD was the initial dialytic treatment for 61% of children. One-year mean patient survival rates for children starting CAPD in 1981 and 1982 were similar to survival rates achieved with hospital hemodialysis. Technique survival was only 50% at 1 year and 30% at 2 years. Peritonitis was the main reason for abandonment of CAPD. Forty percent of children remained peritonitis free after 6 months and 26% after 1 year. The peritonitis rate was one episode per 6.8 months in 1982. Growth rates of prepubertal children on CAPD and on hemodialysis did not differ, after taking into account the fact that growth was better in younger children, most of whom were treated by CAPD. Growth retardation was observed in both patients on CAPD as well as those on hemodialysis. Finally, graft and patient survival rates after transplantations in children on CAPD were lower than in children on hemodialysis, but the difference was not significant.

References

1. Donckerwolcke RA, Chantler C, Broyer M, et al (1980) Combined report on regular dialysis and transplantation of children in Europe, 1979. Proc Eur Dial Transplant Assoc 17:87–115
2. Broyer M, Donckerwolcke RA, Brunner FP, et al (1981) Combined report on regular dialysis and transplantation of children in Europe, 1980. Proc Eur Dial Transplant Assoc 18:60–87
3. Donckerwolcke RA, Broyer M, Brunner FP et al (1982) Combined report on regular dialysis and transplantation of children in Europe, 1981. Proc Eur Dial Transplant Assoc 19:61–91
4. Broyer M, Donckerwolcke R, Brunner F, et al (1983) Combined report on regular dialysis and transplantation of children in Europe, 1982. Proc Eur Dial Transplant Assoc 20:79–107

Indications for CAPD and CCPD in Children

R. N. Fine

Introduction

The renewed interest in the use of peritoneal dialysis as a therapeutic modality for children with end-stage renal disease (ESRD) was stimulated by the description of Popovich et al. [1] in 1976 of a "novel portable/wearable equilibrium peritoneal dialysis technique" which was labeled continuous ambulatory peritoneal dialysis (CAPD). This technique utilized instillation of dialysate into the peritoneal cavity four to five times daily for periods of 4–8 hours. Since the dialysate/plasma (D/P) ratio for most small molecules is less than one up to 4 hours after instillation of dialysate into the peritoneal cavity and the D/P for large molecules does not approach one until 8 hours or more of dialysis, it was shown that long-dwell peritoneal dialysis was an effective clinical dialytic modality. However, the initial use of glass bottles containing dialysate required eight to ten interruptions of the system daily and led to a significant incidence of peritonitis.

In 1978, Oreopoulos et al. [2] introduced the use of plastic bags filled with dialysate. Following the instillation of dialysate into the peritoneal cavity, the empty plastic bag was folded and attached unobtrusively either to the abdominal wall or conveniently to the patient's clothing and then used for efflux of the spent dialysate after the 4- or 8-hour dwell period. The availability of the plastic bags led to a decreased incidence of peritonitis and significantly increased the acceptability of CAPD as an alternative dialytic modality.

The lack of plastic bags filled with appropriate dialysate volumes for pediatric patients inhibited the general use of CAPD in children until mid-1980. At that time, commercially prepared dialysate became available in varied volumes, and the use of CAPD as a viable dialytic modality became a reality for infants and children. During the past 4 years, the use of CAPD as a primary dialytic modality in children has increased markedly, and currently, as many as 90% of children requiring dialysis in pediatric facilities utilize this dialytic method.

In an attempt to reduce further the number of daily connections and disconnections, thereby reducing the incidence of peritonitis, Diaz-Buxo et al. [3] rearranged the diurnal and nocturnal dwell times with the use of a cycling machine. Three 3-h exchanges were delivered at night during sleep by the cycler and one long-dwell daytime exchange was inserted into the peritoneal cavity at the end of the nocturnal cycling period. This variation of long-dwell peritoneal dialysis, called continuous cycling peritoneal dialysis (CCPD) led to reduced peritonitis rates in adult patients and was subsequently used in pediatric patients.

The indications for the use of CAPD and CCPD in pediatric patients with ESRD will be discussed in the context of our experience in the Division of Pediatric Nephrology at the UCLA Center for the Health Sciences between August 1980 and February 1984.

Experience with CAPD and CCPD at UCLA

Patient Population

During the 3 1/2-year period under discussion, 68 patients (35 males and 33 females), aged 3 months to 21 years, or their parents were trained for CAPD and/or CCPD. Of the 68 patients who have undergone CAPD/CCPD at UCLA, 42 chose CAPD/CCPD as an initial dialytic therapy, 13 elected CAPD/CCPD following failure of a renal allograft, 10 switched from hemodialysis, and 3 were converted from intermittent peritoneal dialysis to CAPD/CCPD. Seven of the ten patients were switched from hemodialysis to CAPD/CCPD for medical indications primarily involving excessive weight gain between dialysis, with predialysis hypertension and profound hypotension during ultrafiltration. Three patients electively switched from hemodialysis to CAPD/CCPD.

Of the 68 patients, 63 (93%) were primarily trained for CAPD, and five (7%) were primarily trained for CCPD. Primary CCPD training was undertaken because of single working parents, the presence of other small children in the household which prevented the parent from undertaking the CAPD daytime exchanges, and maternal psychoses. Three of the five children who were primarily treated with CCPD were under 1 year of age.

Of the 63 patients initially treated with CAPD, 24 (38%) were ultimately converted to CCPD. The medical and nonmedical reasons for conversion to CCPD are indicated in Table 1. In the adolescent patient performing the CAPD exchanges, the reluctance to undertake the exchanges at school was a primary factor leading to the conversion to CCPD.

Training

If the child was younger than 12 years of age, at least one responsible adult was trained to perform the CAPD or CCPD procedure. Ideally, both parents, or one parent and another relative or responsible adult were trained to perform the procedure. The reason for training two adults was to reduce the responsibility on the primary caretaker and to decrease the incidence of burnout. We requested that the secondary caretaker undertake performance of the procedure at least once a week in order to maintain facility with the technique. As is detailed in a companion article in this volume (see Hall et al.), the incidence of complications, especially peritonitis, was decreased when two adults were involved in providing care.

Children over 12 years of age and adolescents were taught to perform the CAPD or CCPD procedure themselves. Training was initiated only after technical dexterity and judgment were assessed to be adequate in this group of patients. In all cases, at least one responsible adult was also trained to perform the technique so that if the patient was incapacitated, performance of the procedure could be continued.

Table 1. Reasons for conversion to CCPD in 24 pediatric patients

Nonmedical	14 (58%)
Parental dialysis	
Single working parent(s)	2
Daytime exchange cumbersome	1
Self-dialysis	
Reluctance to performe exchange at school	11
Medical	10 (42%)
More than four exchanges required	4
Hyperkalemia	1
Ultrafiltration	3
Reduced dialysate volume required	3
Hydrothorax	1
Repeated hernias	1
Dialysate leak	1
Repeated episodes of peritonitis	2
Hypotension	1

Procedure

Four daily exchanges at intervals of 4–6 hours during the daytime and 8–10 hours at night were prescribed for CAPD. Occasionally, a fifth, and rarely, a sixth exchange was required when four exchanges were ineffective in preventing hyperkalemia or providing adequate ultrafiltration, or perioperatively following catheter insertion or other abdominal surgical procedures, when reduced exchange volumes were desirable.

The volume of dialysate (Dianeal, Travenol Laboratories, Deerfield, Ill.) per exchange approached 50 ml/kg and was adjusted to the commercially available dialysate volumes in plastic bags. Occasionally, the volume per exchange was reduced and the number of exchanges increased to accommodate the sense of fullness experienced by the patient.

Dialysate was available in three dextrose concentrations: 1.5%, 2.5%, and 4.25%. The dextrose concentration of the exchanges was adjusted to provide adequate ultrafiltration and limit fluid accumulation without impinging upon the patient's dietary habits. In general, a 4.25% dextrose solution was used for the overnight exchange in order to minimize dialysate reabsorption during the long-dwell period.

Four to five 2-hour overnight exchanges with a cycler (AMP 80/2 Cycler, Delmed, Freehold, N.J.) and one daytime dwell with a volume of one-half of that used for the overnight exchanges was precribed for CCPD. Occasionally, no daytime dwell was prescribed in order to reduce abdominal fullness and increase appetite during the day. The volume of dialysate for the cycler exchanges could be adjusted at 125 ml increments and therefore tailored more precisely to the patients' needs. Increased volumes in the supine position at night were easily tolerated. It was possible to adjust the dextrose concentration of the cycler dialysate to almost any desired concentration by mixing a combination of the three available dextrose concentrations.

Indications for CAPD and CCPD

Patients who require initiation of CAPD and/or CCPD can be divided into three categories: (a) patients who present ESRD de novo; (b) patients undergoing hemodialysis who either desire switching to CAPD and/or CCPD or who are not thriving on hemodialysis; and (c) patients who require reinitiation of dialysis following allograft failure.

Ideally, when infants, children, or adolescents with chronic renal disease approach ESRD, a dialogue is initiated with the patient and/or parent regarding the available options. In most instances, successful transplantation is proposed as the optimal therapeutic modality for such patients with ESRD. However, we have rarely proceeded with transplantation without an initial period of dialysis. This format minimizes the urgency of transplantation and reassures the patient and/or parent that life can be sustained if the allograft is lost. Pretransplant dialysis also optimizes the patient's clinical status and assures dialysis access if posttransplant dialysis is required.

In our experience, the choice of CAPD/CCPD as the initial dialytic modality by patients and/or parents is dictated by: (a) the desire to perform the procedure at home; (b) the minimal interruption of usual "life-style" required to undertake this form of dialysis; (c) the minimal risk involved in performing the procedure itself; (d) the avoidance of the need for a vascular access – a "back-up" vascular access is not routinely inserted; and (e) the anticipated minimal need for dietary restrictions. CCPD is primarily chosen over CAPD by parents who are unavailable to perform the daytime exchanges and by patients attending school who are unwilling to perform the procedure at school.

Medical indications for choosing CAPD/CCPD include: (a) the lack of technical problems in comparison to hemodialysis in infants and small children; (b) the avoidance of vascular access and the need for repetitive venipuncture in the infant and child; (c) the desire to optimize nutritional intake by minimizing dietary restrictions; and (d) improved control of hypertension in the oligoanuric patient. CCPD is medically indicated in the infant or young child who will require more than four CAPD exchanges daily to control the biochemical abnormalities associated with uremia and/or facilitate adequate ultrafiltration.

Patients or parents of children undergoing hemodialysis may desire switching to CAPD/CCPD primarily because of the convenience of performing the procedure at home. In such instances, CAPD/CCPD is chosen over home hemodialysis because of the simplicity of the technique. The desire to avoid repetitive venipuncture and decrease the onerous dietary limitations are additional factors which precipitate the switch to CAPD/CCPD.

The lack of available vascular access, repetitive dietary indiscretion leading to life-threatening hyperkalemia and hypertension, and repetitive profound hypotension when attempting ultrafiltration during hemodialysis are the medical indications dictating the conversion from hemodialysis to CAPD/CCPD.

A child and/or his family requiring initiation of dialysis following graft failure is generally aware of the dialytic options from previous experience. The reasons for choosing CAPD/CCPD are similar to those outlined above.

The potential for transplantation should not influence the choice of dialytic therapy. Our experience, as well as that of others [4], has indicated that there are no significant risks to transplantation in the child undergoing CAPD/CCPD. If required, posttransplant peritoneal dialysis can proceed without difficulty. The incidence of peritonitis in such a situation is rare, despite the concomitant use of immunosuppressive drug therapy, and treatment is similar to that used for nonimmunosuppressed patients. It has been our policy to leave the peritoneal access in place for 3–6 months post transplant or until the adequacy of allograft function is assured.

From our experience to date, it appears that CCPD is advantageous in school-aged children who are uncomfortable with peer pressure associated with the need for an exchange during school hours. In addition, CCPD has the advantage over CAPD in the infant or young child who is unable to tolerate the dialysate volumes required to correct the metabolic consequences of uremia and/or allow adequate ultrafiltration without the need to perform more than four daily CAPD exchanges. More than four CAPD exchanges is a burden that few parents can tolerate for a prolonged period of time.

References

1. Popovich RP, Moncrief JW, Decherd JB, et al (1976) The definition of a novel portable/wearable equilibrium peritoneal dialysis technique (Abstract). Trans Am Soc Artif Intern Organs 5:64
2. Oreopoulos DG, Robson M, Izatt HS, et al (1978) A simple and safe technique for continuous ambulatory peritoneal dialysis (CAPD). Trans Am Soc Artif Intern Organs 24:484
3. Diaz-Buxo JA, Walker PJ, Farmer CD et al (1981) Continuous cyclic peritoneal dialysis (Abstract). Kidney Int 19:145
4. Stephanidis CJ, Balfe JW, Arbus GS, Hardy BE, Churchill BM, Rance CP (1983) Renal transplantation in children treated with CAPD. Perit Dialys Bull 3:5

Comparison of CAPD and CCPD in Children

R. J. Hogg, G. M. Lum, and W. Arnold, (For the Southwest Pediatric Nephrology Study Group) *

Introduction

The optimal choice of chronic dialysis therapy for uremic children continues to be a subject of great interest and concern. Although technical aspects of dialysis in children have improved significantly over the past ten years, continued efforts to minimize complications and increase therapeutic benefits for the pediatric patient remain a considerable challenge. The major aim of dialysis in children should be the use of well-tolerated, simple procedures that produce an improved state of well-being in the patient and, most importantly, allow for normal growth and development. The techniques of continuous, long-dwell peritoneal dialysis (continuous ambulatory [CAPD] or continuous cycling [CCPD] peritoneal dialysis) have of late received a great deal of attention and application [1–8], and the reported therapeutic benefits of CAPD and CCPD have led to an evaluation of these two techniques in children with end-stage renal disease (ESRD). Recent reports have revealed variable results in children treated with CAPD [9–15] and indicate that evaluation of greater numbers of children is needed to determine the actual benefits to be gained for children undergoing the different forms of prolonged-dwell peritoneal dialysis. The present report summarizes the collaborative studies of the pediatric nephrologists who comprise the Southwest Pediatric Nephrology Study Group and addresses specific questions regarding the relative efficacy of CAPD and CCPD in a large series of children. These include:
1. The relative frequency of infectious complications – particularly bacterial peritonitis – in patients treated with CAPD or CCPD

* Southwest Pediatric Nephrology Study Group (SPNSG Central Office: University of Texas Health Science Center at Dallas, Room G3.254, 5323 Harry Hines Boulevard, Dallas, TX 75235, U.S.A.). Director: Ronald J. Hogg. Clinical Coordinators: Shane Roy, III, Luther Travis, James Wenzl. Statistician: Joan S. Reisch. Data Manager: William Fox; Administrative Secretary: Kaye Green. SPNSG Centers and clinicians participating in this study: Baylor College of Medicine, Houston: Phillip L. Berry, L. Leighton Hill, Sami A. Sanjad; Tulane University Medical Center, New Orleans: Frank G. Boineau, John E. Lewy; University of Arkansas, Little Rock: Watson C. Arnold; University of Colorado, Denver: Gary M. Lum; University of Louisiana at Shreveport: W. Frank Tenney; University of Oklahoma Medical Center, Oklahoma City: James R. Matson, James E. Wenzl; University of Tennessee, Memphis: Shane Roy, III, F. Bruder Stapleton; University of Texas Health Science Center at Dallas: Billy S. Arant, Jr., Ronald J. Hogg, Mark T. Houser, Ruben Meyer, H. Leslie Moore; University of Texas Health Science Center at Houston: Eileen Brewer, Susan B. Conley, Gilbert Rose; University of Texas Medical Branch, Galveston: Ben H. Brouhard, Alok Kalia, Luther B. Travis; University of Texas Health Science Center at San Antonio: Michael Foulds; Fred A. McCurdy. Preparation of this study and manuscript: Ronald J. Hogg, Gary M. Lum, Watson C. Arnold.

2. The ability of the two modalities to maintain acceptable biochemical and hematologic profiles
3. The extent to which growth may be achieved in children treated with the two
   forms of treatment and evaluated over periods of 6 months or more

Material and Methods

Data were obtained from 11 pediatric renal centers on 82 children who were 18
years of age or less and had received CAPD or CCPD at home for a minimum of 3
months. Ten of the patients received courses of both CAPD and CCPD, each of
which has been analyzed separately. All laboratory studies were performed in the
clinical laboratories of the participating institutions. Data were obtained on the
rates of peritonitis, exit site infections, and catheter life expectancy for each form of
prolonged-dwell peritoneal dialysis. Growth data were analyzed only for children
who had been on CAPD or CCPD for 6 months or longer. Children over 14 years of
age were excluded from this analysis.

Growth velocity index (GVI) in each child was obtained from the formula:

$$GVI = \frac{\text{actual growth velocity of patient (GV)}}{\text{normal growth velocity for chronological age (GVCA)}} \times 100 \, .$$

A *standard deviation score* (Z score) was calculated using the formula:

$$\frac{\text{Patient's height (cm)} - \text{normal height at 50th percentile for age (cm)}}{\text{Standard deviation of height for age (cm)}}$$

using normal data obtained from the National Center for Health Statistics 10-State
Survey [16]. All data were calculated on the basis of one chronological year of
growth. The standard deviation scores represent the deviation from normal growth
of the children at the beginning and end of the periods of observation on CAPD or
CCPD. Changes in growth rate were calculated by ΔS.D. Hence, a positive ΔS.D.
indicates accelerated growth during peritoneal dialysis. Comparisons were made between males and females on CCPD and CAPD, between each modality of therapy,
and between age groups.

Differences between CAPD and CCPD periods were analyzed by a variety of
statistical methods including t tests, Chi-square analysis, Spearman's correlation
testing, Pearson's correlation testing, and Fisher's exact test (when appropriate).
Statistical significance was defined as a P value equal to or less than 0.05.

Results

A total of 92 treatment periods, 63 periods of CAPD and 29 of CCPD, were evaluated. Demographic characteristics of the patients in the two groups showed no differences. Although the children treated with CCPD were slightly older (10.2 years

compared with 7.7 years), this difference was not statistically significant. There was no difference in either the duration of the treatment interval on each modality of prolonged-dwell peritoneal dialysis or in the volume of dialysis solution used in each cycle. The original renal disorders that led to ESRD were comparable in the two groups of patients, with the combination of obstructive uropathy, reflux nephropathy, and renal dysplasia accounting for approximately 40% of the children on dialysis. Another 37% of the patients had ESRD secondary to glomerular diseases. There were no differences in the biochemical profiles between children on CAPD and CCPD with the exception of the serum creatinine level, which was somewhat higher in the CCPD patients (10.1 as compared with 7.7 mg/dl; $P < 0.01$). The higher serum creatinine concentrations in the patients on CCPD may be a reflection of the older age of this group of patients. It should be noted that in the ten children who received a course of both CAPD and CCPD, there were no differences in the hematologic and biochemical profiles between the two types of dialysis.

Peritonitis

The rate of peritonitis in the total population (177 total episodes of clinical peritonitis) was one episode per 4.8 patient months, and there was no significant difference in the rate of peritonitis observed between the CAPD and CCPD patient populations (1/4.6 and 1/5.2 patient months, respectively). The predominant organism responsible for these episodes was *Staphylococcus aureus* (more than one-third of the cases), whereas there were 21 episodes of apparent "sterile peritonitis," where cultures were obtained but no organism was identified. Catheter placement was performed by surgeons in most patients, and although the catheter life tended to be longer in the CCPD patients, this difference was not significant. As stated previously, ten of the children evaluated in this study were treated with separate courses of CAPD and CCPD. CAPD was the first form of therapy in seven and the second form in three patients. The total number of episodes of peritonitis in these patients was not significantly different for the two modalities of treatment (CAPD, 1/6.3 patient months; CCPD, 1/6.6 patient months); however, the rate of peritonitis was higher during the first course of dialysis than during the second (1/4.4 and 1/14 patient months respectively).

Growth

Growth data were available for 53 children (34 CAPD, 19 CCPD) treated for at least 6 months. Growth velocity did not differ significantly between the two modalities of treatment (CAPD, 0.46 ± 0.61 cm/month; CCPD, 0.48 ± 0.40 cm/month). GVCA in CAPD patients (0.58 ± 0.24 cm/month) was somewhat higher than that occurring in CCPD patients (0.50 ± 0.19 cm/month) because the CCPD population was slightly older. Children starting either form of prolonged-dwell peritoneal dialysis were growing at a GVI that was 88 ± 8% of expected, and they were 2.6 ± 1.8 standard deviations below the norm for height. Weight was 75 ± 18% of expected, and the children were 1.5 ± 1.2 standard deviations below the norm for weight at the start of peritoneal dialysis. At the end of a mean of 1.0 ± 0.6 years on prolonged-dwell peritoneal dialysis, the children were growing at the same rate and had the same standard deviation scores. Thus, although these children did not experience "catch-up" growth during a year on peritoneal dialysis, they did maintain their relative position on the growth tables.

This series contained 38 children on prolonged-dwell peritoneal dialysis who were 5 years of age or older and 15 children less than 5 years of age. When the children under 5 years of age were analyzed separately, their growth rate was found to be 89% of expected, and they did not decrease their standard deviation scores. However, when individual patients treated with either CAPD or CCPD were evaluated, it was apparent that, whereas many patients attained excellent growth, there were some in whom minimal or no growth occurred.

Determinants of Optimal Growth in CAPD and CCPD Patients

Patients who were treated with CAPD showed a strong correlation between GVI and serum phosphorus concentrations. Patients with a GVI of less than 80% had a mean serum phosphorus of 4.3 mg/dl, whereas patients with a GVI greater than or equal to 80% had a mean serum phosphorus of 5.7 mg/dl ($P < 0.0001$). A significant correlation was seen also when GVI was compared with blood urea nitrogen (BUN). Children older than 5 years of age with a GVI of less than 80% had a mean BUN of 45 ± 17 mg/dl, while children with a GVI greater than or equal to 80% had a BUN of 73 ± 10 mg/dl ($P = 0.009$). In contrast, children with a GVI of less than 80% had a mean serum creatinine of 11.5 mg/dl, while children with a GVI greater than 80% had a serum creatinine concentration of 8.3 mg/dl ($P = 0.03$).

Discussion

The rationale for cooperative studies of patients on dialysis have been described elsewhere [17] and will not be reiterated in this discussion. The conclusions that may be drawn from our cooperative study pertain to a comparison of two forms of prolonged-dwell peritoneal dialysis in children with ESRD. We have shown that CAPD and CCPD provide equivalent biochemical and hematologic profiles in such children; similar, albeit high frequency rates of peritonitis; and growth rates which, though still inadequate in some children, are equal to or better than growth rates observed in children treated with hemodialysis, particularly in children less than 4 years of age.

The frequency of peritonitis in children treated with prolonged-dwell peritoneal dialysis has been reported to be higher than that seen in comparable series of adults [18, 19], and in our patients, the rate of peritonitis was also high – approximately one episode for every 5 patient months. However, this rate did not differ between children receiving either CAPD or CCPD. As in other studies, our figures were skewed by occasional patients who had multiple episodes of peritonitis, but for whom no alternative form of therapy was available. The organisms that were cultured from dialysis fluid in our children with peritonitis were similar to the spectra that have been observed by other authors and demonstrate the preponderance of skin pathogens [18]. The infrequent demonstration of gram-negative organisms in our patients is also comparable to that reported in other series [19].

The growth rates that were observed in this study in children receiving either form of prolonged-dwell peritoneal dialysis were encouraging. In particular, the finding that children less than 5 years of age grew at a rate comparable to that seen in the older children is important. The biochemical variables associated with improved growth, that is, higher BUN and serum phosphorus concentrations, appear surprising, since Kohaut et al. showed that improved growth in children on CAPD is associated with a reduction in serum parathyroid hormone levels [13]. The relevance of our findings to Kohaut's study cannot be evaluated directly, since we did not determine the role of hyperparathyroidism, but it is postulated that the increased BUN and serum phosphorus levels associated with higher growth rates seen in our children probably represent an improved nutritional status. Those children ingesting adequate substrate grew more normally and have higher BUN and phosphorus concentrations. Unfortunately, due to the lack of uniformity of dietary observations within our different centers, we were unable to make comparisons between calorie and protein intakes and other parameters.

The results of this study demonstrate that CAPD and CCPD provide adequate and comparable methods of interim treatment for children with ESRD. Although renal transplantation will remain the optimal therapy for children with ESRD, it is concluded that both forms of prolonged-dwell peritoneal dialysis have the potential for providing a satisfactory alternative when successful renal transplantation is not possible. The decision regarding the choice, of CAPD or CCPD as the primary form of therapy should be made on the basis of patient, parent, and physician preference, since there does not appear to be any major medical difference between the two forms of therapy.

Acknowledgments. The Southwest Pediatric Nephrology Study Group acknowledges support from the National Kidney Foundation of Texas, Abbott Laboratories, American Medical Products, American McGaw, B-D Drake Willock, Cutter Labs, Hoffman-LaRoche, Inc., Mead Johnson, Merck and Co., Inc., Ross Laboratories, E. R. Squibb, Southwest Airlines, Travenol Labs, and the Upjohn Company.

References

1. Nolph KD, Popovich RP, Moncrief JW (1978) Theoretical and practical implications of continuous ambulatory peritoneal dialysis. Nephron 21: 117–122
2. Popovich RP, Moncrief JW, Nolph KD, Ghods AJ, Twardowski ZJ, Pyle WK (1978) Continuous ambulatory peritoneal dialysis. Ann Intern Med 88: 449–456
3. Popovich RP, Moncrief JW, Nolph KD (1978) Continuous ambulatory peritoneal dialysis. Artif Organs 2: 84–86
4. Lacke C, Senekjian HO, Knight TF, Frazier M, Hatlelid R, Kozak M, Baker P, Weinman EJ (1981) Twelve months' experience with continuous ambulatory and intermittent peritoneal dialysis. Arch Intern Med 141: 187–190
5. Nolph KD, Sorkin M, Rubin J, Arfania D, Prowant B, Fruto L, Kennedy D (1980) Continuous ambulatory peritoneal dialysis: three-year experience at one center. Ann Intern Med 92: 609–613

6. Randerson DH, Farrell PC (1981) Clinical assessment of CAPD. Dial Transplant 10:389
7. Oreopoulos DG (1980) An update on the continuous ambulatory peritoneal dialysis (CAPD). Int J Artif Organs 3:231–234
8. Diaz-Buxo JA, Walker PJ, Chandler JT, Farmer CD, Holt KL (1981) Advances in peritoneal dialysis: continuous cyclic peritoneal dialysis. Contemp Dial Nov 23
9. Kohaut EC (1981) Continuous ambulatory peritoneal dialysis: a preliminary pediatric experience. Am J Dis Child 135:270–271
10. Balfe JW, Vigneaux A, Willumsen J, Hardy BE (1981) The use of CAPD in the treatment of children with end-stage renal disease. Perit Dial Bull 1:35–37
11. Fennell RS, Orak JK, Hudson T, Garin EH, Irvani A, Van Deusen WJ, Howard R, Pfaff WW, Walker RD, III, Richard GA (1984) Growth in children with various therapies for end-stage renal disease. Am J Dis Child 138:28–31
12. Baum M, Powell D, Calvin S, McDaid T, McHenry K, Mar H, Potter D (1982) Continuous ambulatory peritoneal dialysis in children: comparison with hemodialysis. N Engl J Med 307:1537–1542
13. Kohaut EC (1983) Growth in children treated with continuous ambulatory peritoneal dialysis. Int J Pediatr Nephrol 4:93–98
14. Salusky IB, Lucullo L, Nelson P, Fine RN (1982) Continuous ambulatory peritoneal dialysis in children. Pediatr Clin North Am 29:1005–1012
15. Stefanides CJ, Hewitt IK, Balfe JW (1983) Growth in children receiving continuous ambulatory peritoneal dialysis. J Pediatr 102:681–685
16. Hamill PVV, Drizd TA, Johnson CL, Reed RB, Roche AF (1977) NCHS growth curves for children, birth-18 years, United States. National Center for Health Statistics 43-5, Hyattsville (Vital and health statistics, Series 11, Data from the National Health Survey, no 165). [DHEW Publication No. (PHS) 78-1650]
17. Wineman RJ (1983) Rationale of the National Cooperative Dialysis Study. Kidney Int 23 (Suppl 13):8–10
18. McClung MR (1983) Peritonitis in children receiving continuous ambulatory peritoneal dialysis. Pediatr Inf Dis 2:328–332
19. Fine RN, Salusky IB, Hall T, Lucullo L, Jordan SC, Ettenger RB (1983) Peritonitis in children undergoing continuous ambulatory peritoneal dialysis. Pediatrics 71:806–809

CAPD in Acute Renal Failure: Clinical Experience in Children

F. C. B. Abbad and S. L. B. Ploos van Amstel

The initiation of early dialysis in the treatment of acute renal failure (ARF) in children leads to a clear reduction in the mortality rate [1–4]. Because of the catabolic state characterizing ARF, early and frequent dialysis is commonly required [5–8]. Hemodialysis (HD) is relatively easy to perform in older children ($\geq$ 3 years), but in the younger child, it remains complicated despite recent technical improvements [9, 10]. Thus, peritoneal dialysis (PD) is the therapy of choice in the majority of young pediatric patients with ARF. Despite the initiation of PD, the catabolic situation in the anuric stage of this disease is a significant problem even with intravenous or oral hyperalimentation, because of the necessity of restricting fluid intake and imposing dietary restrictions [11, 12]. In the small child, it is especially difficult to obtain an anabolic situation because fluid and dietary restrictions are stringent. Moreover, pediatric patients generally will not cooperate in the oral administration of the unattractive diet necessary during the oligoanuric phase of ARF. Continuous ambulatory peritoneal dialysis (CAPD) offers an attractive alternative because dietary restrictions are minimal.

Methods and Patients

Nine young patients with ARF (five girls, three boys), 3 weeks to 2.9 years of age, and three older children (two girls, one boy), 6.4 to 12.4 years of age, were treated with CAPD in the Pediatric Department of the University Hospital of Amsterdam (Table 1). Ten of the 12 children (seven girls, three boys) with hemolytic uremic syndrome (HUS) were referred to us. The youngest child, a girl of 3 weeks, initially had the clinical features of cardiac failure and overhydration, but the clinical and biochemical findings characteristic of HUS developed within a week of admission. Patient 8 had acute tubular necrosis following severe dehydration, and patient 12 had a complex nephritis with a severe pulmonary pneumococcal infection.

Keeping in mind the possibility of spontaneous remission of ARF in young patients with HUS [13, 14], we initially used a stiff catheter (Trocath) for acute PD during the first 48 hours after admission. This catheter was inserted on the ward through puncture under local anesthesia. Thereafter, the catheter was removed in view of the risk of infection caused by contamination and leakage of the catheter [9]. If the patient remained anuric through the next 48 hours, we initiated CAPD. For this purpose, a Tenckhoff catheter was surgically implanted in the peritoneal cavity under general anesthesia. This procedure was used in patients 1 to 6, with the exception of patient 4. The latter had been operated upon elsewhere with the pre-

Table 1. Children with ARF treated with CAPD

Patient	Sex	Age (years)	Cause of ARD	Total oligo-anuria[a] (days)	Treatment (days)	Periods of peritonitis (n)	Catheter problems (n)
1	f	0.7	HUS	17	31	1	1
2	f	2.2	HUS	14	20	1	1
3	m	2.9	HUS	12	10	–	–
4	m	1.4	HUS	13	13	1	–
5	f	0.1	HUS	27	33	1	1
6	f	1.9	HUS	10	13	–	–
7	m	1.8	HUS	11	9	–	–
8	m	0.9	ATN	14	9	–	–
9	f	1.5	HUS	11	15	–	–
10	f	6.4	HUS	4	9	–	–
11	f	12.4	HUS	2	10	–	–
12	m	8.0	CN	6	10	–	–

HUS, hemolytic uremic syndrome; ATN, acute tubular necroses; CN, complex nephritis.
[a] ≤400 ml/m² body surface/day.

sumptive diagnosis of intussusception. A healthy appendix was removed. Because of the recent laparatomy, surgical insertion of the Tenckhoff catheter was considered safer than insertion of the stiff catheter.

After November 1982, however, we inserted a Tenckhoff catheter surgically under general anesthesia as soon as possible, i.e., within 24 hours of admission (patients 7–11). Of course, in order to carry out this procedure, it is imperative that no contraindications to general anesthesia be present. Due to their poor clinical condition, patients 8 and 12 were treated with intermittent peritoneal dialysis (IPD) and HD respectively prior to general anesthesia.

During the first 24 h of the CAPD procedure, our usual regimen of frequent exchanges of dialysis fluid (every 20–30 min) was maintained in order to prevent clogging of the catheter. Thereafter, the fluid was exchanged four times a day; in children under 1.5 years, six exchanges per day were used. The volume of fluid per exchange was gradually increased from 15 ml/kg to 30–40 ml/kg body weight. The exchanges were done by the nursing staff of our Pediatric ward. The plastic bags, containing commercially available dialysate (Dianeal) are prepared by our hospital pharmacy to fit the size of the child. During this regimen, the diet was truly free with only a slight restriction of fluid intake. This encouraged a normal protein intake. The CAPD treatment was continued until a creatinine clearance of at least 20 ml/min/1.73 m² was reached in order to be able to maintain the same degree of dietary freedom after CAPD was discontinued and the catheter removed.

Results

Table 1 indicates that the total duration of oligoanuria (including the period before admission to our department) varied from 11 to 27 days (average, 14.3 days) in the first nine patients (under 3 years). In these nine patients, CAPD treatment varied from 9 to 31 days (average, 17.0 days), depending upon the time required for the creatinine clearance of 20 ml/min/1.73 m² body surface area to be reached.

Peritonitis was seen in four patients. In three patients, leakage of peritoneal fluid while using pediatric catheters with unattached cuffs was implicated. In patient 4, signs of peritonitis disappeared after removal of a contaminated catheter. Relevant clinical and laboratory data during CAPD are shown in Table 2. There was no significant loss in body weight. The youngest child, patient 5, showed an almost normal increase in weight of 100 g/week. It was possible to maintain a plasma urea level of 8–15 mmol/l throughout the treatment period. Plasma electrolytes were normal in all children. Plasma bicarbonate was normal, with the exception of patient 5 during the first 2 days of CAPD. Serum albumin levels were acceptable (30–34 g/l) in the younger children ($\leqq$ 3 years of age), as were the blood glucose levels (4–8 mmol/l). Patients 1 to 5 were discussed extensively at the EDTA meeting of 1982 [15].

Discussion

In ARF, early and frequent dialysis is accpeted therapy. In adults and older children, frequent HD is commonly used. Even in experienced hands, however, HD is difficult to perform in the young child. An external shunt is usually required, and the smaller the child, the bigger the problems regarding technique, clotting of the shunt, and hemodynamics of the procedure [16, 17]. It is clear that PD is easier to use in children below 15 kg body weight. CAPD offers a number of advantages over IPD. First of all, repeated punctures of the peritoneal cavity are not necessary [18]. Furthermore, immobilization, an absolute necessity with the stiff catheter used during IPD, is not required in CAPD [19]. Thirdly, in contrast to both IPD and HD, there are no dietary restrictions because the fluids and electrolytes are continuously balanced [20]. These advantages clearly apply to both the younger and the older child. The condition of our patients improved rapidly and full mobilization was rapidly permitted. Normal activities were encouraged in order to enhance psychological development and stimulate appetite. Nevertheless, total caloric intake was still subnormal for age in some patients (Table 2), but glucose absorption from the dialysate added a considerable number of calories to the daily dietary intake [21–23].

Despite the use of dialysate containing high concentrations of glucose (2.27% or 3.86%), especially during the anuric stage, blood glucose levels did not exceed 8 mmol/l. Periods of overhydration were observed in the smaller children (patients 1 and 5, once and twice respectively). Short-dwell-time dialysis was applied for 12 hours in each patient in order to achieve a more effective ultrafiltration of fluid. The latter was possible because of the high glucose absorption from the dialysate [24, 25]. The commercially available dialysate (Dianeal) was used without problem. On one occasion (patient 5), we had to exchange the lactate anion of the dialysate for bicarbonate as a buffer. This occurred in the first 2 days of CAPD during a period of extreme metabolic acidosis. Poor physical condition, i.e., circulatory problems and catabolism, caused a chronic metabolic acidosis, and these circumstances led to an impairment in the capacity for lactate breakdown. Blood levels of lactate and pyruvate were not measured.

Table 2. Clinical and laboratory findings during CAPD

Patient	Age (years)	Weight (kg)		Fluid intake (ml/day)		Average protein intake (g/day)	Average oral caloric intake (cal/day)	Plasma urea mmol/l		Serum albumin g/l	
		Initial	Final	Initial	Final			Initial	Final	Initial	Final
1	0.7	7.0	6.9	700	800	2.5	500	33	2.5	27	31
2	2.2	12.3	12.2	500	750	2.5	1330	32	10	34	32
3	2.9	14.8	14.8	500	750	2.5	1390	32	10	33	37
4	1.4	13.2	13.4	250	750	1	600	50	8.0	29	32
5	0.1	2.8	3.2	300	400	2	250	16	3.0	31	33
6	1.9	9.9	10.0	500	800	2.5	700	46	12	33	32
7	1.8	9.7	9.9	500	750	1.5	600	40	9.4	32	33
8	0.9	10.9	9.5	300	700	1.3	600	19	15	32	32
9	1.5	10.8	11.0	500	800	2	700	33	10	31	37
10	6.4	26.0	26.4	800	1400	1.5	1100	28	9	36	37
11	12.4	35.8	34.9	1000	2000	1.5	1300	34	12	31	33
12	8.0	21.3	22.6	600	1200	1.3	1200	32	10	33	39

Table 3. Children with HUS younger than 3 years 1975 – 1984

Patients (n)	IPD/HD 7	CAPD 8
Mean age (years)	2.45	1.56
Mean creatinine clearance ≥ 20 ml/min/1.73 m² (elapsed time, days)	23.8	22.3
Mean duration of hospitalization (days)	68.1	34.5

Peritonitis occurred once in four of the 12 children (patients 1, 2, 4, and 5). In three cases (patients 1, 2 and 5), peritonitis was caused by leakage of the catheter that occurred while using the pediatric Tenckhoff catheter with unattached cuffs. Detaching the catheter from the cuff at the peritoneal exit site always led to leakage of dialysate and peritonitis.

It might be possible to reduce the risk of infection in infants by using 2-liter stock bags rather than small 100-ml bags because the number of bag-changes could then be reduced to one a day. By weighing the bag before and after exchange, the in- and outflow volume of the dialysate can be measured.

We do not consider omentectomy necessary. Apart from the above-mentioned technical difficulties, there were no other problems related to the catheter. IPD or HD may still be necessary in order to improve the clinical condition of some patients prior to general anesthesia. We compared two groups of patients with HUS (Table 3), who had been treated with two different types of dialysis – IPD and CAPD. There was no significant difference between the two groups regarding age or the period of time necessary to reach creatinine clearance of 20 ml/min/1.73 m². There was, however, a considerable difference between the two groups when we compared the time of recovery after a creatinine clearance of 20 ml/min/1.73 m² was reached. There was a strong indication that the physical condition of the patients in the CAPD group improved faster than that of the IPD/HD group. However, because the group was too small, these data are not statistically significant. A prospective study of a larger group will allow more conclusions to be drawn in the future.

Conclusion

CAPD appears to be a practical type of dialysis, especially for the young child with ARF. With proper precautions, it can be performed on a pediatric ward by trained nursing staff. In our series of 12 children, we were able to overcome the catabolic situation characterizing ARF in a more acceptable way, while allowing full nutrition and an attractive diet [26]. Furthermore, it is our impression that CAPD is psychologically less traumatic.

Peritonitis was not a frequent problem. The use of catheters with preattached cuffs should be used, as these diminish the risk of leakage and peritonitis. As soon as a creatinine clearance of 20 ml/min/1.73 m² has been reached, the procedure can be discontinued.

References

1. Kaplan BS, Katz J, Krawitz S et al. (1971) An analysis of the results of therapy in 67 cases of the hemolytic-uremic syndrome. J Pediatr 78:420–425
2. Tune BM, Laevitt TJ, Gribbe TJ (1973) The hemolytic-uremic syndrome in California: A review of 28 non-heparinized cases with longterm follow-up. J Pediatr 82:304–310
3. Gianantonio CA, Vitacco M, Mendilaharzu J et al. (1973) The hemolytic-uremic syndrome. Nephron 11:174–192
4. Kaplan BS, Thompson PO, De Chadarevian JP (1976) The hemolytic-uremic syndrome. Ped Clin N Amer 23:761–777
5. Teshan PE, Baxter CR, O'Brien TF et al. (1960) Prophylactic hemodialysis in the treatment of acute renal failure. Ann Intern Med 53:992–1016
6. Burns RO, Henderson LW, Hager EB et al. (1962) Peritoneal dialysis clinical experience. N Engl J Med 267:1060–1066
7. Eckberg M, Holmberg L, Denneberg T (1977) Hemolytic-uremic syndrome. Results of treatment with haemodialysis. Acta Pediatr Scand 66:693–698
8. Gomperts ED, Lieberman E (1980) Hemolytic-uremic syndrome. J Pediatr 97:419–420
9. Day RE, White RHR (1977) Peritoneal dialysis in children. Arch Dis Child 52:56–61
10. Buselmeier TJ, Kjellstrand CM (1973) A-V shunts and fistulae in neonates, infants and children. Proc Eur Dial Transpl Assoc 10:511–515
11. Gianantonio CA, Vitacco M, Mendilaharzu J et al. (1962) Acute renal failure in infancy and childhood. J Pediatr 61:660–678
12. Oreopoulos DG, Khanna R, McCready W et al. (1980) Continous ambulatory peritoneal dialysis in Canada. Dial Transplant 9:224–226
13. Gianantonio CA, Vitacco M, Medilaharzu J et al. (1968) The hemolytic uremic syndrome. J Pediatr 72:757–765
14. Young Sorrenti L, Lewy PR (1978) The hemolytic uremic syndrome. Am J Dis Child 132:59–62
15. Abbad FCB, Ploos van Amstel SLB (1982) Continuous ambulatory peritoneal dialysis in small children with acute renal failure. Proc Eur Dial Transpl Assoc 19:607–613
16. Lorentz WB, Hamilton RW, Disher B et al. (1981) Home peritoneal dialysis during infancy. Clin Nephrol 15:194–197
17. Fine RN (1982) Peritoneal dialysis update. J Pediatr 100:1–7
18. Lankish PG, Tönnis HJ, Fernandez-Redo E et al. (1973) Use of the Tenckhoff catheter for peritoneal dialysis in terminal renal failure. Br Med J 4:712–713
19. Heal MR, England AG, Goldsmith HJ (1973) Four years' experience with indwelling silastic canulae for long-term peritoneal dialysis. Br Med J 4:596–600
20. Madden MA, Zimmerman SW, Simpson DP (1981) Longitudinal comparison of intermittent versus continuous ambulatory peritoneal dialysis in the same patients. Clin Nephrol 16:293–299
21. Gagnadoux MF, Hernandez MA, Broyer M et al. (1977) Alternative de l'hémodialyse iterative chez l'enfant. Arch Fr Pediatr 34:860–875
22. Etteldorf JN, Dobbins WT, Sweeney NJ et al. (1962) Intermittent peritoneal dialysis in the management of acute renal failure in children. J Pediatr 60:327–339
23. Blumenkrantz NJ, Schmidt RW (1981) In: Nolph KD (ed) Peritoneal dialysis. Nijhoff, The Hague, pp 275–308
24. Balfe JW, Vigneux A, Willumsen J et al. (1981) The use of CAPD in the treatment of children with end stage renal disease. Perit Dial Bull 1:35–38
25. Alexander ISR, Tseng CH, Maksym KA et al. (1981) Clinical parameters in CAPD for infants and children. In: Moncrief JW, Popovich RP (eds) CAPD update 1981. Masson, New York, p 195
26. Oreopoulos DG, Khanna R, Dombros N (1981) Progress in peritoneal dialysis. Proceedings of the 8th international comgress of nephrology, Athens, pp 715–722

Glucose Metabolism in Uremia: Effect of Hemodialysis and CAPD

R. H. K. Mak and C. Chantler

Introduction

Ernst Neubauer [1], a German physician, was the first to report fasting hyperglycemia in patients with advanced nephritis. However, until the survival of patients with end-stage renal disease was improved by dialysis and transplantation, little attention was given to metabolic abnormalities in uremia. With an increasing number of children in terminal renal failure surviving into adult life, the poor growth of such patients has become a major clinical problem. It has been postulated that disturbances of glucose and energy metabolism may be associated with the abnormalities in protein and lipid metabolism as well as various aspects of endocrine function resulting in decreased anabolism. Two indirect pieces of evidence may be taken in support of this hypothesis. First, a number of dysmorphic syndromes presenting with poor growth, such as Turner's syndrome. Lawrence-Moon-Biedl syndrome, and Down's syndrome [2], also exhibit abnormal glucose metabolism. Secondly, with intensive insulin therapy in juvenile insulin-dependent diabetic patients, normalization of blood glucose has been accompanied by the correction of the metabolic abnormalities in protein and lipid metabolism [3]. The latter metabolic disturbances are very similar to those demonstrated in children with uremia. Furthermore, with the correction of these metabolic abnormalities, growth was significantly improved [4].

Glucose Metabolism in Uremic Patients

Glucose Intolerance in Uremia

The principal characteristics of impaired glucose metabolism in uremic patients are fasting hyperglycemia and abnormal oral and intravenous glucose tolerance tests. That is, the peak glucose concentration is elevated after an oral or intravenous glucose load, and return to fasting levels is delayed. Such intolerance to glucose occurs in more than 50% of patients with uremia [5–10]. DeFronzo et al. [11] reviewed the literature in 1973 and suggested that it is possible to distinguish two groups of uremic patients on the basis of glucose metabolism. The first group had normal glucose decay constants and high plasma insulin levels during glucose tolerance tests, whereas a second group had decreased glucose decay constants and normal or diminished insulin levels.

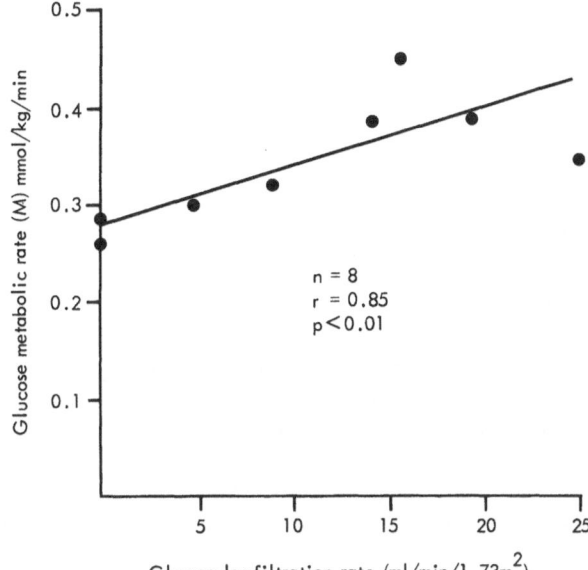

Fig. 1. Relationship between glucose metabolic rate (M) and glomerular filtration rate in eight pubertal children with uremia

There is a paucity of information on glucose metabolism in children with chronic renal failure. EL-Bishti et al. [12] used the intravenous glucose tolerance test and demonstrated glucose intolerance in 16 children with uremia on regular hemodialysis. Mak et al. [13] employed a more sophisticated method, the hyperglycemic clamp technique, and confirmed the same abnormality in children with various degrees of chronic renal failure, also noting a positive correlation between renal function and glucose metabolic rate as measured during the clamp technique (Fig. 1).

Insulin Resistance in Uremia

Peripheral insensitivity to the hypoglycemic action of insulin in uremia is well-supported by clinical and laboratory evidence [11]. Insulin resistance in uremia could result either from abnormal hepatic glucose metabolism (augmented production or impaired uptake) or from impaired glucose uptake by peripheral tissues, i.e., muscle and adipose tissue.

Rubenfeld and Garber [14] studied 13 uremic adults and found increased basal glucose production compared with controls but did not examine the ability of insulin to suppress hepatic glucose production. However, methodological problems, such as using tritiated glucose labeled in the two position (which is known to overestimate glucose turnover because of futile cycles) and failure to demonstrate equilibrium in their tritiated glucose specific activity curves, made interpretation of their results difficult. DeFronzo et al. [15] measured hepatic glucose metabolism in uremic subjects with hepatic venous catheterization and tritiated glucose labeled in the three position. They found both normal hepatic glucose production in the basal state and normal suppression during hyperinsulinemia, where insulin levels were similar to those used during the hyperglycemic and euglycemic clamp techniques as well as during glucose tolerance tests. He also found that hepatic glucose uptake was not different in uremic subjects when compared with controls, both in the basal state and during hyperinsulinemia.

If hepatic glucose metabolism is normal, the site of insulin resistance must reside in the peripheral tissues, i.e. muscle and adipose tissues. Westervelt [16, 17] performed forearm perfusion studies and showed that glucose and phosphate uptake in forearm muscles in response to exogenous insulin was decreased in patients with uremia. DeFronzo et al. [18] measured whole-body and leg glucose uptake simultaneously using the euglycemic clamp technique and femoral venous and arterial catheterization in uremic subjects and demonstrated the same degree of impairment in glucose uptake of the whole body (56% lower than controls) and the leg alone (60% lower than controls). These results suggest that the major sites of insulin resistance reside in muscle and adipose tissues.

Insulin sensitivity is best assessed in vivo by the euglycemic clamp technique, with measurement of hepatic glucose production by either hepatic venous catheterization or tritiated glucose infusion. These invasive studies are, however, not ethically permissible in children. DeFronzo et al. [19] have nevertheless demonstrated that the ratio of glucose metabolic rate to mean insulin levels obtained during the hyperglycemic clamp technique is virtually identical to the same ratio obtained during the euglycemic clamp studies carried out in both normal subjects and uremic patients. Furthermore, they showed that hepatic glucose production as discussed above was almost totally suppressed during these studies [15]. Mak et al. [13], using the hyperglycemic clamp, demonstrated insulin resistance with a positive correlation between insulin sensitivity and renal function in children with uremia (Fig. 2).

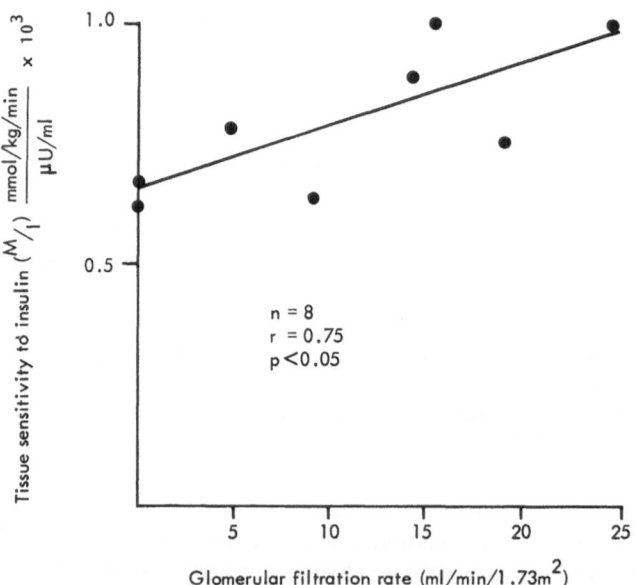

Fig. 2. Relationship between insulin sensitivity (M/I) and glomerular filtration rate in eight pubertal children with uremia

Cellular Mechanism of Insulin Resistance

Little is known concerning the cellular mechanisms contributing to insulin resistance in uremic subjects. Gambhir et al. found a reduction in insulin binding to red blood cells of uremic subjects, which nonetheless increased to levels above control values after initiation of regular hemodialysis [20]. Smith and DeFronzo [21] studied insulin dose response curves in uremic subjects using the euglycemic clamp technique with simultaneous measurement of insulin binding to monocytes. They concluded that the site of insulin resistance must be postreceptor in origin. This concept is supported by in vitro evidence reported in the study of Maloff and Lockwood, who observed normal insulin binding, but decreased glucose transport and impaired intracellular glucose metabolism in adipocytes from rats with uremia [22].

An abnormality in the enzyme regulation of key metabolic pathways in glycolysis, Kreb's cycle, or oxidative phosphorylation could account for the abnormal glucose metabolism in uremia. Westervelt [16] and Cohen and Horowitz [23] suggested impaired phosphorylation of glucose. Metcoff et al. [24] demonstrated decreased activity of rate-limiting glycolytic enzymes. Renner and Heintz [25] showed that glucose utilization diminishes via the Kreb's cycle but increases via the pentose phosphate shunt. Glaze et al. [26] demonstrated uncoupling of oxidative phosphorylation by uremic serum.

Factors Causing Insulin Resistance

The cause of peripheral tissue insensitivity to insulin is not clear. Three mechanisms are possible.

Abnormal Form of Insulin

A higher proportion of proinsulin, which is biologically less active than insulin, could account for the elevated immunoreactive insulin levels following glucose loads and the impaired hypoglycemic caction of endogenous immunoreactive insulin in uremia. However, this cannot account for the tissue insensitivity to exogenously administered insulin.

Circulating Insulin Antagonists

Elevated levels of growth hormone [27], glucagon [28, 29], glucocorticoids [12, 30], adrenaline [31], prolactin [32], and parathyroid hormone [33] are known to be antagonistic to the hypoglycemic action of insulin. Although these hormones have all been incriminated in the pathogenesis of insulin resistance in uremia, the supporting evidence is at present inconclusive. Significant improvement in insulin sensitivity following the initiation of hemodialysis [19, 34] has not been accompanied by significant reduction in the levels of most of these hormones.

Metabolic End Products

Several observations suggest that the accumulation of uremic toxins may be responsible for the impairment in insulin sensitivity. Mak et al. [13] noted a positive correlation between renal function and insulin sensitivity in children with uremia. When uremic serum was incubated with or infused into tissues from control animals, glucose utilization was inhibited [35, 36]. Metabolic acidosis can cause insulin resistance [37], but nonacidotic uremic patients still exhibit abnormal glucose metabolism [13]. Since insulin resistance can be improved either with dialysis [8, 15, 19, 38] or a low protein diet [39], it is possible that a dialyzable breakdown product from protein metabolism could be responsible. Davidson et al. [40] found no difference in the effect of pre- and postdialysis serum on insulin stimulated glucose uptake in the rat diaphragm. However, Dzurik et al. [36] and recently, Maloff and Lockwood [22] have independently isolated low-molecular-weight peptides from uremic serum which inhibit glucose utilization in either muscle or adipose tissues. Other protein breakdown products such as creatinine, urea, guanidinosuccinic acid, and methylguanidine have all been incriminated as the uremic toxin causing insulin resistance, but the supporting evidence is unconvincing.

Insulin Secretion in Uremia

Insulin responses following oral and intravenous glucose administration in uremic patients have been variable [11]. The early insulin response has been reported to be either normal, increased, or decreased. The late insulin response is uniformly elevated. These results suggest that abnormalities in insulin secretion may be present in some uremic patients. DeFronzo et al. [11] postulated that, although insulin resistance is found in most patients with uremia, there might be two different populations distinguishable with respect to insulin secretion and glucose tolerance. The first group could compensate for their insulin resistance by hyperinsulinemia and thereby maintain normal glucose tolerance. In the other group, there could be an inhibition of insulin secretion superimposed on peripheral insulin antagonism, resulting in glucose intolerance.

There is recent evidence to support the view that parathyroid hormone inhibits insulin secretion in uremia. Akmal et al. [41] showed that glucose intolerance did not develop in previously thyroparathryoidectomized uremic dogs and that insulin levels in these uremic dogs without hyperparathyroidism were much higher than in uremic dogs with intact thyroids and parathyroids. They concluded that parathyroid hormone might inhibit insulin release, but they were not able to exclude the effect of thyroidectomy. Mak et al. [42] suppressed hyperparathyroidism medically with a combined regime of high-dose phosphate binders and dietary phosphate restriction in eight children with uremia who were not on dialysis. The change in their glucose metabolism, as measured by the hyperglycemic clamp technique, is shown in Fig. 3. Following treatment, glucose metabolic rate (M) increased by 34%, insulin response (I) increased by 32%, but insulin sensitivity did not change. Compared with corresponding normal values, these patients were glucose intolerant (low M) before treatment and became glucose tolerant (normal M) after treatment. They were in-

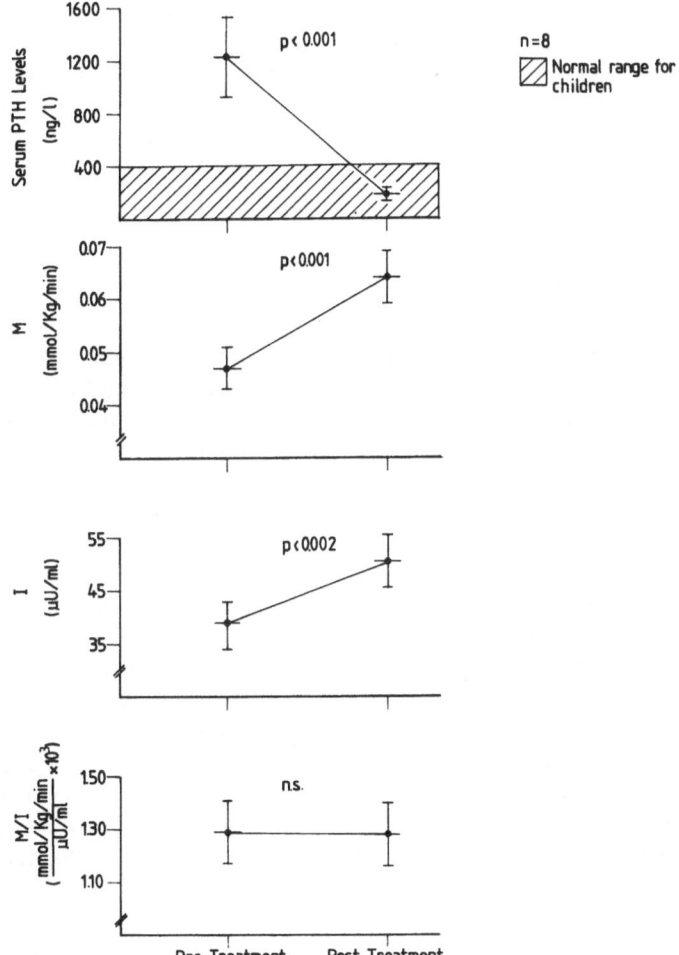

Fig. 3. Changes in glucose metabolism in eight children with uremia before and after medical correction of hyperparathyroidism

sulin resistant (low M/I) before treatment and remained so after treatment. With suppression of hyperparathyroidism, insulin secretion increased and restored glucose tolerance.

Effects of Dialysis on Glucose Metabolism in Uremic Patients

Hemodialysis

It is not surprising that removing waste products accumulated with decreasing renal function by hemodialysis causes an improvement in some of the metabolic disturbances in patients with end-stage renal failure. Hampers et al. [8] performed intravenous glucose tolerance tests in patients with uremia just before and after an intensive period of hemodialysis and reported improvement in their glucose metabolism. DeFronzo et al. [19, 38] employed the hyperglycemic and euglycemic clamp techniques and showed significant improvement in glucose tolerance and insulin sensitivity in uremic patients after initiation of hemodialysis. Their glucose metabolic rate and insulin sensitivity did not, however, return to normal values. El-Bishti et al. [12] studied glucose metabolism in 14 children on regular hemodialysis with intravenous glucose tolerance tests and concluded that they were glucose intolerant and insulin resistant. Thus, hemodialysis improved glucose metabolism in uremia but did not normalize it.

Mak (unpublished observations) studied six patients (aged 17 ± 2 years) on regular hemodialysis for more than 6 months. Their weight for height index was $107 \pm 3\%$. All were consuming weight-maintaining diets containing at least 200 g of carbohydrate. They consumed no medications other than phosphate binders, vitamin supplements, and sodium bicarbonate. The mean plasma urea and creatinine levels were 30 ± 4 mmol/l and 882 ± 51 µmol/l respectively. The mean serum parathyroid hormone level was 1870 ng/l (normal range, < 450). Blood pH, plasma electrolytes, and liver function tests were normal in all. Controls consisted of six healthy young volunteers (aged 25 ± 3) consuming weight-maintaining diets and no medications. All patients and controls had no evidence or family history of diabetes mellitus. The method used was the hyperglycemic clamp technique. A priming dose of 20% dextrose was given intravenously over 15 min to acutely raise plasma glucose concentration to 7 mmol/l above fasting levels. This concentration was kept constant for 120 min by measuring plasma glucose every 5 min with appropriate variation of the 20% dextrose infusion. Under these steady-state conditions, the mean dextrose infusion from 20–120 min minus urinary losses was taken as the index of glucose metabolic rate (M mmol/kg/min). The mean immunoreactive insulin concentration determined at 10-min intervals from 20–120 min was taken as the index of beta cell response to constant hyperglycemia (I, µU/ml), and the ratio of M/I was taken as the index of tissue sensitivity to insulin.

The uremic adolescents have higher fasting blood glucose concentrations (5.4 ± 0.3 mmol/l) than controls (4.9 ± 0.2 mmol/l), although this difference was not statistically significant. Fasting insulin concentrations were also higher in uremics (14 ± 2 µU/ml) but not significantly different from controls (11 ± 2 µU/ml). A summary of the hyperglycemic clamp studies in uremic and control subjects is shown in Table 1. The glucose metabolic rate (M) and insulin sensitivity (M/I) were significantly lower in patients on hemodialysis, indicating glucose intolerance and insulin resistance. Insulin secretion however, was normal. This could be related to the high levels of parathyroid hormone which might inhibit compensatory increases in insulin levels to restore glucose tolerance. The latter hypothesis has been tested in adult patients on hemodialysis. Mak et al. [43] have studied six patients (aged 26 ± 3 years) on regular hemodialysis just before and 4 weeks after they underwent subtotal parathyroidectomy for uncontrollable hyperparathyroidism. The changes in glucose metabolism as measured by the glucose clamp technique are shown in Fig. 4. Following surgical correction of hyperparathyroidism, glucose intolerance was reversed, with an accompanying increase in insulin secretion but no change in the degree of insulin resistance.

Table 1. Glucose metabolism in patients on regular hemodialysis

	Patients on hemodialysis	Controls	
Number	6	6	
Fasting blood glucose (mmol/l)	5.4 ±0.2	4.9 ± 0.2	N.S.
Fasting insulin (μU/ml)	14 ± 2	11 ±2	N.S.
M (mmol/kg/min)	0.035 + 0.005	0.067 + 0.020	P<0.05
I (μU/ml)	52 ±10	44 ±9	N.S.
M/I $\left(\dfrac{mmol/kg/min}{\mu U/ml} \times 10^3 \right)$	0.70 ± 0.07	1.54 ±0.12	P<0.01

N.S., not significantly different by unpaired *t* test.

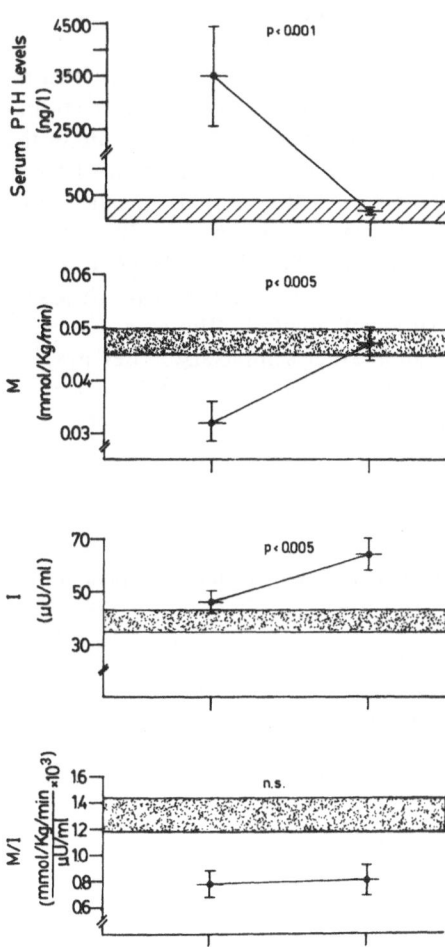

Fig. 4. Changes in glucose metabolism in 6 patients on regular hemodialysis before and after parathyroidectomy (*PTx*)

CAPD

The constant presence of glucose in the peritoneum during CAPD may have profound effects on glucose metabolism. Persistent hyperglycemia and hyperinsulinemia may possibly down-regulate insulin receptors, thus further impairing insulin sensitivity in uremic patients on CAPD. On the other hand, better clearance of waste products and/or uremic toxins by CAPD may remove the cause of insulin resistance in these patients. One difficulty in studying these patients is the definition of a truly fasting state because of the continous absorption of glucose from the dialysate. It would be ideal to study patients who have missed an overnight exchange and undergone a 12-hour fast and who do not have any dialysate in the peritoneum during the study.

Mak (unpublished observations) studied five patients (15 ± 3 years) on CAPD for more than 6 months. The patients had been consuming weight-maintaining diets containing more than 200 g of carbohydrate and had not been receiving medication apart from phosphate binders, vitamin supplements, and sodium bicarbonate. The mean plasma urea and creatinine levels were 27 ± 2 mmol/l and 822 ± 43 μmol/l respectively. Plasma electrolytes, blood pH, and liver function tests were all normal. They had no evidence or family history of diabetes mellitus. Controls have been described above. The patients were studied after missing an overnight exchange, which meant that there was no dialysate in the peritoneum for 12 h prior to and during the studies. There was no difference between the fasting blood glucose levels of the patients (5.1 ± 0.2 mmol/l) and the controls (4.9 ± 0.2 mmol/l). Fasting insulin levels were also similar: uremics, 12 ± 2 μU/ml, compared with controls, 11 ± 2 μU/ml. The results of the hyperglycemic studies are summarized in Table 2. There were essentially no abnormalities of glucose metabolism in the patients on CAPD compared with controls. These results are preliminary and await confirmation by studies with a larger sample size. They are, however, compatible with reports of improved growth in children on CAPD compared with those on hemodialysis [44]. Also, reports on normalization of metabolic disturbances (pyruvate kinase activity, energy charge, and protein synthesis) in patients on CAPD by Metcoff et al. (see this vol-

Table 2. Glucose metabolism in patients on CAPD

	Patients on CAPD	Controls	
Number	5	6	
Fasting blood glucose (mmol/l)	5.3 ±0.2	4.9 ±0.2	N.S.
Fasting insulin (μU/ml)	13 ±2	11 ±2	N.S.
M (mmol/kg/min)	0.065±0.10	0.067±0.020	N.S.
I (μU/ml)	52 ±5	44 ±9	N.S.
$M/I\left(\dfrac{mmol/kg/min}{\mu U/ml}\times 10^3\right)$	1.33 ±0.20	1.54 ±0.12	N.S.

N.S., not significantly different by unpaired t test.

ume) lend further support to these preliminary observations. If these are confirmed. CAPD may prove to be much more efficient than hemodialysis in correcting metabolic derangements in children with end-stage renal failure.

References

1. Neubauer E (1910) Über Hyperglykaemie bei Hochdruck-Nephritis und die Beziehungen zwischen Glykaemie und Glucosurie beim Diabetes mellitus. Biochem Z 25:285
2. Farquhar JW (1978) Diabetes Mellitus. In: Forfar JO, Arneil GC (eds) Textbook of paediatrics. Churchill Livingstone, Edinburgh, p 1016
3. Tamborlane WV, Sherwin RS, Genel M, Felig P (1979) Restoration of normal lipid and amino-acid metabolism in diabetic patients treated with a portable insulin infusion pump. Lancet 1:1258
4. Rudolf MCJ, Sherwin RS, Markowitz R et al. (1982) Effect of intensive insulin treatment on linear growth in the young diabetic patient. J Paediatr 101:333
5. Perkoff GT, Thomas CL, Newton JC et al. (1958) Mechanism of impaired glucose tolerance in uremia and experimental hyperazotemia. Diabetes 7:375
6. Briggs JD, Buchanan KD, Luke RG, McKiddle MT (1967) Role of insulin in glucose intolerance in uremia. Lancet 1:462
7. Horton ES, Johnson C, Lebowitz HE (1968) Carbohydrate metabolism in uraemia. Ann Intern Med 68:63
8. Hampers CL, Soeldner JS, Doak PB, Merrill JP (1966) Effect of chronic renal failure and haemodialysis on carbohydrate metabolism. J Clin Invest 45:1719
9. Spitz IM, Rubenstein AH, Bersohn I et al. (1970) Carbohydrate metabolism in renal disease. Q J Med 39:201
10. Lowrie EG, Soeldner JC, Hampers CL et al. (1970) Glucose metabolism and insulin secretion in uremic subjects. J Lab Clin Med 76:603
11. DeFronzo RA, Andres R, Edgar P, Walker GW (1973) Carbohydrate metabolism in uraemia, a review. Medicine (Baltimore) 52:469
12. El-Bishti MM, Counahan R, Bloom SR, Chantler C (1978) Hormonal and metabolic responses to intravenous glucose in children on regular haemodialysis. Am J Clin Nutr 31:1865
13. Mak RHK, Haycock GB, Chantler C (1983) Glucose intolerance in children with chronic renal failure. Kidney Int 24 (Suppl 15):22
14. Rubenfeld S, Garber AJ (1978) Abnormal carbohydrate metabolism in chronic renal failure. The potential role of accelerated glucose production, increased gluconeogenisis and impaired glucose disposal. J Clin Invest 62:20
15. DeFronzo RA, Alverstrand A, Smith D et al. (1981) Insulin resistance in uremia. J Clin Invest 67:563
16. Westervelt FB (1969) Insulin effect in uremia. J Lab Clin Med 74:79
17. Westervelt FB (1970) Uremia and insulin responses. Arch Intern Med 126:865
18. DeFronzo RA, Ferrannini E, Hendler R, Felig P, Wahren J (1983) Regulation of splanchnic and peripheral glucose uptake by insulin and hyperglycemia in man. Diabetes 32:35
19. DeFronzo RA, Tobin JD, Rowe JW, Andres R (1978) Glucose intolerance in uraemia: Quantification of beta cell sensitivity to glucose and tissue sensitivity to insulin. J Clin Invest 62:425
20. Gambhir KK, Archer JA, Nerurkar SG, Cruz I, Sanders M (1981) Erythrocyte insulin receptors in chronic renal failure. Nephron 28:4
21. Smith D, DeFronzo RA (1982) Insulin resistance in uremia is mediated by post binding defects. Kidney Int 22:54
22. Maloff B, Lockwood D (1981) Cellular basis for insulin resistance in uremia. Diabetes 30 (Suppl 1):28
23. Cohen BD, Horowitz HI (1968) Carbohydrate metabolism in uremia inhibition of phosphate release. Am J Clin Nutr 21:407

24. Metcoff J, Linderman R, Baxter D, Pederson J (1978) Cell metabolism in uremia. Am J Clin Nutr 30:1627
25. Renner D, Heintz R (1972) The inhibition of certain steps of glucose degradation in uremia. In: Kluthe R, Berlyne G, Burton B (eds) Uremia. Thieme, Stuttgart, p 195
26. Glaze RP, Morgan JM, Morgan RE (1967) Uncoupling of oxidative phosphorylation by ultrafiltrates of uremic serum. Proc Soc Exp Biol Med 125:172
27. Batchelor BR, Stern JS (1973) The effect of growth hormone upon glucose metabolism and cellularity in rat adipose tissue. Horm Metab Res 5:37
28. Bilbrey GL, Faloona GR, White MG, Knochel JP (1974) Hyperglycaemia of renal failure. J Clin Invest 53:841
29. Sherwin RS, Bastl C, Finkelstein FD et al. (1976) Influence of uremia and haemodialysis on the turnover and metabolic effects of glucagon. J Clin Invest 57:722
30. Munk A (1971) Glucocorticoid inhibition of glucose uptake by peripheral tissues. Old and new evidence, molecular mechanisms and physiological significance. Perspect Biol Med 14:265
31. Deibert DC, DeFronzo RA (1980) Epinephrine-induced insulin resistance in man. J Clin Invest 65:717
32. Katzen HM, Glitzer M (1968) Insulin antagonists and disturbances in carbohydrate metabolism. In: Dickens F (ed) Carbohydrate metabolism and its disorders, vol 2. Academic Press, London, p 265
33. Kim H, Kalhoff RK, Costrini NV et al. (1971) Plasma insulin disturbances in primary hyperparathyroidism. J Clin Invest 50:2596
34. DeFronzo RA, Tobin J, Boden G, Andres R (1979) The role of growth hormone in the glucose intolerance of uremia. Acta Diabet Lat 16:279
35. Dzurik R, Niederland TR, Cernacek P (1969) Carbohydrate metabolism by rat liver slices incubated in serum obtained from uremic patients. Clin Sci 37:409
36. Dzurik R, Valovicova E (1970) Glucose utilisation during uremia: in vivo study. Clin Chim Acta 30:137
37. DeFronzo RA, Beckles AD (1979) Glucose intolerance following chronic metabolic acidosis in man. Am J Physiol 236:E328
38. DeFronzo RA (1978) Pathogenesis of glucose intolerance in uremia. Metabolism 27 (Suppl 2):1866
39. Snyder D, Pulido LB, Kagan A (1968) Dietary reversal of the carbohydrate intolerance in uremia. Proc Eur Dial Transplant Assoc 5:205
40. Davidson MB, Lowrie EG, Hampers CL (1969) Lack of dialysable insulin antagonist in uremia. Metabolism 18:387
41. Akmal M, Goldstein DA, Multani S, Massry SG (1981) Parathyroid hormone and glucose intolerance in man. Kidney Int 19:194
42. Mak RHK, Turner C, Haycock GB, Chantler C (1983) Secondary hyperparathyroidism and glucose intolerance in children with uraemia. Kidney Int 24 (Suppl 16):5128
43. Mak RHK, Bettinelli A, Turner C, Haycok GB, Chantler C (1984) The influence of hyperparathyroidism on glucose metabolism in uraemia. J Clin Endocrin Metab (in press)
44. Stefanidis CJ, Hewitt IK, Balfe JW (1983) Growth in children receiving continuous ambulatory peritoneal dialysis. J Paediatr 102:681

Lipoprotein Profiles in Plasma and Dialysate of Children on CAPD

U. Querfeld, W. Haberbosch, A. Gnasso, C. C. Heuck, and J. Augustin

Introduction

Alterations of lipid metabolism are consonant with the uremic state. The data of Bagdade [1] and others have indicated that uremic patients frequently have secondary hyperlipoproteinemia; elevated plasma triglyceride (TG) levels and a modest increase in plasma cholesterol (CHOL) level is the predominant pattern. According to the classification of Frederickson, type IV and to a lesser degree, type IIa or IIb hyperlipoproteinemia are most frequently observed.

The incidence of these abnormalities in adult uremic patients varies considerably from 30% [2] to 83% [3]. Studies in adults of lipoprotein fractions (as separated by ultracentrifuge) demonstrate a consistent increase in very-low-density lipoproteins (VLDL), the plasma fraction containing mainly triglycerides. Levels of low-density lipoproteins (LDL) are also frequently elevated, although to a lesser degree, whereas high-density lipoproteins (HDL) show a significant decrease [4].

The composition of these fractions is altered in uremia: VLDL, LDL, and HDL contain an increased percentage of TG and a decreased percentage of CHOL [4]. The decrease of HDL and HDL-CHOL may be of particular importance with regard to the protective function of these lipoproteins. Several large epidemiological studies in different populations demonstrated a low incidence of coronary heart disease in volunteers with high HDL-CHOL levels. In addition, a recent study by Rapoport et al. [5] demonstrated an altered HDL composition in adult uremic patients, with a diminution of HDL-CHOL and apoprotein (Apo) CII in HDL and a relative increase of Apo E in HDL, irrespective of the presence of hypertriglyceridemia.

The pathophysiological mechanisms responsible for these alterations can be summarized as diminished catabolism of VLDL, accompanied by an inappropriately high hepatic production [6]. Clearance of TG-rich lipoproteins measured as postheparin lipolytic activity of hepatic triglyceride lipase (HTGL) and lipoprotein lipase (LPL) was found to be low in uremic patients [7, 8]. In addition, the presence of circulating inactivators [9] of LPL and a deficiency of activators like Apo CII [5] have been postulated. An altered fat absorption from the gut [10] together with a diet rich in carbohydrates and fat may also contribute to these disturbances.

In various studies, children with chronic renal failure exhibited patterns similar to those described in adult patients with predominantly type IV hyperlipoproteinemia [11–14]. In the only study known to us in which different lipoprotein fractions and their lipid composition were measured, Papadopoulou et al. [15] found elevated VLDL and normal LDL in the plasma of children on hemodialysis; HDL were low in patients with a GFR less than 40 ml/min/1.73 m². Thus, disturbances in lipid metabolism in children seem to occur rather early in renal failure.

On *CAPD*, adult patients have increased levels of plasma TG and CHOL due to a rise in VLDL during the first 6 months of treatment, as was shown by Ramos et al. [16]. Other reports confirmed a rise in CHOL and VLDL-CHOL, whereas HDL-CHOL levels were found to be elevated, decreased, or normal in different studies [16, 17]. In children on CAPD, Salusky et al. found high TG and normal CHOL levels in plasma and failed to demonstrate a significant change during a 12-month observation period [18]. Broyer et al. [19] observed high CHOL levels, which were correlated with peritoneal protein loss. Comprehensive studies in children on CAPD, including lipoprotein fractions, apoproteins, and lipolytic activities in plasma, are not yet available. It seems possible that the constantly high glucose absorption from the dialysate might aggravate preexisting alterations of lipid metabolism in uremia [17]. Apoprotein loss into the dialysate could be an additional pathogenetic factor favoring early development of atherosclerosis.

Patients and Methods

Lipid metabolism was investigated in five children undergoing CAPD, aged 4 months–13 years (mean, 5.8 years). The duration of CAPD treatment was 1–5 months (mean, 3.6 months). One patient had diabetes mellitus. The children were not hypoproteinemic, and there were no signs of peritonitis at the time of and at least 6 weeks prior to the investigation. Three children received antihypertensive drugs (Table 1).

After a 12-h fast, TG, CHOL, and phospholipids (PLP) were measured in plasma, using commercially available kits (Boehringer Mannheim, F.R.G.). The lipoproteins were isolated from 10 ml plasma in a Beckmann L8/70 preparative ultra-

Table 1. Clinical data of five pediatric patients undergoing CAPD treatment

	Age (yrs)	Disease	Medication	Months on CAPD	Dialysate volume per day (glucose concentration)	Hyperlipo-proteinemia Phenotype
B. Y.	4/12	Shock after birth	Propranolol Dihydralazine	4	5×175 ml (4.25%)	IIb
B. M.	13 2/12	Obstructive uropathy	0	5	4×1000 ml (1.5%)	IV
E. M.	1	Infantile polycystic disease	0	4	4×175 ml (1.36%)	IV
H. G.	3 5/12	H. U. S. Diabetes mellitus	Propranolol Dihydralazine Furosemide	1	5×300 ml (2.3%) +5 u. Insulin	IIa
H. S.	11 4/12	Schönlein-Henoch nephropathy	Propranolol	4	4×1500 ml (2.3%)	IIb

centrifuge at 4 °C by sequential flotation at densities of 1.006 for VLDL (50 000 rpm, 18 h), 1.019 for intermediate-density lipoproteins (IDL) (50 000 rpm, 18 h), 1.063 for LDL (50 000 rpm, 18 h), and 1.21 for HDL (65 000 rpm, 48 h), using Beckmann Quick Seal tubes (16 mm × 76 mm) and a Beckmann 70.1 Ti Rotor. The HDL were separated into two density subclasses: 1.063–1.125 (HDL$_2$) and 1.125–1.21 (HDL$_3$). The densities were adjusted with solid KBr and measured with a Heraeus-Paar DMA 45 densitometer. To determine lipid concentrations immediately, 700 µl of the lipoprotein fractions were used, while the remainder was extensively dialyzed against distilled water (Visking Dialysis Tubings type 8/32, Serva, Heidelberg, F.R.G.) and lyophilized. Delipidation of the samples followed in the same tubes with 2 ml × 5 ml of ethanol/ ether (3:1, v/v) for 20 h and 4 h and finally with 5 ml of ether for 1 h at −18 °C.

The separation and quantification of apolipoproteins was performed by isoelectric focusing on 7% acrylamide ultrathin (0.3 mm) flat gels in 6 M urea and 2% ampholynes. Apolipoproteins were dissolved in a buffer containing 6 M urea and 0.1 M tris-HCL (pH 8.3) and focused for 3 h at 1000 V, amperage free. The protein bands in the gels were fixed by 10% trichloroacetic acid for 10 min, stained in 1% Light Green (Serva, Heidelberg, F.R.G.) for 15 min, and destained in 7% acetic acid for 50 min. The quantification was performed by densitometric determination of the stained protein bands, using a LKB 2202 Ultra-Scan Laser Densitometer. The peaks were compared with standards of known concentration. Apo B was determined by immunodiffusion on NOR-partigen plates (Behringwerke AG, Marburg, F.R.G.). LPL and HTGL were determined by immunoassay after heparin injection.

Total amounts of protein, lipids, and apoproteins were also determined in concentrated dialysate (after an overnight dwell time of 12 h). Apo A and Apo B in dialysate were additionally measured by immunodiffusion on partigen plates. The results of the plasma values were compared with those of ten healthy control children (mean age, 12 y) examined under the same conditions as the CAPD patients as well as with data published for healthy American children aged 0–14 y [20].

Results

All patients had hyperlipoproteinemia: type II a in one, type II b in two, and type IV in two patients (Table 1). Total levels of CHOL and TG in plasma were highly elevated, but PLP levels were normal (Fig. 1). In the VLDL and IDL fractions, TG and CHOl, but not PLP were elevated (Fig. 2, 3). The LDL fraction showed increased amounts of TG, but normal CHOL and PLP concentrations (Fig. 4). In the HDL$_2$ fraction, TG and CHOL levels were similar to those of the controls, but the PLP concentration was low (Fig. 5). In the HDL$_3$ fraction, TG levels were elevated, but CHOL and PLP concentrations were similar to the controls (Fig. 6). Parallel to its content in HDL$_2$ and HDL$_3$, HDL-CHOL as measured by precipitation was in the normal range (Fig. 7). This is a remarkable finding, considering the consistently reported low HDL-CHOL levels in adult uremic patients and in adults and children on hemodialysis. Low activity of HTGL and of LPL in plasma was apparent in three and four children on CAPD, respectively (Fig. 7). Apo AI levels in the HDL$_2$ frac-

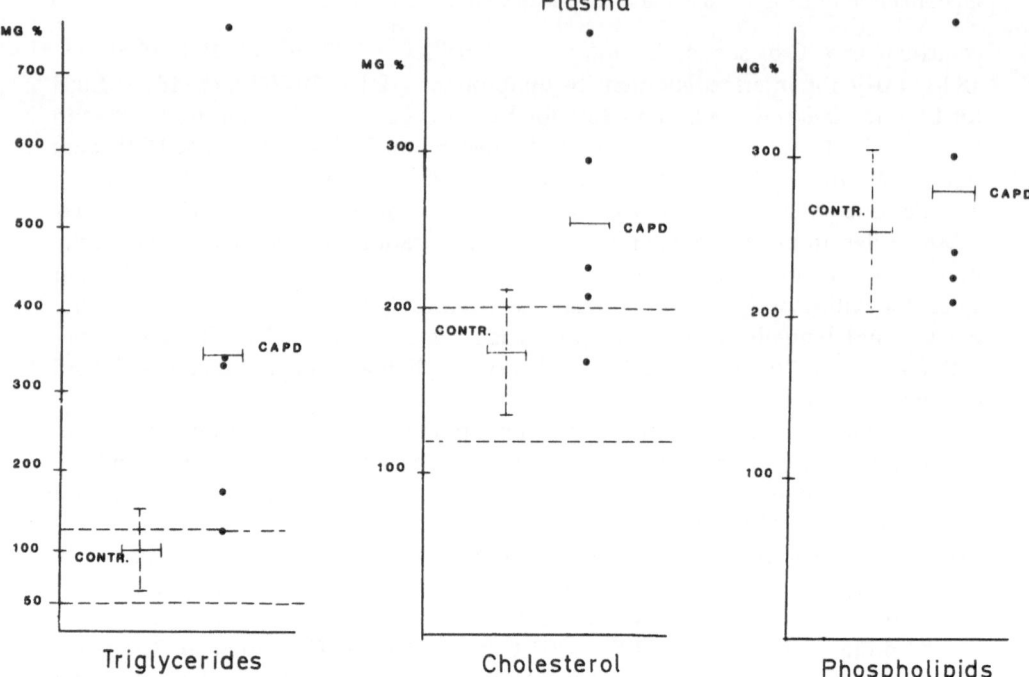

Fig. 1. Total triglycerides, cholesterol, and phospholipids in plasma of five patients (*CAPD*) and controls (*contr.*). *Horizontal broken lines* indicate the 5th and 95th percentile of values for healthy American children of comparable age [20].

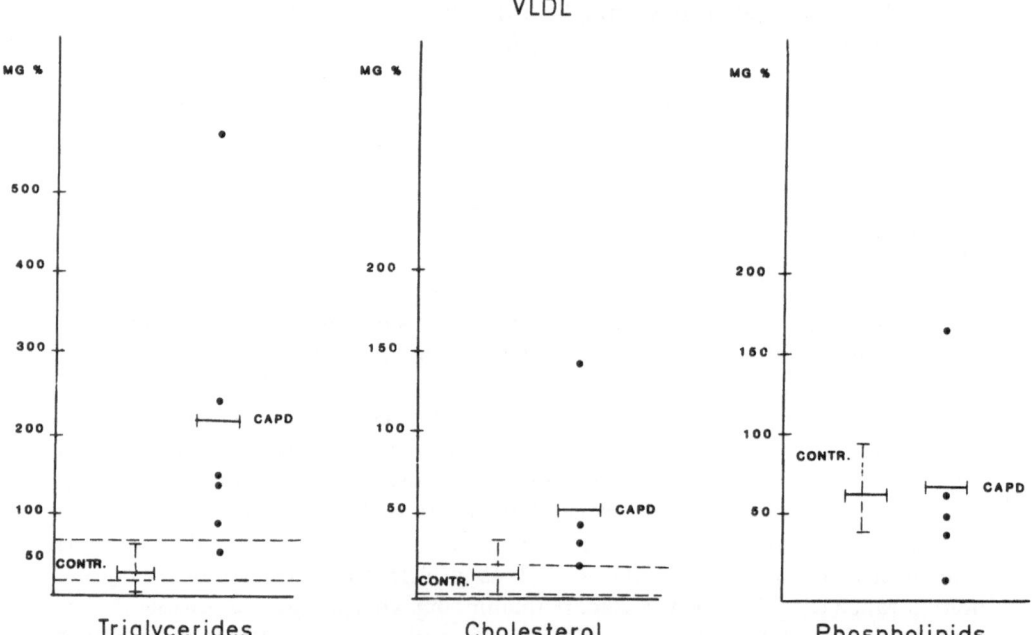

Fig. 2. Plasma concentrations of triglycerides, cholesterol, and phospholipids in the very-low-density lipoprotein fraction (*VLDL*) of five patients (*CAPD*) and controls (*contr.*). *Horizontal broken lines* indicate the 5th and 95th percentile of values for healthy American children of comparable age.

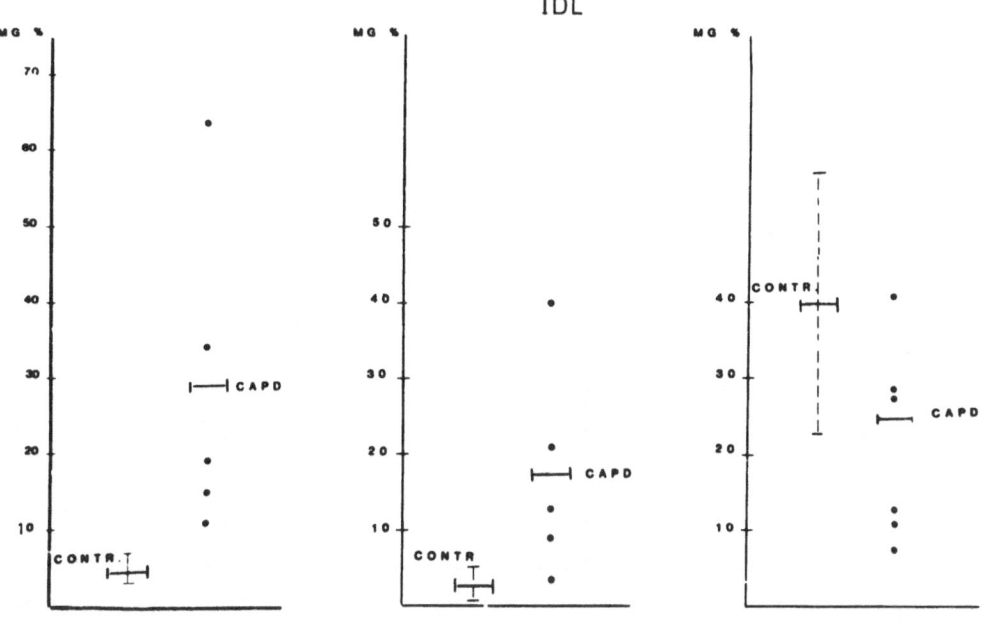

Fig. 3. Plasma concentrations of triglycerides, cholesterol, and phospholipids in the intermediate density lipoprotein fraction (*IDL*) of five patients (*CAPD*) and controls (*contr.*).

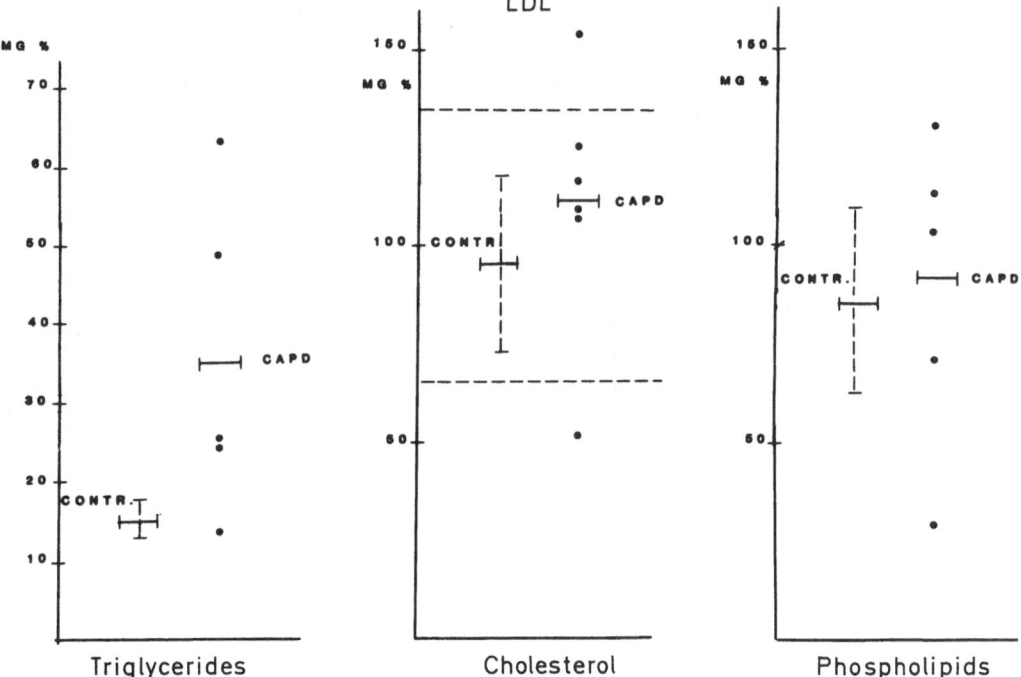

Fig. 4. Plasma concentrations of triglycerides, cholesterol, and phospholipids in the low-density lipoprotein fraction (*LDL*) of five patients (*CAPD*) and controls (*contr.*). *Horizontal broken lines* indicate the 5th and 95th percentile of values for healthy American children of comparable age (cholesterol).

HDL 2

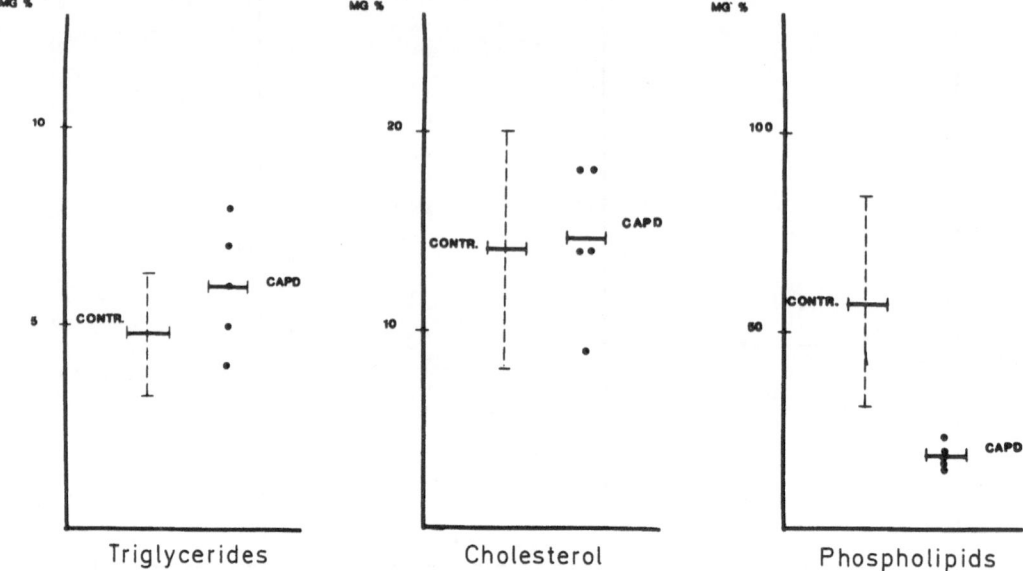

Fig. 5. Plasma concentrations of triglycerides, cholesterol, and phospholipids in the high-density lipoprotein fraction 2 (*HDL₂*) of five patients (*CAPD*) and controls (*contr.*).

HDL 3

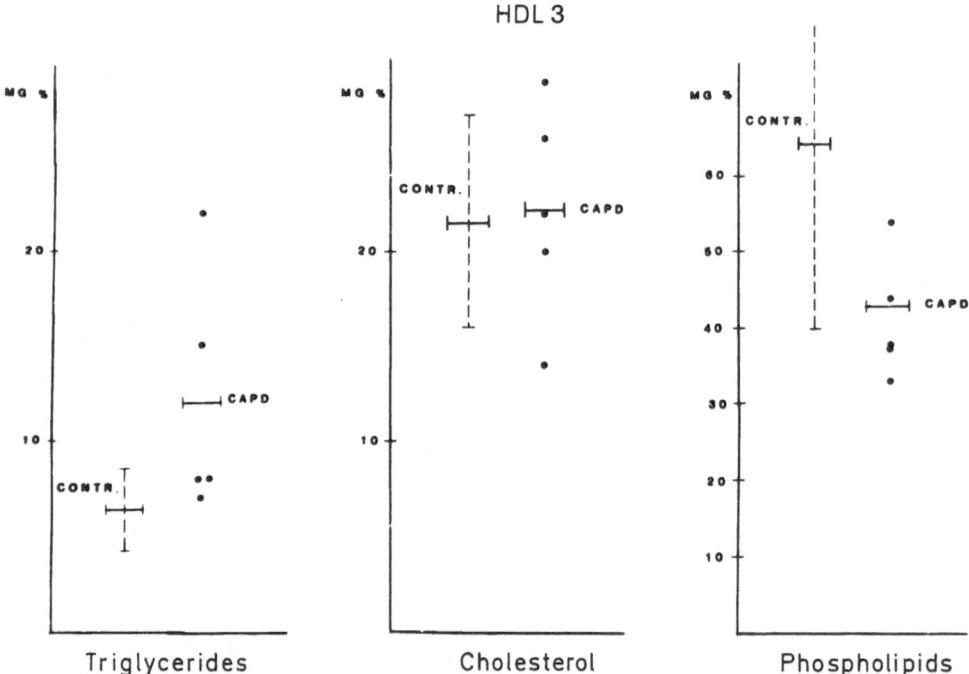

Fig. 6. Plasma concentrations of triglycerides, cholesterol, and phospholipids in the high-density lipoprotein fraction 3 (*HDL₃*) of five patients (*CAPD*) and controls (*contr.*) measured by precipitation. *Horizontal broken lines* indicate the 5th and 95th percentile of values for healthy American children of comparable age.

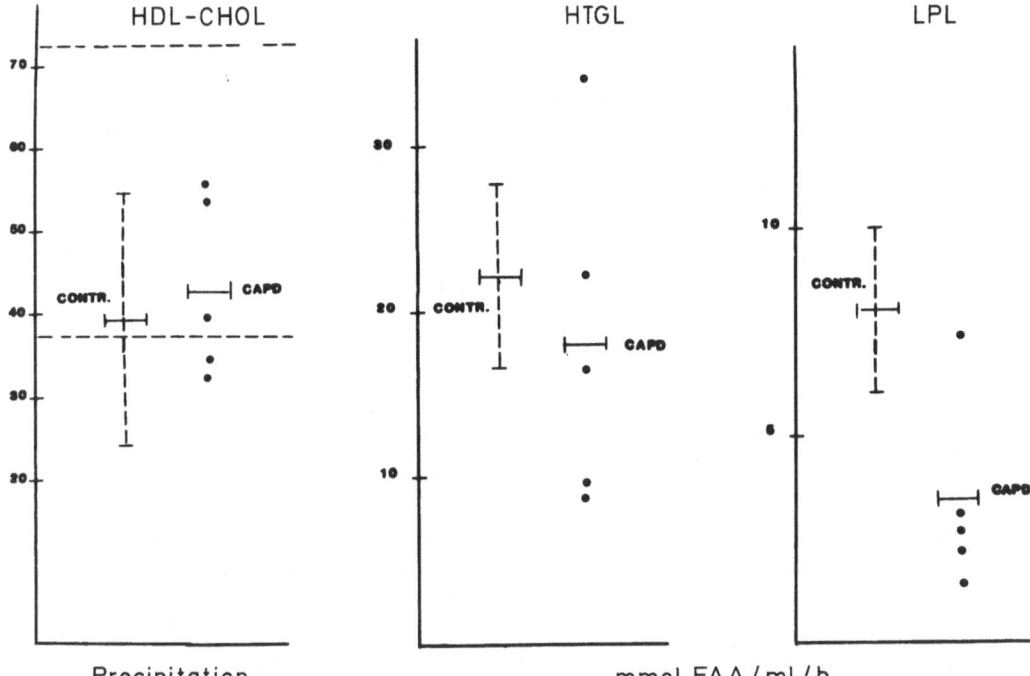

Fig. 7. Concentration of *HDL-CHOL* and activity of hepatic triglyceride lipase (*HTGL*) and lipoprotein lipase (*LPL*) in plasma of five patients (*CAPD*) and controls (*contr.*).

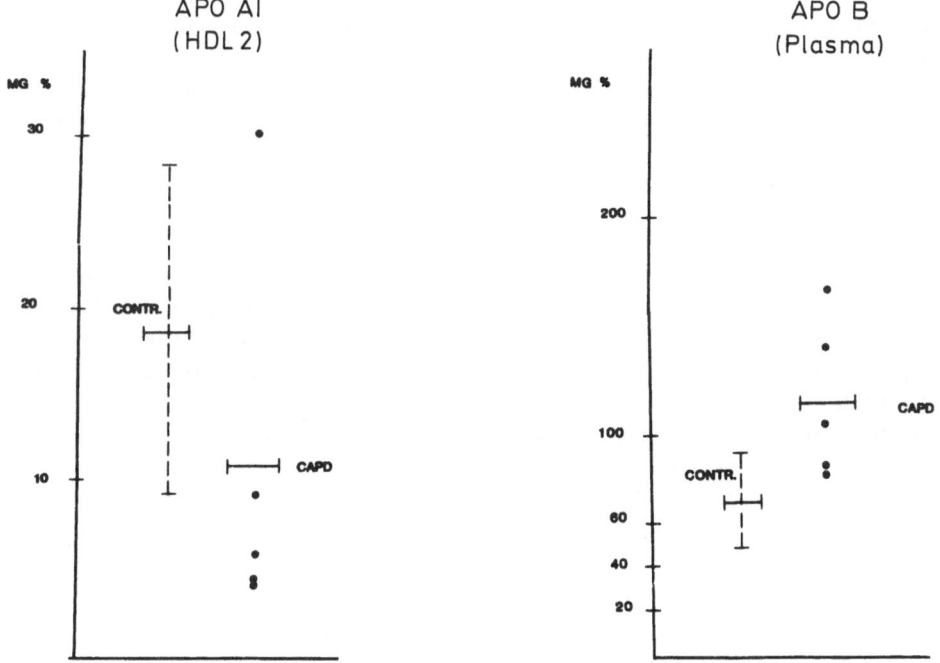

Fig. 8. Concentration of apoprotein AI (*Apo AI*) in the high-density lipoprotein fraction 2 (*HDL₂*) measured by isoelectric focusing (*left*) and concentration of apoprotein B (*Apo B*) in plasma measured by immunodiffusion (*right*).

tions were usually low (Fig. 8). Plasma Apo B was elevated in three of five patients (Fig. 8). All C apoproteins showed increased levels in the VLDL fraction.

Total protein in the dialysate averaged 1.46 g/l/12 h. Small amounts of TG (87 ± 74 mg/l/12 h) and PLP (21 ± 7 mg/12 h) could be detected in all patients. CHOL was found only in the dialysate of the diabetic patient (14 mg/l/12 h). Traces of Apo AI and AII were demonstrated by immunodiffusion on partigen plates in the dialysate. The elimination of Apo AI was calculated to be 10 mg/l/12 h. No Apo B was found in the dialysate. The presence of other apoproteins could be demonstrated in the dialysate by isoelectric focusing, but quantification was not possible due to the extremely low concentrations.

Discussion

In this pilot study, which does not permit statistical analysis because of the small number of patients, we demonstrate that all children on CAPD have marked alterations in plasma levels of lipoproteins and that small, variable amounts of lipids and apoproteins are lost in the dialysate. Factors such as drug therapy and physical activity which may influence these results could not be further evaluated.

The findings in the one diabetic patient who had the most severe disturbances of lipid metabolism may have possibly contributed to the high mean values in the entire group. No relationship was found between plasma lipid levels and age, time on CAPD, or protein loss in the dialysate. This is in contrast to the observations by Broyer et al. [19], who found plasma CHOL, and TG elevations that were more pronounced in the younger CAPD patients with increased protein losses. The hyperlipoproteinemia in our patients was mainly due to the marked elevation of TG; all lipoprotein fractions except HDL_2 contained increased amounts of TG. This may be explained by diminished lipoprotein catabolism stemming from decreased activity of LPL in plasma; however, the chronic glucose load from the dialysate may be an additional factor. Mean HTGL activity was normal in CAPD children, in contrast to the results in adult uremic patients [8] in whom reduced activity was found. Plasma CHOL in our patients was clearly elevated and mainly appeared in the VLDL and IDL fractions, whereas the IDL and HDL mean values for CHOL were in the normal range. PLP were low in the HDL and IDL fractions. Decreased levels of Apo AI were observed in HDL, whereas concentrations of Apo B (in plasma) and C in VLDL were elevated.

Considering the high incidence and early appearance of atherosclerotic lesions reported in adult patients with uremia [17] and the similar pattern of hyperlipoproteinemia in pediatric patients, the latter may be prone to develop premature atherosclerosis [13]. Whereas hypertriglyceridemia per se is not believed to represent a significant risk factor for atherosclerosis, combined hyperlipoproteinemia, especially of type II, is known to produce early atherosclerotic complications. All our patients except one presented combined hyperlipoproteinemia. HDL-CHOL levels in the patients were within the normal range. It is of special interest that HDL-Apo AI levels were decreased in four out of five patients because Maciejko et al. [21] recently demonstrated that Apo AI levels are of higher discriminatory value than HDL-CHOL levels in determining patients with atherosclerotic coronary artery disease. Long-term studies of CAPD patients are needed to further evaluate the significance of the loss of Apo AI and/or other apoproteins into the dialysate.

References

1. Bagdade JD, Porte D jr, Biermann DL (1968) Hypertriglyceridemia: a metabolic consequence of chronic renal failure. N Engl J Med 279:181–185
2. Ponticelli C, Gianluigi B, Cantaluppi A et al. (1978) Lipid abnormalities in maintenance dialysis patients and renal transplant recipients. Kidney Int 13:572–578
3. Cramp DG, Trickner TR, Varghese Z et al. (1977) Plasma lipoprotein patterns in patients receiving dialysis therapy for chronic renal failure. Clin Chim Acta 76:233–236
4. Bagdade JD, Casaretto A, Albers J (1976) Effects of chronic uremia, hemodialysis and renal transplantation on plasma lipids and lipoproteins in man. J Lab Clin Med 87:37–48
5. Rapoport J, Aviram M, Chaimovitz C et al (1978) Defective high density lipoprotein composition in patients on chronic hemodialysis. N Engl J Med 299:1326–1330
6. Heuck CC, Ritz E (1980) Hyperlipoproteinemia and renal insufficiency. Nephron 25:1–7
7. Bagdade JD (1970) Uremic lipemia. An unrecognized abnormality in triglyceride production and removal. Arch Intern Med 126:875–881
8. Mordasini R, Frey F, Flury W et al. (1977) Selective deficiency of hepatic triglyceride lipase in uremic patients. N Engl J Med 297:1362–1366
9. Murase T, Cattran DC, Rubenstein B, et al (1975) Inhibition of lipoprotein lipase by uremic plasma, a possible cause of hypertriglyceridemia. Metabolism 24:1279
10. Drukker A (1981) Lipid metabolism in chronic renal failure. In: Gruskin AB, Norman ME (eds) Pediatric nephrology. Martinus Nijhoff, The Hague, pp 326–333
11. Pennisi AJ, Heuser ET, Mickey MR, et al (1976) Hyperlipidemia in pediatric hemodialysis and renal transplant patients (associated with coronary artery disease). Am J Dis Child 130:957–961
12. El-Bishti M, Counahan R, Jarrett RJ, et al (1977) Hyperlipidemia in children on regular haemodialysis. Arch Dis Child 52:932–939
13. Gambert P, Lallement C, Andre JL, et al. (1981) Cholesterol content of serum lipoprotein fractions in children maintained on chronic hemodialysis. Clin Chim Acta 110:295–300
14. Berger M, James GP, Davis ER, et al. (1978) Hyperlipidemia in uremic children: response to peritoneal dialysis and hemodialysis. Clin Nephrol 9:19–24
15. Papadopoulou ZL, Sandler P, Tina LU, et al. (1981) Hyperlipidemia in children with chronic renal insufficiency. Pediatr Res 15:887–891
16. Ramos JM, Heaton A, McGurk JG, et al. (1983) Sequential changes in serum lipids and their subfractions in patients receiving continuous ambulatory peritoneal dialysis. Nephron 35:20–23
17. Cattran DC (1983) The significance of lipid abnormalities in patients receiving in dialysis therapy. Perit Dial Bull 3:329–332
18. Salusky IB, Kopple JD, Fine RN (1983) Continuous ambulatory peritoneal dialysis in children. Twenty months' experience. Kidney Int 24 Suppl 15:101–106
19. Broyer M, Niaudet P, Champion G, et al. (1983) Nutritional and metabolic studies in children on continuous ambulatory peritoneal dialysis. Kidney Int 24 (Suppl 15):106–110
20. The Lipid Research Clinics Programme Epidemiological Committee (1979) Plasma lipid distribution in selected North-American population: The lipid research clinics programme prevalence study. Circulation 61:302
21. Maciejko J, Holmes DR, Kottke BA, et al. (1983) Apolipoprotein AI as a marker of angiographically assessed coronary artery disease. N Engl J Med 309:385–389

Protein Losses During Peritoneal Dialysis in Children

R. Drachman, P. Niaudet, A.-M. Dartois, M. Broyer,
with the technical assistance of M. Lothon

Introduction

During peritoneal dialysis, some blood proteins including bound substances, are lost via the peritoneal membrane. There is considerable interpatient variability in protein loss, but the factors responsible for this variation have not been elucidated. The aim of this study is to examine the factors which may influence the ability of the peritoneal membrane to restrict protein leakage and to evaluate the consequences of these losses.

Methods

The study group included 23 children and adolescents (13 boys and 10 girls), treated by peritoneal dialysis (PD) as the initial and only therapy for terminal renal failure. The age at initiation of dialysis ranged from 2½ to 17 years, 9 months (mean, 9.8 ± 5.2 years) and time on PD ranged from 7 to 44 months (mean, 18.7 ± 11 months). The 23 children underwent three types of PD: Continuous ambulatory peritoneal dialysis (CAPD), intermittent cycling peritoneal dialysis (ICPD) using an automatic cycler system during the night without a daytime dwell, and intermittent ambulatory peritoneal dialysis (IAPD) using standard bags during the day without instillation of fluid of night. Of the 23 children, 15 underwent CAPD only, while two received ICPD only; four children were treated by ICPD and two with IAPD after an initial period of CAPD which varied from 4 to 31 months. When comparing the mean age of patients treated by IAPD, ICPD, and CAPD, there is no difference; in addition, these methods of treatment have often been used sequentially in the same patient.

Peritoneal dialysis was performed through a permanent Tenckhoff catheter. All dialysate solutions were commercially available, containing lactate and standard concentrations of electrolytes, calcium, and magnesium. Hyperosmolar solutions were used occasionally. The dialysate volume was 35–50 ml/kg of body weight (BW) per cycle, and the number of exchanges ranged from two to five a day. All studies were done in the absence of any signs or symptoms of peritonitis. However, in five children, dialysate protein losses were measured during episodes of peritonitis (n, 8). Protein losses incurred during peritonitis episodes were determined up to the 40th day, but only the results obtained during the first 3 days of clinical infection are reported in this paper.

Total protein concentration of the dialysate effluent was measured per 24 hours once a month by the Biuret colorimetric method [1]. Electrophoresis of dialysate proteins was performed on cellulose acetate. Blood samples were obtained monthly for electrophoresis of protein (on cellulose acetate) and determination of total proteins, albumin, and globulins in serum. Prealbumin, transferrin, thyroxin-binding globulin (TBG), IgA, IgG, and IgM in serum were measured every 3 months by radial immunodiffusion [2]. The plasma concentration of free amino acids was measured twice a year by column chromatography with lithium buffers [3].

Dietary intake was assessed in 19 children every 3 months by means of a survey carried out over a 3-day period.

Results

Daily peritoneal protein losses for children under 6 years of age were greater than for older children: 0.24 ± 0.04 g/kg/day as compared with 0.17 ± 0.06 ($P < 0.05$) (Table 1). Serum albumin was lower in the younger children, though not significantly (Table 1). A linear correlation was found between peritoneal protein loss and the serum albumin level. Protein intake was 2.1 ± 0.67 g/kg/day ($124 \pm 24\%$ of the recommended dietary allowances [RDA]), but there was no correlation between serum albumin level and protein or energy intake. Protein losses remained stable in individual patients free of peritonitis, but interpatient variation was as high as 260%. Albumin and immunoglobulins accounted for 75% to 85% of the total protein losses.

Children lost less protein while undergoing ICPD and/or IAPD than while on CAPD: 0.215 ± 0.065 g/kg BW/day on CAPD compared with 0.133 ± 0.037 g/kg/day on ICPD or on IAPD (Table 2). There was no significant difference in peritoneal clearances of creatinine and urea with the various modes of treatment.

Peritoneal protein loss was not affected by the duration of dialysis, the number of exchanges per day, the dialysate volume, or the outflow volume (Table 3). Changes in dialysate glucose concentration were not associated with variations in protein loss. The latter varied from 0.182 ± 0.074 g/kg BW/day to 0.374 ± 0.084 ($P < 0.001$) g/kg BW/day during peritonitis and returned to baseline values within 10–35 days (mean, 25 days) (Tables 3 and 4) following recovery from the infection.

Table 1. Peritoneal protein loss and serum albumin level in 23 children correlated with age

	Children < 6 years of age (n, 8) (mean ± SD)	Children > 6 years of age (n, 15) (mean ± SD)
Peritoneal protein loss (kg/day)	0.24 ± 0.044	0.17 ± 0.063 [a]
Serum albumin (g/l)	29.8 ± 2.89	35.0 ± 4.2 [b]

Correlation between peritoneal protein losses and serum albumin level: $r = -0.392$; $P < 0.05$.
[a] $P < 0.05$.
[b] not significant.

Table 2. Peritoneal protein losses, serum albumin and immunoglobulin levels in children undergoing CAPD, ICPD, and/or IAPD

	Normal values	CAPD (mean ± SD)	ICPD/IAPD (mean ± SD)
Peritoneal Protein losses g/kg/day		0.215 ± 0.065	0.133 ± 0.037[a]
Serum albumin g/l	35 – 50	33.7 ± 4.8	39.0 ± 3.7[b]
IgG g/l	6.8 – 11.8	6.74 ± 1.32	10.76 ± 2.34[a]
IgA g/l	0.56 – 1.34	1.00 ± 0.126	1.80 ± 1.2[a]
IgM g/l	0.50 – 1.14	2.01 ± 0.65	1.33 ± 0.65[a]

[a] $P < 0.01$.
[b] not significant.

Table 3. Influence of some factors on peritoneal protein loss

	Modification of protein loss
– Duration of PD (7 – 44 months)	no
– Number of exchanges/day (2 – 5)	no
– Dialysate volume ml/kg/day (94 – 256)	no
– Use of hyperosmolar solution. % of dialysate/day (0 – 45)	no
– Peritonitis: one episode per 35.8 patient months	yes (but only for a period of up to 10 – 37 days after peritonitis

Table 4. Influence of peritonitis on peritoneal protein losses

Patient number	Usual protein loss g/kg/day	Protein loss during peritonitis g/kg/day	Time necessary to achieve baseline (days)
4	0.16	0.42	32
7	0.30	0.48	35
12	0.23	0.39	28
18	0.09	0.22	21
20	0.13	0.36	10
Mean ± SD	0.182 ± 0.074	0.374 ± 0.087[a]	25.2

[a] $P < 0.001$.

Serum concentrations of TBG and transferrin were in the normal range, but prealbumin was elevated (Table 5). Serum IgG and IgA concentrations were significantly higher in children undergoing ICPD and IAPD, while serum IgM concentrations were higher in children undergoing CAPD (Table 2).

Many of the various amino acids remained elevated after 1 year of PD (Table 6). Cystine and lysine achieved almost normal levels, but as a whole, the total pool of free amino acids per liter of plasma remained unchanged after 6 months of CAPD,

Table 5. Serum thyroxine-binding globulin (TBG), prealbumin, and transferrin levels in children undergoing PD

	Normal values	Values in children undergoing PD (mean ± SD)
TBG (mg/l)	15 – 35	20.37 ± 6.51 (range: 14 – 30)
Prealbumin (mg/l)	0.25 ± 0.1	0.40 ± 0.08 (range: 0.22 – 0.52)
Transferrin (g/l)	2 – 4	2.64 ± 0.43 (range: 1.96 – 3.76)

Table 6. Serum free amino acids before start of PD and after 1 year of PD

Amino acid	Normal values (mean ± SD in μmol/l)	At onset of PD (mean ± SD in μmol/l)	One year after onset of PD (mean ± SD in μmol/l)
Aspartic acid	5.7 ± 0.7	24.1 ± 1.1	25.0 ± 2.3
Hydroxy-proline	14.9 ± 1.4	32.5 ± 6.0	29.6 ± 3.6
Glutamine	381.1 ± 24.3	567.2 ± 45.7	525.7 ± 27.7
Proline	112.7 ± 7.6	232.7 ± 32.5	202.3 ± 15.7
Glycine	151.4 ± 8.2	304.6 ± 18.6	246.7 ± 15.6
Citrulline	15.5 ± 2.1	76.1 ± 15.7	80.0 ± 7.1
Leucine	49.1 ± 11.4	93.1 ± 7.4	76.3 ± 3.5
Ornithine	29.6 ± 1.3	49.9 ± 7.3	43.5 ± 5.3
Cystine	35.4 ± 3.1	60.0 ± 11.8	42.0 ± 5.6
Lysine	107.7 ± 5.4	159.2 ± 27.8	126.3 ± 10.0
Essential/Nonessential	0.49 ± 0.03	0.35 ± 0.02	0.32 ± 0.01

and the decrease was not significant after 1 year. The ratio of essential to nonessential amino acids was only minimally changed by PD (Table 6).

Discussion

The function of the peritoneal membrane is paradoxical: the system sieves electrolytes and small neutral solutes while allowing protein loss. There is considerable interpatient variability in protein loss associated with PD [4–6]. Some investigators have attempted to determine which factors influence protein leakage into the peritoneal cavity [7], including the chemical composition of the dialysate solution used for dialysis and the presence of drugs in the dialysate [8, 9]. Other authors have demonstrated that the dialysate protein concentration increases with the use of hypertonic solutions [4, 5] and with the number of cycles performed per day [5]. According to our data, the changes in dialysate glucose concentration were not associated with variations in protein loss, and peritoneal protein losses were not affected by the duration of dialysis, the number of exchanges per day, or the inflow and outflow volumes. Our study confirms previous observations that the major factor influencing protein loss is peritonitis [4, 10]. However, our data show that children lose less protein while undergoing ICPD or IAPD than while undergoing CAPD and that serum IgG and IgA concentrations were significantly higher in children on the intermittent types of PD (Table 2).

Peritoneal protein losses were greater in younger than in older children (Table 1), and the serum albumin level was lower in the younger children, although not significantly.

Our data concerning serum proteins considered to be representative indicators of malnutrition are not consistent. TBG and transferrin remained in the normal range, whereas prealbumin was above normal. An assessment of the peritoneal loss of these molecules is required to understand the relationship between these proteins and nutritional status.

Plasma concentrations of free amino acids are almost constantly altered in uremic patients, and CAPD failed to improve these abnormalities significantly [11, 12]. However, studies comparing the influence of the different types of peritoneal dialysis on plasma free amino acides are not available.

Some authors have suggested that activation of the alternative pathway of complement may cause variation in protein loss during PD [13]. Such activation could be involved in the increased protein loss which occurs during peritonitis. Whether or not enough complement activation occurs in uncomplicated PD to be a major contributor to the usual protein loss remains to be determined. The hypothesis of heteroporosity of the peritoneum [14] could account for many characteristics of the peritoneal membrane. Our data showing a decrease in protein losses during IAPD and ICPD suggest that the prolonged exposure of the peritoneum to dialysate solution is responsible for membrane lesions and that periods of rest provide a shorter exposure time as well as an opportunity for some recovery.

The mechanism of peritoneal protein loss and its considerable variability require further investigations. For the time being, it seems preferable to us to use ICPD and IAPD rather than CAPD to avoid excessive protein loss, particularly in young children.

References

1. Gornall AG, Bardawill CJ, David MM (1949) Determination of serum proteins by means of the Biuret reaction. J Biol Chem 177:751–766
2. Mancini G, Carbonara AO, Heremans JF (1965) Immunochemical quantitation of antigens by single radial immuno-diffusion. Immunochemistry 2:235–254
3. Delaporte C, Jean G, Broyer M (1978) Free plasma and muscle amino acids in uremic children. Am J Clin Nutr 31:1647–1652
4. Blumenkrantz MJ, Gahl GH, Kopple JD, Kamdar AV, Jones MR, Kessel M, Coburn JW (1981) Protein losses during peritoneal dialysis. Kidney Int 19:593–602
5. Rubin J, Nolph KD, Arfania D, Prowant B, Fruto L, Brown P, Moore H (1981) Protein losses in continuous ambulatory peritoneal dialysis. Nephron 28:218–221

6. Broyer M, Niaudet P, Champion G, Jean G, Chopin N, Czernichow P (1983) Nutritional and metabolic studies in children on continuous ambulatory peritoneal dialysis. Kidney Int 24 (Suppl 15): S106–S110
7. Nolph KD, Ghods AJ, Brown P, Vanstone J, Miller FN, Wiegman DL, Harris PD (1977) Factors affecting peritoneal dialysis efficiency. Dial Transplant 6:52–63
8. Miller FN, Nolph KD, Sorkin MI, Gloor HJ (1983) The influence of solution composition on protein loss during peritoneal dialysis. Kidney Int 23:35–39
9. Rubin J, Nolph KD, Arfania D, Miller FN, Wiegman DL, Joshua IG, Harris PD (1979) Clinical studies with non vasoactive peritoneal dialysis solution. J Lab Clin Med 93:910–915
10. Strauch M, Walzer P, Henning GE, Poettger G, Christ H (1967) Factors influencing protein loss during peritoneal dialysis. Trans Am Soc Artif Intern Organs 13:172–177
11. Giordano C, Esposito R, de Pascale C, De Santo NG (1966) Dietary treatment in renal failure. Proceedings of 3rd international congress of nephrology 1966, Washington, Karger, Basel, pp 214–219
12. Giordano C, De Santo NG, Capodicasa G (1981) Amino acid losses during CAPD in children. Int J Pediatr Nephrol 2:85–88
13. Miller FN, Hammerschmidt DE, Anderson GL, Moore JN (1984) Protein loss induced by complement activation during peritoneal dialysis. Kidney Int 25:480–485
14. Nolph KD, Miller FN, Pyle WK, Popovich RP, Sorkin MI (1981) An hypothesis to explain the ultrafiltration characteristics of peritoneal dialysis. Kidney Int 20:543–548

Amino Acid Dialysis in Children on CAPD

J. W. Balfe, R. M. Hanning, and S. H. Zlotkin

Introduction

Children with chronic renal failure (CRF) grow poorly and are frequently malnourished. Inadequate dietary intake is only one of several factors which have been implicated in the etiology of the growth failure [1–3], yet its relevance may be significant. Nutritional management of CRF usually involves the restriction of protein, phosphate, sodium, and potassium, which severely limits nutrition and food selection for these often anorectic patients. With the introduction of continuous ambulatory peritoneal dialysis (CAPD), more liberal diets may be prescribed.

CAPD as applied to children has become increasingly popular since it was first introduced at our institution in 1978. Currently, over 40% of Canadian dialysis patients under 15 years of age are managed by CAPD [4], and at our hospital, 75% receive CAPD. Despite its popularity and the more permissive diet it makes possible, CAPD has failed to normalize growth [1] and reverse the malnutrition of CRF [5]. Indeed, a number of nutrition-related problems have been identified in infants and children undergoing CAPD.

Dextrose traditionally has been used as the osmotic agent in peritoneal dialysis solutions. Approximately 77% of the dextrose is absorbed during the course of a dialysis exchange [6, 7], with absorption being relatively greater on a per kilogram body weight basis in younger as opposed to older children and children as opposed to adult dialysis patients [7]. While dextrose absorbed from dialysate provides up to 21% of a child's caloric intake [8], resultant episodes of elevated blood glucose may contribute to the decreased appetite [6] and the hypertriglyceridemia [9] observed in CAPD patients.

In addition, protein and amino acids are lost in the dialysate. These losses amount to 8–10 g of protein [10–12] and 2–3.5 g of amino acids [10, 13] per day in adult CAPD patients and are relatively greater on a per kilogram body weight basis in infants and children [7, 14]. Considering also the increased amounts of protein and amino acid required for growth, these losses in the young and often anorectic CAPD patients may be critical. It is unlikely that they may be easily replaced by increased dietary intake, as has been suggested for adults [15].

Dombros et al. found that amino acid losses in effluent dialysate are in proportion to their plasma concentrations. It therefore appears that CAPD neither improves nor worsens the abnormal plasma amino acid profile of uremia [12].

It may be that dextrose is not the ideal dialysate osmotic agent, especially for infants and children, and thus, the use of alternatives such as xylitol and sorbitol have been investigated [16]. More recently, the use of amino acids has been proposed [17, 18].

Amino acid dialysis was a very new concept when we began our studies of the efficacy and short-term metabolic consequences of amino acid dialysis in children in 1982. As early as 1968, Gjessing demonstrated that amino acids can be absorbed across the peritoneum [20]. Kobayashi et al. [21] and Jackson et al. [22] reported that it is possible to give amino acids via the peritoneal cavity to counteract amino acid losses occurring during dialysis. Oreopoulos et al. formulated amino acid solutions with osmolalities comparable to the traditional dextrose dialysis solutions used for CAPD patients [23]. Trials of amino acid dialysis in rabbits and one adult patient by Oreopoulos et al. as well as our own experience with one infant indicate that amino acids are effective osmotic agents that show promise in the reversal of hypoprotein-emia and hypertriglyceridemia [24].

Our patient was a 6-month-old female with end-stage renal disease (ESRD) and anuria from congenital oxalosis. She required repeated infusions of albumin to cor-rect hypoalbuminemia and edema. It was decided to start her on dialysate contain-ing 1.5 g% dextrose and 1.0 g% amino acids (Travasol, Baxter-Travenol). Initially, all four exchanges contained amino acids; however, because of worsening azotemia, with blood urea nitrogen levels (BUN) of 120–130 mg/dl we reduced the rate to one exchange with amino acids a day. The remaining three exchanges were carried out with regular dextrose dialysate. Plasma total protein and albumin levels normalized over the ensuing months without the need for albumin infusions. In addition, growth improved despite an increase in the BUN level (basal BUN was 20 mg/dl, increased to 70–80 mg/dl).

These early studies suggested that amino acid dialysis solutions would be as ef-fective as dextrose-containing solutions in removing excess fluid and metabolic waste products and yet, would prevent the transient hyperglycemia and reverse the net loss of amino acids associated with dextrose dialysis.

It appears that amino acids are absorbed by diffusion [25], and thus it might also be possible to normalize the plasma and/or intracellular amino acid profile by alter-ing the dialysis solution amino acid composition and thereby improving nitrogen balance [26] and growth [27].

Patients and Methods

Protocol

Between February 1982 and June 1983, 19 patients with ESRD (age, 0.5–19 years) participated in a short-term trial comparing amino acid with dextrose dialysis. Pa-tients were studied over the course of four single, fasted, morning dialysis ex-changes, using each of four dialysate solutions in a randomly selected order. The four test solutions comprised dextrose solutions at two concentrations, 2.5% and 4.25% (Dianeal, Baxter-Travenol), and amino acid solutions at approximately 1.1% and 2.0% concentrations, whose osmolalities were comparable to those of the dex-trose solutions (Table 1). Each patient acted as his own control.

Blood and peritoneal fluid aliquots were sampled over the course of the 5-h dialysis exchange (at 0, 0.5, 1.0, 1.5, and 5.0 h). The blood glucose, amino acid, elec-

Table 1. Dialysate solutions[a]

2.5% glucose 1.1% amino acid (Travasol-based) 1.3% amino acid (Vamin-based) }	osmolality 384
4.25% glucose 2.0% amino acid (Travasol-based) 2.3% amino acid (Vamin-based) }	osmolality 463

[a] All dialysate solutions and Travasol from Baxter-Travenol (Deerfield, Illinois), Vamin from Pharmacia.

trolyte, urea, creatinine, and insulin responses to the amino acid and glucose solutions were compared. Amino acid and glucose absorption from the respective dialysis solutions and losses in effluent dialysate were assessed. Changes in peritoneal fluid osmolality, urea, and creatinine concentrations were monitored, and total protein, amino acid, albumin, and insulin losses were quantified.

Amino Acid Solutions

The first nine patients were studied using amino acid solutions based on Travasol (Baxter-Travenol), and solutions based on Vamin (Pharmacia) were used on the latter group of ten children as described in Table 2. The plasma amino acid response to different amino acid concentrations and profiles were then assessed.

Follow-up Studies

A subsample of patients were restudied using a similar protocol at a 3-month follow-up period. The response to an amino acid dialysis exchange was also studied in the fed state. The blood glucose and amino acid levels at the time of peak absorbance from both the gastrointestinal tract and the peritoneal cavity were then determined and potential amino acid toxicities and imbalances identified.

We have found that maximal glucose and amino acid absorption from dialysate occurs within 1 h of the exchange. Gastrointestinal absorption rates for nutrients are variable, depending on the age of the child and the nutrient density and composition of the meal. In order to maintain uniform nutrient density and composition, a nutritionally complete food supplement (Ensure, Ross Laboratories) was used in a fixed volume per kilogram body weight for each subject. A short pilot study showed that maximal plasma glucose and amino acid levels occur about 1.5 hours after the ingestion of this liquid meal.

Results

The results of these studies have been reported in abstract form [18, 19]. In general, our studies support the findings of Oreopoulos et al. in adults [17].

Table 2. Composition of dialysate solutions

Dialysate		4.25% glucose (Baxter-Travenol)	2% Amino Acid (Travenol-based)	2% Amino Acid (Vamin-based)
Composition per liter				
Dextrose, hydrous g		42.5	–	–
Na	mEq/L	132	132	132
Ca	mEq/L	3	3	4
Mg	mEq/L	1.5	1.5	2
Cl	mEq/L	102	113	108
Lactate	mEq/L	35	26	29
Acetate	mEq/L		13	
Na bisulfate	mEq/L		1	
L Leucine	mg		1238	1511
L Phenylalanine	mg		1238	1568
L Methionine	mg		1158	542
L Lysine	mg		1158	1112
L Isoleucine	mg		957	1112
L Valine	mg		917	1226
L Histidine	mg		877	684
L Threonine	mg		837	855
L Tryptophan	mg		360	285
L Alanine	g		4.15	0.855
Amino acetic acid	g		4.15	–
L Arginine	mg		2075	941
L Proline	mg		837	2309
L Tyrosine	mg		80	143
L Cyteine/Cystine	mg			399
L Aspartic Acid	mg			1169
L Glutamic Acid	mg			2565
L Glycine	mg			599
L Serine	mg			2138

Amino acids appear to be effective osmotic agents in a dialysate solution and provide satisfactory fluid, urea, and creatinine removal. Amino acid dialysate solutions maintain normal blood glucose levels and result in net amino acid absorption.

The elevation of certain plasma amino acids at the end of a 5-hour dialysis exchange with either Travasol- or Vamin-based solutions suggested that modification of the dialysate amino acid profiles used in these studies was needed. It is appreciated, however, that the abnormalities in plasma amino acids in uremia do not always reflect the larger intracellular amino acid pool [28]. The findings of Alvestrand et al. [26, 29] that oral amino acid supplements can correct plasma and muscle amino acid abnormalities and appear to improve nitrogen utilization in untreated uremic patients is encouraging.

The success of the short-term studies has led us to consider the long-term use of amino acid dialysis in infants and children on CAPD. Using a new amino acid solution, we are currently assessing the daily use of one amino acid dialysis exchange as opposed to dextrose dialysis alone in a 3 month, randomized, cross-over design trial.

Amino acids administered via the peritoneal dialysate solution may provide the needed nutritional support for infants and children on CAPD and ultimately enhance growth.

References

1. Stefanidis CJ, Hewitt IK, Balfe JW (1983) Growth in children receiving continuous ambulatory peritoneal dialysis. J Pediatr 102:681–685
2. Hsu AC, Kooh SW, Fraser D, Cumming WA, Fornasier VL (1982) Renal osteodystrophy in children with chronic renal failure: an unexpectedly common and incapacitating complication. Pediatrics 70:742–750
3. Holliday MA, Chantler C (1978) Metabolic and nutritional factors in children with renal insufficiency. Kidney Int 14:306–312
4. Canadian Renal Failure Register (1982) report. Kidney Foundation of Canada
5. Salusky IB, Fine RN, Nelson P, Blumenkrantz MJ, Kopple JD (1983) Nutritional status of children undergoing continuous ambulatory peritoneal dialysis. Am J Clin Nutr 38:599–611
6. Grodstein GP, Blumenkrantz MJ, Kopple JD et al. (1981) Glucose absorption during continuous ambulatory peritoneal dialysis. Kidney Int 19:564–567
7. Balfe JW, Vigneux A, Willumsen J, Hardy BE (1981) The use of CAPD in the treatment of children with end stage renal disease. Perit Dial Bull 1:35–38
8. Potter DE, McDaid TK, McHenry K, Mar H (1981) Continuous ambulatory peritoneal dialysis (CAPD) in children. Trans Am Soc Artif Intern Organs 27:64–67
9. Moncrief J, Pyle W, Simon P, Popovich R (1981) Hypertriglyceridemia, diabetes mellitus and insulin administration in patients undergoing CAPD. In: Moncrief JW, Popovich RP (eds) CAPD update: continuous ambulatory peritoneal dialysis. Proceedings of an international symposium, Austin, Texas, 1980, Chap 22. Masson, New York, pp 143–165
10. Kopple JD, Blumenkrantz MJ (1983) Nutritional requirements for patients undergoing continuous ambulatory peritoneal dialysis. Kidney Int 24 (Suppl 16):S295–S302
11. Katirzoglou A, Oreopoulos DG, Husdan H et al. (1980) Reappraisal of protein losses in patients undergoing CAPD. Nephron 26:230–233
12. Rubin J, Nolph KD, Arfania D et al. (1981) Protein losses in continuous ambulatory peritoneal dialysis. Nephron 28:218–221
13. Dombros N, Oren A, Marliss GB et al. (1982) Plasma amino acid profiles and amino acid losses in patients undergoing CAPD. Perit Dial Bull 2:27–32
14. Giordano C, De Santo NG, Capodicasa G et al. (1981) Amino acid losses during CAPD in children. Int J Pediatr Nephrol 2:85–88
15. Kopple JD, Blumenkrantz MJ, Jones MR et al. (1982) Plasma amino acid levels and amino acid losses during continuous ambulatory peritoneal dialysis. Am J Clin Nutr 36:395–402
16. Wu G (1982) Osmotic agents for peritoneal dialysis solutions. Perit Dial Bull 2:151–154
17. Oreopoulos DG, Marliss E, Anderson GH et al. (1983) Nutritional aspects of CAPD and the potential use of amino acid containing dialysis solutions. Perit Dial Bull (Suppl 3):10–15
18. Hanning RM, Balfe JW, Zlotkin SH (1983) The efficacy of amino acid vs glucose dialysis in children on continuous ambulatory peritoneal dialysis (Abstract). Ped Res 17:1590
19. Balfe JW, Zlotkin SH, Hanning RM (1984) Amino acid vs glucose dialysis in children on continuous ambulatory peritoneal dialysis. Perit Dial Bull [Suppl 4]:3
20. Gjessing J (1968) Additional of acids to peritoneal-dialysis fluid. Lancet II:812
21. Kobayashi K, Manji T, Hiramatsu S et al. (1979) Nitrogen metabolism in patients on peritoneal dialysis. Contrib Nephrol 17:93–100
22. Jackson M, Thomas D, Talbot S, Lee H (1979) Prevention of amino acid losses during peritoneal dialysis. Postgrad Med J 5:533–536
23. Oreopoulos DG, Crassweller P, Katirtzoglou A et al. (1979) Amino acids as an osmotic agent (instead of glucose) in continuous ambulatory peritoneal dialysis. In: Legrain M (ed) Continuous ambulatory peritoneal dialysis. Proceedings of an international symposium, Paris. Excerpta Medica, Amsterdam, pp 335–340
24. Oreopoulos DG, Balfe JW, Khanna R et al. (1981) Further experience with the use of amino acid containing dialysate (amino-dianeal) in peritoneal dialysis. In: Moncrief JW, Popovich RP (eds) CAPD update: continuous ambulatory peritoneal dialysis. Proceedings of an International Symposium, Austin, Texas, 1980. Masson, New York, pp 109–115

25. Williams PF, Marliss EB, Oreopoulos DG et al (1982) Amino acid absorption following intraperitoneal administration in CAPD patients. Perit Dial Bull 2:124–129
26. Alvestrand A, Fürst P, Bergström J (1982) Plasma and muscle free amino acids in uremia: influence of nutrition with amino acids. Clin Nephrol 18:297–303
27. Broyer M, Jean G, Dartois AM, Kleinknecht C (1980) Plasma and muscle free amino acids in children at the early stages of renal failure. Am J Clin Nutr 33:1396–1401
28. Alvestrand A, Fürst P, Bergström J (1983) Intracellular amino acids in uremia. Kidney Int 24:9–16
29. Alvestrand A, Ahlberg M, Fürst P, Bergström J (1983) Clinical results of long-term treatment with a low protein diet and a new amino acid preparation in patients with chronic uremia. Clin Nephrol 19:67–73

Dietary Survey in a Group of Children Treated with CAPD

A.-M. Dartois and M. Broyer

Introduction

CAPD is now applied in many specialized units as a treatment of first choice for uremic children. While this method has obvious advantages for pediatric patients that are detailed elsewhere in this symposium, such aspects as nutrition remain controversial. Dietary constraints are less severe for CAPD than for hemodialysis, and that could allow higher intakes and a better nutritional status. On the other hand, the ascites associated with CAPD could decrease appetite, and loss of protein from the peritoneum exerts a further negative influence on nutritional status. There are almost no data available on the dietary intake of children on CAPD [1]. Therefore, the aim of this study is to determine the dietary intake in such patients by means of dietary surveys.

Patients and Methods

The study analyzed 17 children treated with CAPD for periods of longer than 1 year. Six of the children had a statural age of between 2 and 4 years, six between 4 and 6 years, and five between 11 and 12 years. Chronological age was between 3 and 19 years. All patients had a prescribed diet.

Dietary Prescriptions

The amount of protein to be included in the diet was calculated according to the statural age. It was suggested the children be given 100% of the US RDA, 1980, plus the anticipated dialysate protein losses, which amounted to a supplement of 2–4 g/day (see Drachman et al., this volume). The protein allowance was increased in the case of infection or poor nutritional status. A maximum percentage of high-biological-value protein was required: 100% for infants, 80%–90% for small children, and at least 70% for the older children.

As for energy intake, the aim was to give the amount adapted to physiological needs and activities. It was generally possible for infants and toddlers to eat the quantities recommended for normal children. For patients aged 1–6 years, we prescribed 90% of the RDA, and for 7- to 10-year-old children, 80%. We were not able to make the older children consume more than 60%–75% of the RDA [2].

Saturated fats were replaced as much as possible by polyunsaturated ones.

Sodium allowance was often free or slightly restricted to 1 or 2 mmol/kg BW per day, depending upon the type of kidney disease. Potassium was restricted to 2–2.5 mmol/kg BW per day. It should be recalled that a "normal" diet for a 1-year-old child contains 3–6 mmol/kg/day [4].

Phosphorus was limited to 500–800 mg/day. Understanding of and compliance with the dietary prescription, was assessed by a dietary diary, which was complemented by interviews with the dietitian.

Dietary Survey

There is no perfect technique for evaluating food consumption. We have used the method of the dietary diary complemented by interviews [3]. The procedure was carried out in three stages. The first stage consisted of an initial interview to explain to the child and his mother (or a surrogate) the reason for the survey and how to complete the dietary questionnaire. Secondly, the child and his mother recorded the child's entire food intake for a period of 3 days. The families usually refused to record more than 3 or 4 days of dietary information, and in addition, longer studies are not more informative [4, 5]. We also devised a special questionnaire to determine the quantities of household measures or, preferably, weighed portions. Third, a final interview ended the investigation. During the interview, the dietitian usually discovered some omissions while checking the exact quantities consumed, the type of fat and sugar used, the composition of dishes or recipes served, or whether the amounts recorded corresponded to fresh or cooked food. In the case of foreign families, the dietitian had to become familiar with the particular dietary customs of the country involved.

This method requires much attention and cooperation on the part of the patient and parents. All omitted or inaccurate details are sources of error when converting the food portions eaten into weight measures. The fat intake was always a stumbling block unless the child ate it separately. How closely the recorded intake corresponds to actual food consumption remains difficult to assess because even the very fact of recording the intake in one way or another introduces some bias in the analysis [6]. Unfortunately, there is no way to check actual energy intake.

For the present study, the following data have been calculated: total and animal proteins, fats, carbohydrates, water, and energy. We do not give data detailing the nature of the fat and carbohydrate intake here. We have also studied sodium, potassium, calcium, and phosphorus intake. The data calculation has been performed with the data from the French food composition tables [7], together with values provided by the food industry and, occasionally, the English [8] or German [9] tables.

Results

Reliable dietary assessments were obtained for a total of 212 days, which amounts to 2–4 days every 3 months for all 17 patients. Dietary assessment for six other patients

Table 1. Recommended dietary intake as suggested by the Food and Nutrition Board 1980 [2]

	Age (years)	Protein (g/day)		Energy kcal/day
	1– 3	23 ⎫		1300
	4– 6	30 ⎪ 7%		1700
Boys	11–14	45 ⎬ energy intake		2700
Girls	11–14	46 ⎭		2200

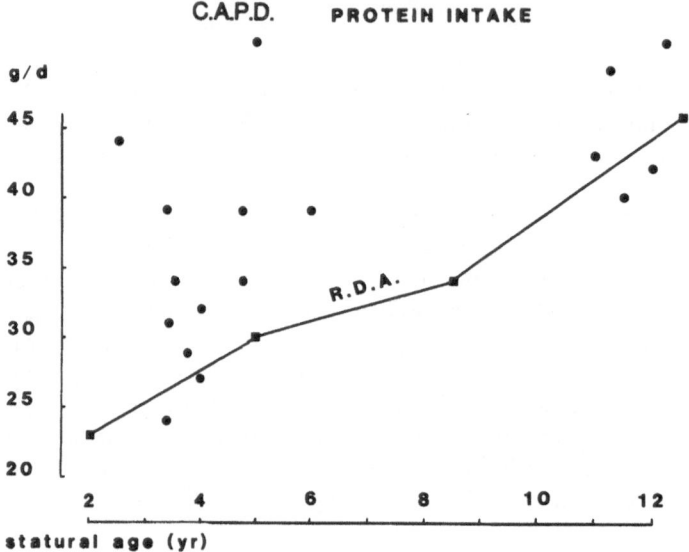

Fig. 1. Protein intake of children according to age. The *solid line* depicts the RDA

on CAPD proved impossible due to language difficulties with foreign families or to noncompliance with survey conditions. Protein intake is compared with the American recommendations in Table 1 [2]. The young CAPD patients consumed 128% of the American RDA, the older children 106%. The 2- to 6-year-old children had an average of 2.5 g/kg BW/day (range, 1.9–4 g) of protein, amounting to 35 g (range, 51–24 g), or 0.34 g/cm. The 11- to 12-year-old children consumed an average of 1.5 g/kg BW/day, totaling 42–50 g/day (Fig. 1), or 0.31 g/cm of protein (see Table 2). The energy derived from protein corresponded to 15% of energy from food alone and 11% of the total energy intake (food plus dialysate). Three-quarters of the total amount of proteins were from animal sources.

Energy Consumption

Energy consumption was also compared with the American recommendations [2].

Using a dialysate solution containing 80 mmol/l of glucose, the mean remaining concentration in the outflow was 10–15 mmol/l in the CAPD patients and

Table 2. Mean daily protein intake in children on CAPD

	Statural age (years)	Patients (n)	Protein intake		% Energy	
			g/day	% RDA	Without dialysate	With dialysate
	2 – 4	6	33.5	128 ⟨131	12	10.5
	4 – 6	6	37.0	128 ⟨125		
Boys	11 – 12	3	50.0	106 ⟨116	14	12
Girls	11 – 12	2	42.5	106 ⟨96		

Table 3. Mean daily energy intake in children on CAPD

	Statural age (years)	Patients (n)	Without dialysate		With dialysate	
			kcal	% RDA	kcal	% RDA
	2 – 4	6	1242	75 ⟨84	1347	83 ⟨94
	4 – 6	6	1104	75 ⟨65	1234	83 ⟨73
Boys	11 – 12	2	1267	58 ⟨52	1485	69 ⟨61
Girls	11 – 12	3	1435	58 ⟨64	1734	69 ⟨77

20–25 mmol/l in intermittent ambulatory peritoneal dialysis (IAPD) patients undergoing 12 h of dialysis. Consequently, the mean glucose uptake was 65–70 mmol/l and 55–60 mmol/l respectively, providing an energy supplement of 200 kJ and 167 kJ or 48 kcal/l and 40 kcal/l of dialysate, respectively. Depending on the volume of exchanges, this energy varied from 63 to 337 kcal/day, with an average intake per kilogram BW of between 25 and 46 kJ (6–11 kcal). Actual energy intake was generally much higher in the younger child, with a mean value of 84%, 65%, and 58% respectively of RDA for the statural age groups 2–4, 4–6, and 11–12 years of age. These figures were higher after taking into account the energy from the dialysate, with a mean value of 94%, 73%, and 69% of RDA, respectively. For the 2-to 4-year-old statural age group child, a mean total intake of 106 kcal/kg BW or 13.9 kcal/cm was obtained, while for the 4- to 6-year-old statural age group, a mean total intake of 77 kcal/kg BW or 11.6 kcal/cm was obtained. Older children had a mean total energy intake of 43 kcal/kg, or 9.95 kcal/cm, for boys and 51 kcal/kg, or 11.8 kcal/cm, for girls (Table 3, Fig. 2). The energy intake of normal French children varies from 12 to 15 kcal/cm [10].

The breakdown of energy into fat and carbohydrates followed the pattern generally observed in western countries. The diet was very rich in fat, around 45% of the total energy intake, part of which consisted of polyunsaturated fats (oils and margarines). Carbohydrate consumption decreased with chronic peritoneal dialysis.

We have also compared the energy consumed during CAPD with that consumed during intermittent cycling peritoneal dialysis (ICPD) performed at night. After 3–5 months of ICPD, three out of five patients had an increase in appetite (consuming 85% versus 75% of RDA), one remained unchanged, and one had decreased intake (62% versus 69% RDA after 11 months of ICPD).

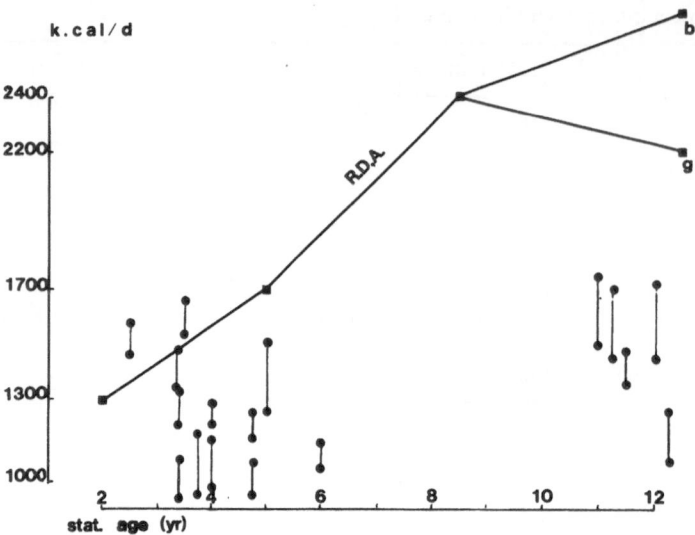

Fig. 2. Energy intake of children according to age. The range observed in individual patients is shown as a *vertical bar;* the *solid line* depicts the RDA; *b,* boys; *g,* girls

Water and Electrolytes

Fluid intake was free for 14 out of 17 patients and limited to 65–60 ml/kg BW per day for the others.

Sodium intake was free for eight patients, very limited for three patients (0.5 mmol/kg), and slightly limited for four patients (1–1.8 mmol/kg BW).

Potassium consumption was between 18 and 61 mmol/day, or 1–3.4 mmol/kg BW.

Phosphorus intake varied from 317 to 1007 mg/day, with an average of 650 mg/day.

Conclusion

This study reports original data from one specific center on the dietary intake of children on CAPD following specific dietary prescriptions. The first observation to be made is that the children on CAPD and/or their families complied well with the dietary prescriptions, as this survey found that intakes corresponded rather closely to the prescriptions.

Protein intake was around or above the US RDA; however, considering the peritoneal protein losses the children suffered, this was not sufficient in some cases.

With regard to energy intake, the data are disappointing, since only a few children younger than 4 years of statural age ingested energy at levels corresponding to the US RDA. It appears nevertheless that it was possible to improve energy intake in some patients by using ICPD with abdomen at rest during the day.

Comparison with dietary intake during hemodialysis shows no obvious differences [4]. However, the energy intake was probably less in the older children on CAPD.

In conclusion, children on CAPD are generally in good compliance with the dietary prescriptions and ingest proteins at the levels prescribed by the US RDA. The energy intake is low, especially in the older children. Regular dietary surveys facilitate the checking of compliance and permit adaption of the dietary prescriptions.

Appendix: Guidelines for Completing Food Intake Records

1. Choose 3 or 4 days of which 1 or 2 should be nonworking or nonschool days.
2. Record everything that the child has consumed: food and drink at meals and between meals.
3. Specify the form or type of food consumed:
   - Powdered milk, liquid milk (evaporated or not, sweetened or not); whole, half, or full cream; skimmed or flavored milk
   - Any special milk
   - Yoghurt and soft cheeses: indicate fat content as well as whether natural, flavored, or made from whole milk
   - Cheese: specify the type of cheese
   - Meat, fish: specify whether lean or fatty
   - Bread and biscuits: indicate whether white or wholemeal
   - Salted and sweet biscuits: give the brand
   - Vegetables: state whether cooked or fresh
   - Fruits: indicate whether fresh or cooked, prepared with or without sugar
   - Fruit juices: fresh, frozen, canned, sweetened; give the brands
   - Margarine and oils: state kind used (peanut, corn olive, grape seed, soya, sunflower, or other)
4. Indicate as accurately as possible the amount consumed: In teaspoons or tablespoons, level or rounded, for sugar, jam, butter, margarine, oils, vegetables, flour, stewed fruit
   - In glasses, teacups, bowls, ladles for liquids
   - In centimeters (cm) for three-dimensional portions (length, width, thickness)
   - In portions (e.g., 1/6th of a Camembert, knob of sausage)
5. State the method of preparation or cooking, sauces, flavorings (e.g., boiled, grilled, roasted, fried, sautéed, served with homemade or commercial sauces).
   If necessary give the recipes, stating the proportion eaten by the child.
6. Include all sweets and drinks consumed; note the brands and amounts, and do not forget sugar or sugar-containing foods added to drinks, yoghurts, or on bread.

References

1. Warren GS, Conley SB (1983) Nutritional considerations in infants on continuous peritoneal dialysis. Proc Eur Dial Transplant Assoc 12:263–264
2. National Research Council, Food and Nutrition Board (1980) Recommended dietary allowances, 9th edn. National Academy of Sciences, Washington, DC
3. Hackett AF, Augg-Gunn AJ, Appleton DR (1983) Use of a dietary diary and interview to estimate the food intake of children. Hum Nutr Appl Nutr 37 A:293
4. Broyer M, Dartois AM (1973) Analyse de la consommation alimentaire des enfants traités par hémodialyse chronique. Arch Fr Pédiatr 30:647–654
5. Gersovitz M, Madden JP, Smiciklas-Wright H (1978) Validity of the 24-h dietary record and seven-day record for group comparisons. J Am Dietet 73:48
6. Marr JW (1971) Individual dietary surveys. Purposes and methods. World Rev Nutr Diet 13:205
7. Randoin L, Legallic P, Dupuis Y, Bernardin A (1978) Tables de composition des aliments, 6th edn. Lanore, Paris
8. Paul AA, Southgate DAT (1978) McCance and Widdowson's the composition of foods, 4th edn. HMS Office, London
9. Souci SW, Fachmann W, Kraut H (1981) Food composition and nutrition tables, 2nd edn. Wissenschaftliche Verlagsgesellschaft, Stuttgart
10. Boggio V, Klepping J (1981) Caractéristiques de la ration alimentaire de l'enfant. Arch Fr Pédiatr 38:679–686
11. Dartois AM, Broyer M (1983) Diététique et néphrologie pédiatrique. In: Royer P, Habib R, Mathieu H, Broyer M (eds) Néphrologie pédiatrique, 3rd edn. Flammarion, Paris, pp 568–590
12. Vermeil G, Dartois AM, Dufraysseix M (1983) L'alimentation de la naissance à 3 ans, vol 1. Doin, Paris

The Management of the Infant on CAPD

E. C. Kohaut, S. R. Alexander, and O. Mehls

Introduction

Swan and Gordon [1] reported the use of peritoneal lavage in five children with renal failure. In the early 1960s, reports by Segar et al. [2] and Etteldorf et al. [3] popularized this form of therapy in children. In 1967 Levin and Winklestein [4] reported the use of intermittent peritoneal dialysis (IPD) in the treatment of a pediatric patient with chronic renal failure. However, due to the lack of a permanent peritoneal access, repeated punctures were required and dialysis was only done monthly in conjunction with vigorous dietary management, which was the main mode of therapy. The development of a chronic peritoneal access device by Palmer, which was refined by Tenckhoff [5], coupled with the development of automated cycling machines by Boen [6], provided the capability to treat patients with chronic renal failure with IPD. Counts et al. [7] initiated an IPD program in children in Seattle, and since then other centers [8–10] have described similar programs.

Intermittent peritoneal dialysis was never used extensively in the treatment of children with chronic renal failure. Of the 823 children under the age of 15 years who were alive on dialysis in the member countries of the European Dialysis and Transplant Association on 31 December 1979, only 38 (4.6%) were being treated with peritoneal dialysis [11]. Popovich et al. [12] first described a new form of peritoneal dialysis called continuous ambulatory peritoneal dialysis (CAPD). The authors recognized that the peritoneal membrane was inefficient, but demonstrated that if dialysis were done continuously, adequate dialysis clearances of solute could be obtained. They then designed a system that was wearable and portable so that convenient, continuous dialysis could be provided. This form of dialysis reached prominence after the publication in 1978 of the combined experiences of Moncrief and Nolph [13]. In 1980 the first preliminary reports of the use of CAPD in children appeared in abstract form [14]. In 1981, more extensive experience was reported [15, 16], and the following year, Baum et al. [17] presented definitive data demonstrating that CAPD was an attractive alternative to hemodialysis in the pediatric population. The possibility that CAPD could be used in very young infants has previously been suggested by a number of authors [14–16]. In this paper, we will describe our experiences in the treatment of ten infants who were less than 3 months of age at the initiation of CAPD.

Patient Population

Ten infants were started on CAPD at less than 3 months of age. Three had renal failure secondary to renal dysplasia, three had obstructive uropathy, three had acute renal failure without recovery, and one had renal aplasia. Eight infants were started on therapy in the first month of life; one at age 6 weeks; and one at age 10 weeks. All of the infants had a creatinine clearance of less than 5 ml/min/1.73 m². Eight of the ten infants were started on CAPD because of inability to control fluid and electrolyte abnormalities with vigorous medical management. Two infants were started on CAPD due to failure to thrive, despite vigorous medical management which included nutritional supplementation.

Methods

Therapy was initiated after placement of a Tenckhoff catheter, utilizing the procedure described by Alexander and Tank [18]. Initially, double cuff catheters were used; however, the last eight infants had a catheter implanted with only the peritoneal cuff placed. Originally, the catheter was placed in the midline. However, as experience was gained, we found that a catheter placed at the lateral edge of the rectus muscle was more effective.

Dialysate exchange volume used in this group of patients varied anywhere from 600 cc/m² per exchange to 1200 cc/m² per exchange. As previously reported [19], dialysate volume can be a major determinant of ultrafiltration. Six of these ten patients had residual urine output and the need for a large amount of ultrafiltration was not only unnecessary but undesirable; therefore, lower dialysate volumes could be used. However, in the four anuric infants, dialysate volumes approaching 1200 cc/m² were required before adequate ultrafiltration could be obtained. The majority of the infants were treated utilizing a dialysate solution containing 2.5% dextrose. Higher dextrose concentrations were used in the four anuric infants when increased ultrafiltration was critical.

Early in our experience, Dianeal 137 was used. When Dianeal PD-2 became available, it was used because it provided both better control of serum magnesium concentration and improved the acid-base balance [20]. In Heidelberg CAPD-4 fluid (Fresenius Co) was used. All infants underwent at least five CAPD exchanges a day. At times, the number of exchanges was increased if required for better control of metabolic parameters. One infant was treated with continuous cycling peritoneal dialysis (CCPD) for 2 months during this study period.

Results

At the time of this report, our experience totals 88 patients months of therapy with CAPD in these ten infants. The current status of these infants is outlined in Table 1. Two of the ten infants died while on CAPD: One died secondary to entrapment of a piece of bowel in a column disk peritoneal catheter, which led to necrosis of that segment of bowel and sepsis. The second infant died due to an inability to effect adequate dialysis because of multiple mechanical problems. Four of the eight surviving infants have been transplanted, one did not need further dialysis after 3 months of CAPD (partial recovery), and three remain on CAPD.

Table 1. Status of ten infants started on CAPD prior to 3 months of age

Died on CAPD	2/10
Transplanted	4/10
Alive on CAPD	3/10
Alive off CAPD	1/10

Table 2. Complications/patient months in neonates and older children

	< 3 months of age at onset of CAPD	> 3 months of age at onset of CAPD	
Total months experience	88	371	
Mortality	1/44	1/185	$P < 0.01$
Peritonitis	1/4	1/7	NS
Significant hypotension	1/6	1/92	$P < 0.01$
Catheter loss[a]	1/3	1/11	$P < 0.01$
Hyponatremia	1/3	1/74	$P < 0.01$

[a] Does not include catheters removed post-transplant or because of changes in treatment modality unrelated to catheter problems or peritonitis.

Important complications seen in this group of infants are tabulated in Table 2 and are compared with our older pediatric patient population. The mortality in the young infants was significantly higher than that seen in our older pediatric patient group. Peritonitis was seen once every 4 patient months in the study population, whereas in the older pediatric patient group the rate was one episode every 7 patient months of therapy. This difference was not significant. Significant hypotension, defined as symptomatic changes in blood pressure which required intravenous fluid therapy, was seen in the infant population at a rate of one episode every 6 patient months. Hypotension rarely occurred in the older patients.

Catheter loss occurred at a significantly higher rate among infants. Catheter loss is defined as those catheters which are lost because of nonfunction, or those catheters that had to be removed because of chronic peritonitis. This figure does not include catheters removed after a successful transplant, or catheters that were removed due to a change in treatment modality unrelated to catheter problems or peritonitis.

Hyponatremia (serum sodium < 130 mEq/l) was a common problem in the infant population, and occurred at a rate of one episode every 3 patient months, while in our older population it was rarely observed – one episode every 74 patient months. As shown in Table 3, the daily obligatory loss of sodium by ultrafiltration in a uremic infant exceeds by far the sodium intake from basic formula (amounting to 1–2 mEq/kg/day). In the non-sodium-depleted infant (situation A) the obligatory loss is about 10 mEq/kg/day. In the situation of sodium depletion (situation B), sodium absorption from the dialysate does not fully compensate for the loss by ultrafiltration, and the obligatory loss is reduced only to 7 mEq/kg/day.

Table 3. Sodium loss by CAPD in an anuric infant; body weight 4 kg, ultrafiltration (UF) 300 ml/day

	Situation A (non-sodium-depleted)	Situation B (sodium-depleted)
Sodium (mEq/l)		
Serum	139	124
Dialysate before exchange	134	134
Dialysate after exchange	134	126
Sodium loss by UF (mEq/day)	40	38
Sodium absorption from dialysate (mEq/day)	0	10
Na^+ net loss (mEq/day)	40	28

Table 4. Forced feeding

Infants were gavage fed an average of 5.3 days/month. Two infants required constant transpyloric feedings.

Recommendations

Gavage feed during periods of stress

Gavage feeding of sodium supplements if oral intake is inadequate

Constant feedings indicated if infant's intake remains inadequate

Many of these infants were not able to spontaneously maintain adequate nutritional intake. It was our goal that these infants ingest at least 100% of the recommended dietary allowance (RDA) for calories and 4 g/kg/day of protein. When this patient population developed peritonitis or even minor viral infections, their intake dropped dramatically. Early in our experience, we noted that if the infants developed anorexia due to an intercurrent illness, then it took a long time for them to recover. We therefore set a minimum amount of nutrient intake that an infant must consume per day. If the infant did not consume this amount, the patient was gavage fed. This patient population required gavage feeding at an average of 5.3 days/ month. Two of the infants developed prolonged anorexia, coupled with intermittent vomiting, and were placed on chronic transpyloric feedings for a period of 1 and 3 months, respectively (Table 4).

Growth was not as good in this population as it was in our patients who were started on CAPD after 3 months of age. The latter group of patients had a height which averaged −1.62 SD from the mean at the onset of therapy, and had improved to −1.38 SD at the end of therapy. The infants who began therapy at less than 3 months of age had an average length which was −0.72 SD from the mean at the initiation of therapy. At the end of therapy, the average length had declined to −1.95 SD from the mean.

In Table 5, the neurological status of the infants at the end of the treatment period is tabulated. We were able to study five of the eight surviving infants. Neurologi-

Table 5. Neurological assessment

5/8 – Surviving infants studied
2/5 – Normal
2/5 – Normal except for 1- and 2-month delays in gross motor function
1/5 – Three-month delay in all areas
3/5 – Normal CAT scan
1/5 – Normal sonogram
1/5 – Mild cerebral atrophy

cal evaluation was performed by a pediatric neurologist who had no knowledge of the treatment course. Two of the five infants were developmentally normal for age; two were normal except for a 1- to 2-month delay in gross motor function; and one infant had a 3-month delay in developmental parameters. Three of the five infants had a normal cerebral CAT scan. One of the five infants did not have a CAT scan, but had a normal sonogram of the head. One infant had mild cerebral atrophy demonstrated on CAT scan.

Discussion

The aggressive treatment of young infants with renal failure raises many social and moral questions, as well as questions pertinent to the therapy. Previously, the approach to this group of patients was to provide aggressive medical management, and if they survived the first few years of life, to then provide dialysis and, ultimately, renal transplantation. However, this approach has resulted in some significant complications. Betts and Magrath [21] demonstrated that infants born with renal insufficiency had very poor growth in the first year or two of life and that it was nearly impossible to regain subsequently the growth lost during that period. Catch-up growth in these children either during dialysis or following renal transplantation has been difficult to obtain [22]. Therefore, if infants are left untreated during this period of time, even if they do survive, they will almost certainly be dwarfed. Of greater importance is the potential development of serious and permanent neurological dysfunction, as noted by Rotundo et al. [23] in 20 of 23 patients with the onset of renal insufficiency in the first year of life. We believe that such findings support the concept that if normal growth and neurological function is to be obtained in infants with renal insufficiency, therapy should be initiated early.

When we decided to treat young infants with CAPD, we adopted the following criteria for treatment: those infants with renal insufficiency would first be treated with aggressive medical management which would include correction of any acid-base abnormality, control of metabolic parameters, and aggressive nutritional support. If the infant failed to thrive on this therapy, they would then be placed on CAPD. It is of interest that seven infants having a creatinine clearance greater than 5 ml/min/1.73 m² did well. Those with less endogenous renal function failed to thrive and required dialysis.

Therapy for the infant on CAPD is similar to that for the older child and adult, with some notable exceptions. Since the infant cannot reach a fluid source unaided, his thirst mechanism is not operational and fluid intake must be controlled. We have had more problems with low intake than we have had with excessive intake, as suggested by the hypotension seen in these infants. If the infants do not take the prescribed amount of fluid, the remainder must be given by gavage feeding. This daily minimum is calculated by adding estimated insensible losses, residual urine output, and dialysis ultrafiltration. In those infants with minimal residual urine output, we would rather increase ultrafiltration and thus preserve calorie intake, than limit fluid intake. As previously reported [19], adequate ultrafiltration is often dependent on providing a dialysate exchange volume of 1200 cc/m^2. In some infants, it may be impossible to do this because of limited respiratory capacity. In such situations, short dwell times and/or the use of hypertonic dialysate solution may be required to effect ultrafiltration.

Nutritional support has been essential in the management of these young infants. We have used several different formulas, but have had success with that regimen outlined in Table 6. The amount of Propac, a protein supplement, given daily is altered dependent upon the volume of formula delivered, the patient's BUN, and the serum albumin level. One of our older patients on CAPD developed clinical signs of zinc deficiency. Since that time, daily trace element supplementation similar to that given to patients receiving total parenteral nutrition has been prescribed. The daily intake of this formula is strictly monitored by the caretaker. If it is found that the infant has not received the minimum amount of volume required to provide adequate nutrition and maintain salt and water balance, gavage feedings are performed during the evening hours to supplement the oral intake. In two of our patients, this form of intermittent gavage therapy was unsuccessful. In one, ad lib intake was so poor that the infant required gavage feedings twice daily. In the other, the patient would vomit the gavage feeding. Both of these patients were placed on continuous transpyloric feedings at an amount required to maintain nutritional and fluid balance.

The average daily intake of these infants exceeded the RDA for calories. In our older patients, growth has been associated with a protein intake of greater than 2 g/kg/day [24]. However, we found in this population that many of the infants were consuming 4–6 g/kg/day of protein. This is very similar to the amount the average well-fed infant might receive.

Sodium loss in infants on CAPD was first measured by Mehls [25]. Hyponatremia is a complication seen almost exclusively in these youngest CAPD patients, though it can also be seen in older children with a small body size and a high ultrafiltration rate. The basic formula provides a relatively small amount of sodium. In those infants who require significant ultrafiltration, obligatory dialysate sodium losses well exceeded sodium intake. Such infants require oral sodium chloride sup-

Table 6. Infant formula

Base:	Similac 20	20 cal/oz
Additives:	Polycose, one teaspoon/oz	10 cal/tsp
	Propac, 2 – 3 tablespoons/day	4 g/Tbs
	Final calorie content, 32 – 36 cal/oz	

plements up to 10 mEq/kg/day to maintain a normal serum sodium level. A significant sodium depletion may be missed if only the serum sodium is measured. Hyponatremia occurs late with continuous losses of sodium and can be masked by volume contraction. A serum sodium value of 132 mEq/l can be associated with advanced sodium depletion. Therefore, it is of paramount importance to regularly measure the sodium loss in the 24-hour sample of dialysate of infants. Since 24-hour collections are not commonly available, at least a determination of the sodium content of a random dialysate sample should be undertaken. A rule of thumb is that the sodium content of the effluent dialysate should be in the range of the content of the affluent dialysis fluid.

Hyponatremia can also be seen in those patients in whom only a small amount of ultrafiltration is required. However, most of these patients have obstructive uropathy and significant urinary salt losses. These patients also require oral sodium chloride supplements. Occasionally, hyponatremia is seen because of inadequate ultrafiltration of water and subsequent volume expansion.

The maintainance of normal bone metabolism is important to the growth of the patient on CAPD [24]. Our aim was to maintain the serum parathormone level at less than twice the upper limits of normal. To accomplish this, these patients required rather large doses of Rocaltrol, 0.5–2 μg/day. We have also used calcium supplementation, first in the form of calcium gluconate and later in the form of calcium carbonate. Use of aluminum hydroxide phosphate binders was not excessive. The average intake of elemental aluminum in this population was 60 mg/day. Recent concerns [26] regarding chronic aluminum intoxication in infants with renal insufficiency have led us to attempt to eliminate aluminum hydroxide from our treatment regimen.

Previous reported experiences with forms of continuous peritoneal dialysis in the treatment of the very young infant have been limited. Conley et al. [27] treated three infants under 6 months of age with continuous peritoneal dialysis. These investigators did not use traditional CAPD, but rather designed a system using a Y-tubing that allowed multiple (seven to ten) exchanges a day while entering the system only once. This permitted the use of lower dialysate volumes. Conley et al. [27] have provided aggressive nutritional support via constant nasogastric feedings. Two of these patients have been successfully transplanted after reaching appropriate size. The third infant expired. If one takes our series, added to the above experience, the mortality for the treatment of the young infant with forms of continuous peritoneal dialysis is approximately 25%, which is much higher than that seen in older patients. Unfortunately, no control data are available; however, one could assume that the mortality in a similar group of patients left untreated would be higher.

Conclusion

In addition to the usual concerns which need to be addressed in treating older patients with CAPD, the following problems must be dealt with when treating very young infants with this form of therpay:
1. Dialysate and renal sodium and water losses must be measured and replaced daily. The infant must be evaluated if body fluid losses change.

2. Nutritional requirements must be met. We would recommend that at least 100% of the RDA for calories be provided, as well as 4 g/kg/day of protein.
One should not hesitate to institute tube feeding if these requirements are not met with ad lib intake.

3. Acid-base status should be normalized.

4. Renal osteodystrophy should be prevented. This may require larger doses of vitamin D metabolites and/or calcium supplements than previously realized.

5. The use of aluminum hydroxide phosphate binders may be detrimental. Certainly, minimal use is optimal.

The experience described in this report has reinforced our belief that successful treatment of very young infants with ESRD using CAPD and eventual renal transplantation is not only possible but may be the treatment of choice in those infants who do not thrive after vigorous medical management has been instituted. Minimum age and size criteria for the entrance into a pediatric ESRD program are no longer tenable in our view, except perhaps in the most extreme situations. Although it is too early to provide rigid guidelines for the treatment of infants with CAPD, we feel the concerns expressed in this paper must be considered when any infant is treated with CAPD.

Criteria for acceptance into ESRD programs should be no different for infants than for patients in older age groups. Renal transplanation is still the ultimate goal in the treatment of young patients with ESRD. With continued advancement of the understanding of this form of therapy in young infants, it is our hope that CAPD will provide a mechanism to allow these children to reach transplantation while maintaining their full potential for growth and development.

References

1. Swan H, Gordon H (1949) Peritoneal lavage in the treatment of anuria in children. Pediatrics 4:586–595
2. Segar WE, Gibson RK, Rhomy R (1961) Peritoneal dialysis in infants and small children. Pediatrics 27:603–613
3. Etteldorf JN, Dobbin WT, Sweeney MJ, Smith JD, Whittington GL, Sheffield JA, Meadows RW (1962) Intermittent peritoneal dialysis in the management of acute renal failure in children. J Pediatr 60:327–339
4. Levin S, Winklestein JA (1961) Diet and infrequent peritoneal dialysis in chronic anuric uremia. N Engl J Med 277:619–624
5. Tenckhoff H, Schechter H (1968) A bacteriologically safe peritoneal access device. Trans Am Soc Artif Intern Organs 14:181–185
6. Boen ST, Moon C, Curtis PK et al. (1964) Periodic peritoneal dialysis using the repeated puncture technique and automated cycling machine. Trans Am Soc Artif Intern Organs 10:409–414
7. Counts S, Hickman R, Barbaccio A et al. (1973) Chronic home peritoneal dialysis in children. Trans Am Soc Artif Intern Organs 19:157–163
8. Brouhard BH, Berger M, Cunningham RJ (1979) Home peritoneal dialysis in children. Trans Am Soc Artif Intern Organs 25:90–93
9. Feldman W, Baliah T, Drummond K (1968) Intermittent peritoneal dialysis in the management of chronic renal failure in children. Am J Dis Child 16:30–36
10. Day RE, White RHR (1977) Peritoneal dialysis in children. Arch Dis Child 62:56–61
11. Donckerwolcke RA, Chantler C, Broyer M et al. (1979) Combined report on regular dialysis and transplantation of children in Europe. Proc Eur Dial Transplant Assoc 17:89–115

12. Popovich RP, Moncrief JW, Decherd JF, Bomar JB, Pyle WK (1976) The definition of a novel portable, wearable equilibrium peritoneal dialysis technique. Abstr Am Soc Artif Intern Organs 5:64
13. Popovich RP, Moncrief JW, Knolph KD, Ghods AJ, Twardowski ZJ, Pyle WK (1978) Continuous ambulatory peritoneal dialysis. Ann Intern Med 88:449–456
14. Alexander SR, Tseng CH, Maksym KA et al. (1980) Early clinical experience with continuous ambulatory peritoneal dialysis (CAPD) in infants and children. Clin Res 28:131A
15. Kohaut EC (1981) Continuous ambulatory peritoneal dialysis, a preliminary pediatric experience. Am J Dis Child 135:270–271
16. Balfe JW, Vigneux A, Willumsen J, Hardy BE (1981) The use of CAPD in the treatment of children with end stage renal disease. Perit Dial Bull 1:35–38
17. Baum M, Powell D, Calvin S et al. (1982) Continuous ambulatory peritoneal dialysis in children. N Engl J Med 307:1537–1541
18. Alexander SR, Tank ES (1982) Surgical aspects of continuous ambulatory peritoneal dialysis in infants, children and adolescents. J Urol 127:501–504
19. Kohaut EC (1983) Effect of dialysate volume on ultrafiltration in young children. Eur J Pediatr 140:179A
20. Kohaut EC, Balfe JW, Potter D, Alexander SR, Lum G (1983) Hypermagnesemia and mild hypocarbia in pediatric patients on continuous ambulatory peritoneal dialysis. Perit Dial Bull 3:42
21. Betts PR, Magrath G (1974) Growth pattern and dietary intake of children with chronic renal insufficiency. Br Med J 2:189–193
22. Schärer K, Gilli G (1984) Growth in children with chronic renal insufficiency. In: Fine RN, Gruskin AB (ed.): End stage renal disease in children. WB Saunders, Philadelphia, pp 271–290
23. Rotundo A, Nevins TE, Lipton M, Lockman LA, Mauer SM, Michael AF (1982) Progressive encephalopathy in children with chronic renal insufficiency in infancy. Kidney Int 21:686–691
24. Kohaut EC (1983) Growth in children treated with continuous ambulatory peritoneal dialysis. Int J Pediatr Nephrol 4:93–98
25. Mehls O (1984) Hyponatremia in infants on CAPD: presentation at International Symposium on CAPD in Children, May 14–15, 1984, Heidelberg, FRG
26. Andreoli SP, Bergstein JM, Sheppard DJ (1984) Aluminum intoxication from aluminum containing phosphate binders in children with azotemia not undergoing dialysis. N Engl J Med 310:1079–1084
27. Conley SB, Brewer ED, Grady S et al. (1982) Normal growth in very small children on peritoneal dialysis. Program and Abstracts, National Kidney Foundation, December 8–13, 1982, Chicago, Illinois, p 8

Growth of the Patient on CAPD

E. C. Kohaut

Introduction

The maintenance of growth in the child on dialysis remains a challenge to the pediatric nephrologist. Betts and Magrath [1] presented data concerning the natural history of growth in children with renal insufficiency. They demonstrated that growth was most disturbed in those patients who had renal insufficiency present from birth. These patients grew very poorly during the first 2 years of life. Between the ages of 2 and 11 years of age the children grew at near normal rates, but did not regain the growth lost during the first 2 years of life. Therefore, as a group, children with the onset of renal insufficiency during the first 2 years of life remained small, whether treated conservatively or with dialysis.

Since that time many authors [2–6] have demonstrated that while a few patients receiving hemodialysis, intermittent peritoneal dialysis, or renal transplantation have normal growth increments, rarely do they regain the growth lost early in life.

Popovich et al. [7] described a form of dialysis which later became known as continuous ambulatory peritoneal dialysis (CAPD) [8]. Since that time CAPD has been adapted for children. The methods for the use of this dialytic therapy in children have been described by many authors [9–12]. The purpose of this paper is to describe the growth seen in our pediatric end-stage renal disease (ESRD) population treated with CAPD, and to attempt to correlate growth to various biochemical and dietary parameters. Early in our experience with CAPD we noted that this form of dialytic therapy could allow a wider latitude of fluid intake than hemodialysis. This gave us the opportunity to increase dietary intake and liberalize the type of food ingested. We used this opportunity to institute an aggressive nutritional management program. At the same time we began to treat renal osteodystrophy more aggressively. This study was undertaken to examine the effects of the above interventions on growth in this population.

Patient Population (Table 1)

Since 1979 we have treated 42 patients with CAPD, for a total of 449 patient months of therapy. Because of a rather active transplant service, most of our patients remain on CAPD for less than 1 year. The data in this paper only concern 16 patients who have been treated with CAPD for at least 1 year. The longest period of time a patient has been treated with CAPD at our institution is 26 months. The average age of these 16 patients was 7.2 years. Nine patients were white and seven were black.

Table 1. Patient population of study

Average age:	7.2 years	
Race:	9 white	7 black
Sex:	10 males	6 females
Original disease		
Obstructive uropathy	7	
Glomerulopathy	7	
Dysplasia-hypoplasia	2	

There were ten males and six females. Seven had obstructive uropathy, seven had various glomerulopathies, and two were born with dysplastic and/or hypoplastic kidneys. Creatinine clearance was less than 5 ml/m²/min in all patients. Four of the 16 patients were anuric; average urine output in the remaining 12 patients was 316 cc/m²/day.

Methods

Heights or lengths in the nonambulatory patients, were measured by the same person monthly. Three measurements were obtained at each visit, and the average was used for this study. Height velocity was calculated from these measurements. Height velocities were plotted on a Tanner-Whitehouse height velocity chart. Bone age was obtained by the method of Greulich and Pyle [13]. Height velocities were plotted against bone age, not chronological age. Expected height velocity is defined as the height velocity which equals the 50th percentile for a given bone age. Bone age was used rather than chronological age because early in our experience we treated a number of older patients who had not gone through puberty, and in those cases the use of chronological age would have falsely improved our results. Parathormone levels were obtained monthly. The reported parathormone level is an average of three monthly tests. During the study period two different assays for parathormone were performed. Therefore, parathormone levels are reported as a ratio of actual parathormone level to the high normal parathormone level for the assay utilized. Protein and calorie intake was calculated from patient diaries which were kept initially for 3 days, and subsequently for 5 days, prior to each monthly clinic visit. Protein and calorie intake are reported in this study as an average of the nine days, or 15 days, for each 3-month patient period. Blood urea nitrogen and total CO_2 estimations were performed by standard hospital laboratory procedure at each monthly visit. The reported value is an average of the three monthly values.

Results

Growth for the population over the entire year is illustrated in Table 2. Four of the patients grew at greater than 100% of expected height velocity. Eight grew at a value between 80% and 100%, and four grew at a rate less than 80% of expected height

Table 2. Growth of 16 patients treated with CAPD for at least 1 year

No. of patients	% of expected height velocity
4	> 100%
8	80% – 100%
4	< 80%

Table 3. Correlation coefficients between height velocity and biochemical and nutritional variables studied ($n = 68$)

Height velocity vs:	r	P
Control of PTH	– 0.68	< 0.01
Protein intake	– 0.65	< 0.1
Calorie intake	– 0.61	< 0.1
Control of acidosis	– 0.40	< 0.1
BUN	– 0.27	
Total urea clearance	– 0.14	

velocity. The average growth rate for the entire population was 0.62 cm/month. The average expected growth rate was 0.74 cm/month. Another way of expressing growth data is in terms of standard deviations (SD) from the mean for chronological age. This method is widely used in data from the EDTA [6]. At the start of therapy this patient group averaged –1.56 SD from the mean, and at the end of therapy the Z-score improved to an average –1.41 SD from the mean. We then correlated height velocity with the patients' dietary and biochemical data. For this purpose the treatment times for the patients were separated into 3-month periods. There were a total of 68 3-month periods; however, the data were not complete for all of them. Table 3 lists correlation coefficients for each of the biochemical and nutritional variables we examined. For 68 patients periods, the r value must be greater than 0.27 to reach significance (P value less than 0.01). The correlation coefficient of –0.68 for control of parathormone was most significant. Protein intake correlated with growth with an r value of 0.65; caloric intake did so with an r value of 0.61, and control of acidosis with an r value of 0.40. The correlation of height velocity with BUN was almost significant, with an r value of 0.27. This is not surprising since BUN correlated with protein intake with an r value of 0.53. There was no correlation with total urea clearance or remaining renal function as measured by endogenous urea clearance. Total urea clearance did correlate significantly with protein intake.

Discussion

The data presented are extremely difficult to evaluate. There is no doubt that observing growth over a 3-month period could lead to numerous errors. Normal children do not grow evenly over a year, but rather erratically. The height velocities used for references are calculated for a year, and not for 3-month periods. There would also be some question as to whether bone age is valid when the bone age is depressed owing to renal failure. However, if the treatment periods for growth were extended, the data would suffer from other inaccuracies. We could not purposely defer treatment of a high parathormone level for a year, nor could we purposely allow a patient to have inadequate caloric intake, or protein intake, for a year. Realizing the inherent inaccuracies in the methods, we do feel that growth was best correlated in this patient group with control of parathormone level, control of acidosis, and a higher level of protein and caloric intake.

Our approach to the treatment of renal osteodystrophy has been the use of increasing amounts of calcium supplements, and relatively high doses (0.5–2.0 µg/day) of 1,25-dihydroxycholecalciferol. Aluminum hydroxide phosphate binders have also been used. However, because of the use of large amounts of calcium gluconate, and later calcium carbonate supplements, the dose of aluminum hydroxide binders has been kept relatively low. The average intake of elemental aluminum was only 62 mg/kg/day. This has been fortuitous since, lately, aluminum intoxication has also been associated with bone disease [14].

Protein intake also correlated well with adequate growth in this study. It is difficult to interpret whether the protein or the calorie intake is more important since most of the patients who were taking adequate amounts of protein were also taking adequate calories. In fact, protein and calorie intake correlated with an r value of 0.79. Fourteen of the 16 patients treated in this population required protein supplements to maintain an adequate protein intake. The protein supplement we have utilized is Propac, a hydrolyzed whey powder, which has a concentration of 4 g/tbs. The amount given depended on the patient's voluntary protein intake, as well as the serum albumin and later serum transferrin levels. Protein supplements were used in an attempt to increase protein intake to at least 2 g/kg/day in the patient over 1 year of age. In many of our infants on CAPD, protein intake was increased to 4–6 g/kg/day to maintain normal serum transferrin and serum albumin levels. Calorie supplements were also utilized in this patient population. Fourteen of the 16 patients at some point during the study received supplementation with Polycose. The amount of Polycose given was dependent upon the patient's voluntary calorie intake. Polycose was used in an attempt to increase calorie intake to at least 100% of the recommended dietary allowance for age. Intermittent tube feedings were provided to younger patients during periods of anorexia.

The relationship between protein intake, total urea clearance, and blood urea nitrogen is well known [15]. Our patients' protein intake did not correlate with total urea clearance as well as would be expected. This discrepancy could be explained in two ways: 1) that the parents were giving us an inaccurate statement of protein intake, or 2) the patients were anabolic. I think the latter is probably the best explanation in this patient group. Others have also shown that children on CAPD with adequate protein intake maintained positive nitrogen balance [16]. Energy intake has previously been shown to be a major determinant of growth in children with renal failure [17]. Our data would suggest that at least 100% of the RDA be given, and one would speculate whether this figure should even be higher. Increased calorie intake occurred in our patient population not only because of the vigorous use

Table 4. Findings of various studies regarding growth in children on CAPD

Author	Patients (n)	% of height velocity expected		
		100% or greater	70% – 100%	< 70%
Current study	16	4	9	3
Stefanidis et al. [19]	17	6	6	5
Baum et al. [12]	6	Average growth 83% of normal		
Salusky et al. [20]	21	Average growth near normal		

of calorie supplements, but also because the patients received 9–18 calories/kg/day from absorption of glucose from the dialysate. It is also our feeling that the patients enjoyed liberalized dietary intake because salt and water restrictions were not as rigid as they are on hemodialysis. We have always taken the attitude of manipulating dialysis to fit the patient's diet, rather than changing the diet to fit in with the patient's dialysis schedule.

Control of acidosis did not reach significance in our early studies of growth and CAPD [18]. However, with increasing numbers, control of acidosis is a significant determinant of growth in this population.

Conclusion

The data presented indicate that children on CAPD can have normal growth if parathormone and bicarbonate levels are controlled, and adequate protein and calorie intake are established. Our data are in basic agreement with other studies which have looked at growth in this patient population. These studies are tabulated in Table 4.

References

1. Betts PR, Magrath G (1974) Growth pattern and dietary intake in children with chronic renal insufficiency. Br Med J 2:189–194
2. Kleinknecht C, Broyer M, Gagnadoux M et al. (1980) Growth in children treated with long term dialysis. A study of 76 patients. Adv Nephrol 9:133–163
3. Broyer M, Kleinknecht C, Loirat C, Marti-Henneberg C, Roy MT (1974) Growth in children with long term hemodialysis. J Pediatr 84:642–649
4. Chantler C, Carter JE, Bewick M, Counahan R, Cameron JS, Ogg CS, Williams DA, Winder E (1980) 10 years experience with regular hemodialysis and renal transplantation. Arch Dis Child 55:435–445
5. Schärer K, Mehls O, Gilli G (1974) Renal bedingte Skeletterkrankungen und Wachstumsstörungen. Orthopäde 3:58
6. Schärer K, Chantler C, Brunner FP et al. (1976) Combined report on regular dialysis and transplantation of children in Europe, 1975. Proc Eur Dial Transplant Assoc 12:65–108

7. Popovich RP, Moncrief JW, Decherd JF, Bomar JB, Pyle WK (1976) The definition of a novel portable, wearable equilibrium peritoneal dialysis technique. Abstr Am Soc Artif Intern Organs 5:64A
8. Popovich RP, Moncrief JW, Nolph KD, Ghods AJ, Twardowski ZJ, Pyle WK (1978) Continuous ambulatory peritoneal dialysis. Ann Intern Med 88:449–456
9. Alexander ST, Tseng CH, Maksym KA, Campbell RA, Talwalkar YB, Kohaut EC (1981) Clinical parameters in continuous ambulatory peritoneal dialysis for infants and children. In: Moncrief RW, Popovich JW (eds) CAPD update. Masson, New York, pp 195–209
10. Balfe JW, Vigneux A, Willumsen J, Hardy BE (1981) The use of CAPD in the treatment of children with end stage renal disease. Perit Bull 1: 35–38
11. Kohaut EC (1981) Continuous ambulatory peritoneal dialysis. A preliminary pediatric experience. Am J Dis Child 135:270–277
12. Baum M, Powell D, Calvin S, McDaid T, McHenry K, Mar H, Potter D (1982) Continuous ambulatory peritoneal dialysis in children in comparison with hemodialysis. N Engl J Med 307:1537–1542
13. Greulich WW, Pyle SI (1959) Radiologic atlas of skeletal development of the hand and wrist, 2nd edn. Stanford University Press, Stanford
14. Andreoli SP, Bergstein JM, Sheppard DJ (1984) Aluminum intoxication from aluminum containing phosphate binders in children with azotemia not undergoing dialysis. N Engl J Med 310:1079–1084
15. Kassirer JP (1971) Clinical evaluation of kidney function: glomerular filtration. N Engl J Med 285:385–389
16. DeSanto NG, Capodicasa G, Pluvio M, Gilli G, Giordano C (1981) Nitrogen balance and growth in children on CAPD. In: Gahl GM, Kessel M, Nolph KD (eds) Advances in peritoneal dialysis. Proceedings of the 2nd International symposium on peritoneal dialysis, 16–19 June 1981, Amsterdam
17. Holliday MA (1975) Calorie intake and growth in uremia. Kidney Int 7:5, S73–S78
18. Kohaut EC (1983) Growth in children treated with continuous ambulatory peritoneal dialysis. Int J Pediatr Nephrol 4:93–98
19. Stefanidis CJ, Hewitt IK, Balfe JW (1983) Growth in children receiving continuous ambulatory peritoneal dialysis. J Pediatr 102:681–685
20. Salusky IB, Fine RN, Nelson P et al. (1982) Nutritional status of pediatric patients undergoing CAPD. Kidney Int 21:177–181

Thyrotropin-Releasing Hormone and Growth Hormone-Releasing Factor in the Evaluation of Hypophyseal Function in Children Undergoing CAPD

F. Perfumo, M. Giusti, D. Bessarione, F. Ginevri, G. Basile, and R. Gusmano

Introduction

Hormonal abnormalities are a well-known complication of the uremic syndrome, and it is well established that renal failure may be associated with a variety of endocrine disturbances and alterations in "feed-back control" mechanisms [1]. In uremic adults acquired defects in the hypothalamic-pituitary-target organ axis, manifested by glucose intolerance [2], decreased potency and reduced testicular size [3–5], and clinical signs of thyroid dysfunction [6] are well recognized, while in children, particularly prepubertal children, data are minimal [7–10].

The aim of this study was to investigate the hypothalamo-hypophyseal function using the thyrotropin-releasing hormone (TRH) test and the human pancreatic tumor growth hormone releasing factor (GRF) test in prepubertal children undergoing continuous ambulatory peritoneal dialysis (CAPD). While the TRH test has been used previously in order to investigate endocrine function in uremia, studies with the GRF test are lacking.

Studies with hypothalamic extracts have strongly suggested the existence of a substance capable of stimulating growth hormone secretion from the pituitary. Ectopic production of growth hormone releasing factors provides a new source of these peptides. In recent years the extraction, purification, and sequencing of active growth hormone releasing peptides from two pancreatic tumors has been successfully carried out [11, 12]. The structure of the largest of these peptides was formed by 44 amino acids [GRF-(1–44)]. This peptide and two smaller peptides, possibly degradation products, GRF-(1–40) and GRF-(1–37), were present in one tumor [13], while only the 40 amino acid form was isolated from another tumor [12]. Analogues of these peptides have now been synthesized, and it has been shown that the N-terminal 29 residues possess full growth hormone secretagogue activity [12]. The effects of bolus doses of GRF have been recently described in man; they were found to specifically stimulate growth hormone secretion, with no effects on other anterior pituitary function [14]. Nevertheless, the influence of such peptides on secretion in pathological states such as uremia is unknown. We therefore examined these effects in uremic children on CAPD and here report our preliminary data.

Patients and Methods

Eleven patients (nine boys and two girls) ranging in age from 1 to 12.2 years were studied during their CAPD treatment. The duration of CAPD varied between 3 and 24 months at the time of the study. One patient was treated with hemodialysis before CAPD for a period of 12 months; the remaining ten were treated exclusively by CAPD. The patients received four exchanges per day of 35–45 ml/kg/exchange; in four patients the dextrose concentration was 1.5 g/dl in three exchanges and 2.5 g/dl in one exchange, while seven patients received four exchanges/day with 1.5 g/dl. No patient received medication known to alter plasma hormone levels.

Data from these patients were compared with data from a control group (C) of 16 prepubertal children of the same age, all of whom were in good health at the time of the study. The protocol of the study was explained to the parents and written informed consent obtained.

The tests were performed at 9 a.m. after an overnight fast, before the first exchange of the morning, the last exchange having been done 12 h before.

The TRH test was carried out in ten normal controls and ten CAPD patients. An indwelling i.v. catheter was secured so that frequent blood samples could be easily obtained and was kept open with a continuous infusion of isotonic saline. Blood was drawn 30 min before and again immediately before the i.v. injection of 7 µg/kg BW of TRH (Biodata), and 10, 20, 30, 45, 60, 90, and 120 min after injection. The blood was immediately centrifuged at 4 °C, and the serum stored at −20 °C until assayed for thyroid-stimulating hormone (TSH), growth hormone (GH), prolactin (PRL), luteinizing hormone (LH), and follicle-stimulating hormone (FSH).

The GRF test was done in six normal controls and seven CAPD patients. They remained recumbent throughout the study. At 8 a.m. an indwelling catheter was placed in a forearm vein for blood withdrawal and for intravenous injection of 1 µg/kg BW of the peptide at 9 a.m. GRF-(1–40) (CRB Cambridge) was dissolved in sterile isotonic saline, and the solution was then sterilized by filtration (Millipore). The peptide solution was divided into portions, placed in sterile vials, and immediately frozen at −20 °C until the moment of injection (no more than 20 days from the time of preparation). One vial per subject was thawed immediately before the injection, and any unused solution was discarded.

In control subjects, blood was drawn at 0, 15, 30, 45, 60, 75, 90, 105, and 120 min for hormone analysis. In the CAPD patients, in order to spare blood, the time of blood sampling was 0, 30, 60, 90, 120, 150, and 180 min after GRF. The specimens were immediately centrifuged at 4 °C and the serum removed and frozen at −20 °C until assayed for GH, TSH, PRL, LH, FSH, and cortisol. Serum GH (CIS Saluggia), LH, FSH, PRL (DPC Los Angeles), TSH, and cortisol (Biodata Rome) were measured by standard radioimmunoassay technique using the double antibody method. The samples of a given subject were measured in the same assay so that inter-assay variability was avoided. The intra-assay variability coefficient for the different hormones in our laboratory is 3% for GH, 4% for PRL, LH, FSH, and TSH, and 7% for cortisol. All values are expressed as mean ± SEM; statistical analyses were done using the variance analysis.

Results

Baseline Values

Basal values of TSH $(2.74 \pm 0.41 \, \mu U/ml)$, GH $(1.33 \pm 0.23 \, ng/ml)$, and FSH $(2.65 \pm 0.43 \, mU/ml)$ in the CAPD patients were not significantly different from those of controls. PRL basal values were abnormal (> 25 ng/ml) in six out of ten CAPD patients, with a mean value of 99.1 ± 36.4 ng/ml. LH levels were higher in the dialyzed children (5.36 ± 1.15 mU/ml) than in controls ($P < 0.01$).

Response to TRH

TSH (Fig. 1): In normal subjects the maximum TSH values after TRH was observed at 20 min; after this, serum TSH declined toward baseline. In CAPD patients TRH always increased the serum TSH concentration, but the response was delayed and prolonged, and the maximum levels were reached after 30–60 min. Two hours later the TSH level was still elevated. The peak value of the dialyzed children (12.29 ± 1.62 µU/ml) was not significantly different from that of controls (13.75 ± 1.91 µU/ml).

GH (Fig. 2): TRH did not increase serum GH concentration in normal children; while dialyzed children showed a paradoxical rise, with the highest value at 45 min after TRH. At the end of the test the patients showed a mean value near that of controls.

PRL (Fig. 3): The normal rise of PRL following TRH injection was completely blunted in CAPD patients. Normal controls showed a 816.5 ± 176.4% increase with

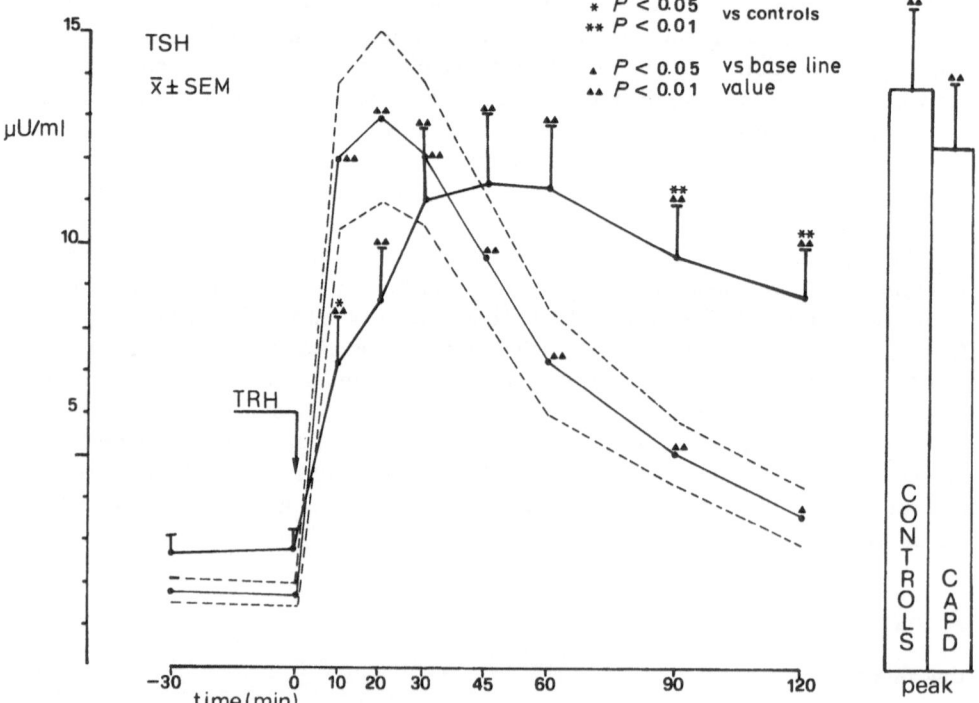

Fig. 1. Response of serum *TSH* to i.v. injection of *TRH*. *Broken lines* represent the range of controls

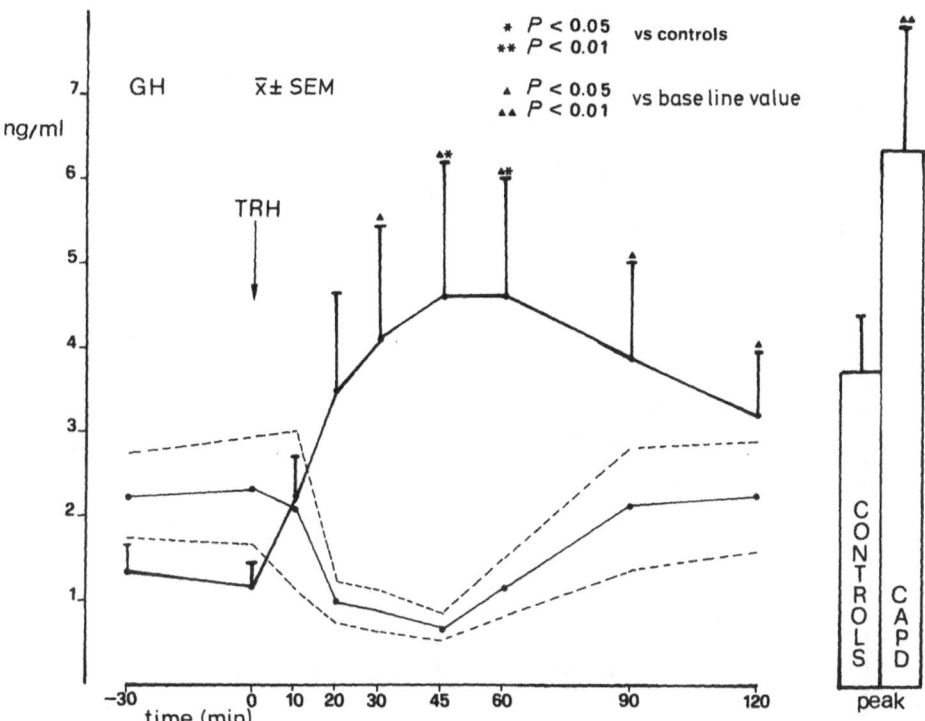

Fig. 2. Response of serum *GH* to i.v. injection of *TRH*. *Broken lines* represent the range of controls

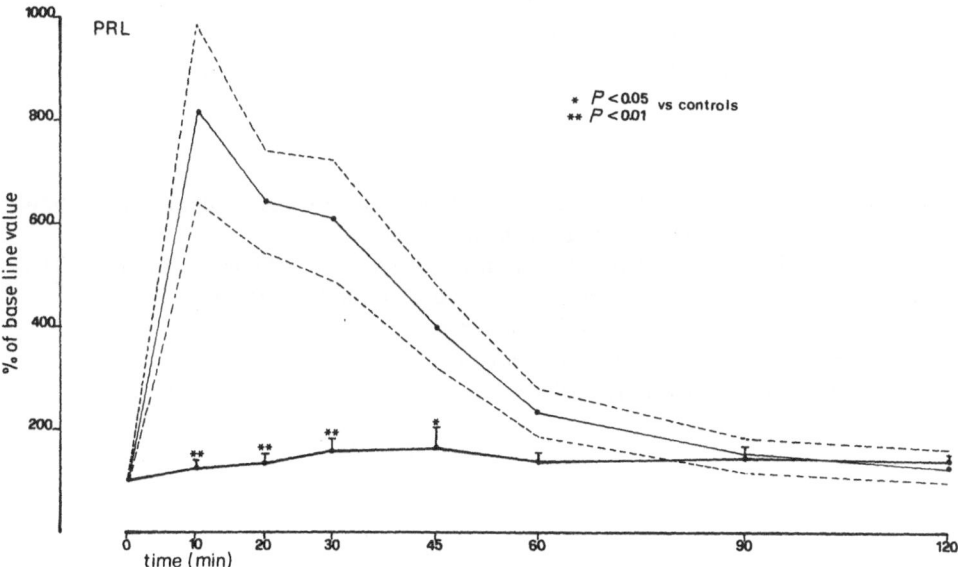

Fig. 3. Response of serum *PRL* to i.v. injection of *TRH*. *Broken lines* represent the range of controls

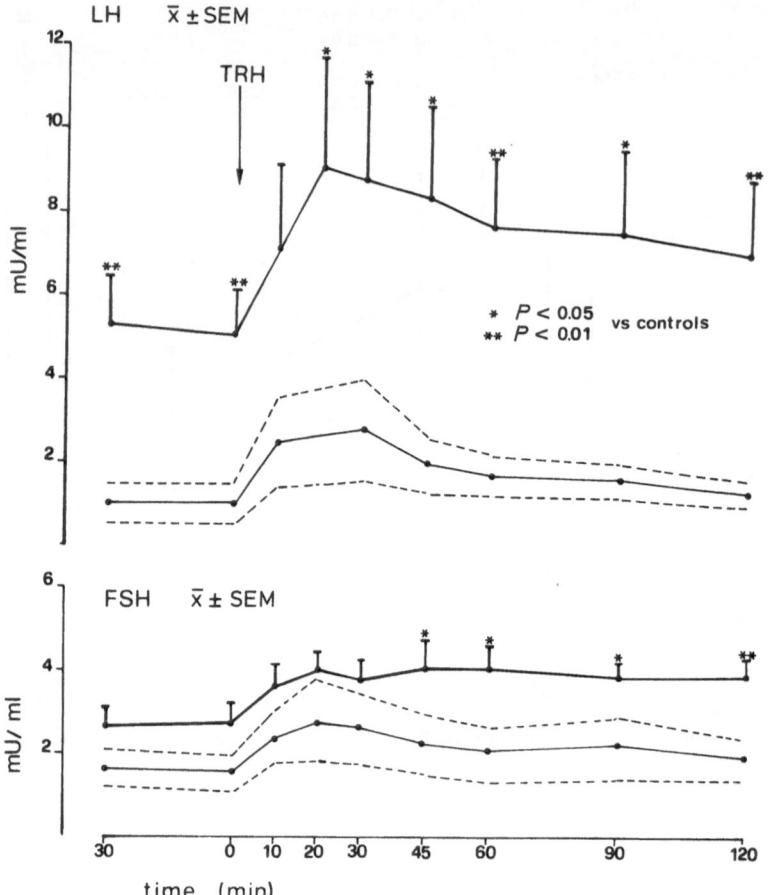

Fig. 4. Response of serum *LH* and serum *FSH* to i.v. injection of *TRH*. *Broken lines* represent the range of controls

respect to base line values 10 min after TRH, whereas the CAPD children exhibited a 166.9 ± 32.5% increase 45 min after the injection.

LH and FSH (Fig. 4): These hormones showed similar behavior after i.v. TRH with an increase in a small percentage of subjects in the two groups:

FSH: 30% of controls, 22% of CAPD patients
LH: 30% of controls, 40% of CAPD patients
LH was constantly elevated in the dialyzed children.

Response to GRF

GH (Fig. 5): After GRF-(1–40) administration, serum GH concentrations were increased in all normal subjects after 15 min, the first time-point studied, and reached a peak 30 min after the injection. All seven dialyzed children showed a significant

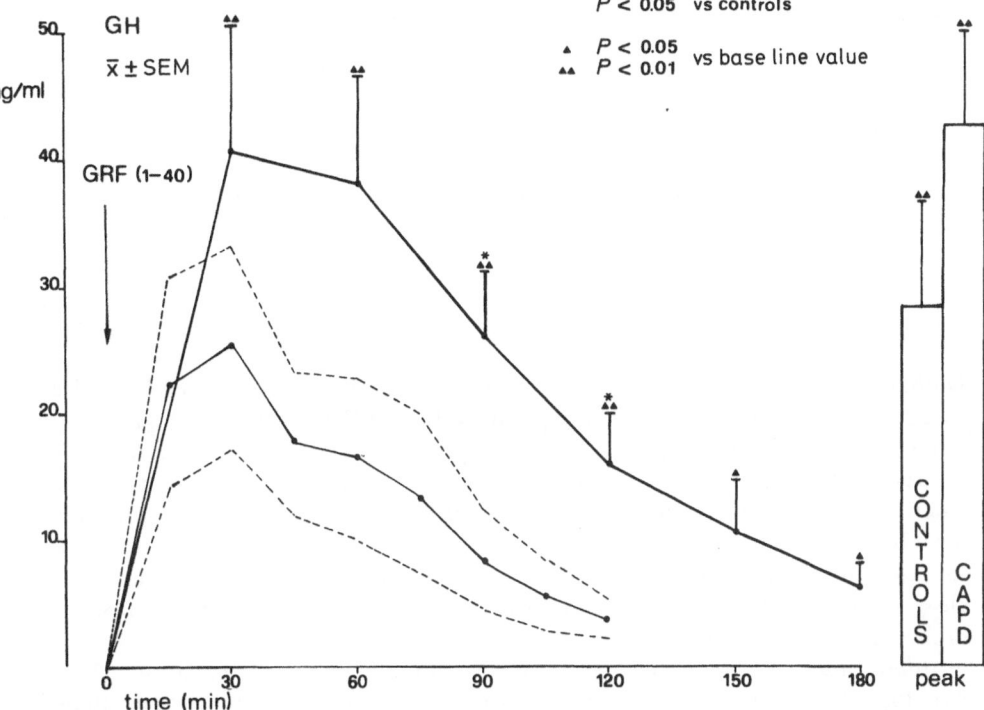

Fig. 5. Response of serum *GH* to i.v. injection of *GRF*-(1–40). *Broken lines* represent the range of controls

Table 1. Responses of anterior pituitary hormones (other than GH) after GRF – (1 – 40) administration in five children undergoing CAPD (mean values ± SEM)

Time (min)	TSH (μU/ml)	PRL (ng/ml)	LH (mU/ml)	FSH (mU/ml)	Cortisol (ng/ml)
0	3.20±0.64	104.9±62.2	4.40±1.61	3.08±1.66	80.5±15.4
30	3.58±0.47	100.0±54.4	6.69±2.06	3.05±1.56	81.2± 7.8
60	3.28±0.33	98.4±52.5	7.35±2.97	3.08±1.31	59.9±12.3
90	3.70±0.59	127.6±80.2	6.08±1.56	3.00±1.18	60.3±10.4
120	3.34±0.34	93.6±48.2	5.87±1.72	2.94±1.64	65.2± 7.1
150	3.24±0.43	72.5±29.9	4.91±1.36	3.16±1.40	61.4± 6.5
180	3.26±0.37	70.9±30.2	6.39±2.07	2.76±1.68	93.8±29.1

increase in GH level 30 min after GRF, with a return toward baseline values at the end of the test. In the dialyzed children the peak value of GH (42.8 ± 7.2 ng/ml) was greater than that of controls (28.2 ± 8.3 ng/ml), but the difference was not significant.

Other Anterior Pituitary Hormones (Table 1): The analysis of these hormones was carried out in five dialyzed subjects. Serum PRL, TSH, LH, FSH, and corticotropin (measured indirectly through plasma cortisol) were not stimulated by 1 µg/kg BW of GRF-(1–40) in patients undergoing CAPD.

Side-Effects

Intravenous administration of 1 µg/kg BW of GRF-(1–40) and 7 µg/kg BW of TRH produced no side-effects in any subject.

Discussion

Our data show that baseline levels of anterior pituitary hormones in uremic children treated by CAPD are normal regarding TSH, GH, and FSH, while a high proportion of them show hyperprolactinemia. There is a generalized increase of serum LH.

The causes of hyperprolactinemia are still unclear and have been discussed elsewhere [9, 15, 16]. Increased baseline values of serum LH and less frequently FSH have been reported in uremic adults [3, 17, 18]. The absence in these patients of a simultaneous increase in baseline values of FSH does not imply a reduced metabolic clearance of gonadotropins [19], and these data could indicate a reduced sensitivity of the regulatory system of the gonads [10].

More interesting are the responses to stimuli for the evaluation of the hypothalamo-hypophyseal function. TRH responses have been previously studied in uremic patients both during conservative treatment and during maintenance hemodialysis, but there are few such data during treatment with chronic peritoneal dialysis, and no data at all regarding the effects of GRF on anterior pituitary hormone secretion in chronic renal failure.

First of all we want to consider the so-called normal responses:

a) TSH secretion following TRH administration has been reported to be blunted in uremic patients during both conservative treatment and maintenance hemodialysis [7, 20, 21]. There are in addition two reports [22, 23] showing that TRH stimulation responses were abnormal in adults on CAPD, indicating an impairment of the hypothalamo-pituitary function and implying that the increased clearance of "middle molecules" known to occur in CAPD does not dramatically improve this axis [22]. Our experience is quite different. TRH increased serum TSH concentration in all CAPD patients with both a delayed and prolonged response. The only abnormality was in the time of response, but not in the magnitude, implying that in children on CAPD some receptorial alteration may be present, but that the hypothalamo-pituitary axis is not severely impaired.

b) GRF-(1–40) stimulated the secretion of GH at a rate that was greater than that of normal controls. From the first time-point studied it was possible to observe a prompt increase in serum GH concentration. The increase of serum GH was greater than that reported in normal adults [14, 24] or in normal children [25], and it seems to indicate an increased sensitivity of receptors to GRF or a greater availability of GH stored inside the cells.

Secondly we would like to consider the existence of an abnormal response to these stimuli:

a) TRH did not increase PRL concentration in children treated by CAPD. The lack of response to TRH does not seem due to reduced synthesis of the hormone, because this pattern was present also in children with normal baseline values of PRL. This behavior could be ascribed to the insensitivity of the receptors of PRL-secreting cells to TRH stimulation [26].

b) TRH does not increase serum GH concentration in normal children, while in uremic children it has been shown that TRH stimulates GH secretion [7, 9]. The same observation is possible for our CAPD patients. This paradoxical response has been observed in other conditions [27]. Therefore, there are several conditions where TSH as well as GH secretion are stimulated by TRH. The mechanism of this abnormal response is not fully understood, but it is possible to postulate some variations within the receptor sites of the GH-secreting cells. Considering the prompt response of GH to GRF, demonstrating a great intracellular availability of GH stored, the same hypothesis could be the explanation for the paradoxical rise of GH after TRH that could be a specific pharmacological stimulus.

Finally we would like to discuss the GRF test in our uremic dialyzed patients. GRF-(1–40) is one of a group of peptides recently isolated from a pancreatic tumor [13] which potently and specifically stimulates growth hormone secretion in vitro and in vivo [13, 28]. There is considerable evidence that this ectopic peptide resembles the hypothalamic growth hormone releasing factor in structure and function [12]. Previous studies have shown that GRF-(1–40) specifically releases GH in man [14]. In general the peak GH response elicited by GRF was much greater than that obtained after insulin-induced hypoglycemia or the glucagon-propanolol test in normal children [25]. This may be due to the fact that insulin-induced hypoglycemia and the glucagon-propanolol test stimulate GH secretion through a central nervous system pathway, whereas GRF acts directly on the pituitary. The effect of GRF can also be considered highly specific because of reports that it does not stimulate the secretion of PRL, TSH, LH, FSH, or corticotropin either in normal or in pathological states [14, 25, 29]. Our preliminary findings seem to confirm these observations. The total lack of side-effects of GRF, together with the possibility of avoiding the danger of hypoglycemia, strongly suggests the use of this peptide instead of insulin or other tests as a routine growth hormone stimulation test.

References

1. Feldman HA, Singer I (1974) Endocrinology and metabolism in uremia and dialysis: a clinical review. Medicine 54:345–376
2. De Fronzo RA, Andres R, Edgar P, Walker WG (1973) Carbohydrate metabolism in uremia: a review. Medicine 52:469–481
3. Guevara A, Vidt DG, Halberg MC, Zorn EM, Pohlman C, Wieland RG (1969) Serum gonadotropin and testosterone levels in uremic males undergoing intermittent dialysis. Metabolism 18:1062–1070
4. Distiller LA, Morley JE, Sagel J, Pokroy M, Rabkin R (1975) Pituitary-gonadal function in chronic renal failure: the effect of luteinizing hormone-releasing hormone and the influence of dialysis. Metabolism 24:711–720
5. Lim VS, Fang VS (1975) Gonadal dysfunction in uremic men: a study of the hypothalamo-pituitary-testicular axis before and after renal transplantation. Am J Med 58:655–662

6. Lim VS, Fang VS, Katz AJ, Refetoff S (1977) Thyroid dysfunction in chronic renal failure. A study of the pituitary-thyroid axis and peripheral turnover kinetics of thyroxine and tri-iodothyronine. J Clin Invest 60:522–534

7. Czernichow H, Dauzet MC, Broyer M, Rappaport R (1976) Abnormal TSH, PRL and GH response to TSH releasing factor in chronic renal failure. J Clin Endocrinol Metab 43:630–637

8. Ijaiya K (1979) TSH and PRL response to thyrotropin-releasing hormone in children with chronic renal failure undergoing haemodialysis. Arch Dis Child 54:937–941

9. Perfumo F, Giusti M, Gusmano R, Giordano G (1982) Study of pituitary secretion using the thyrotropin-releasing hormone test in uremic prepubertal children. In: Bulla M (ed) Renal insufficiency in children. Springer, Berlin Heidelberg New York, p 121

10. Oertel PJ, Lichtwald K, Häfner S, Rauh W, Schönberg D, Schärer K (1983) Hypothalamo-pituitary-gonadal axis in children with chronic renal failure. Kidney Int 24 (Suppl 15):34–39

11. Frohman LA, Szabo M, Berelowitz M, Stachura ME (1980) Partial purification and characterisation of a peptide with growth hormone releasing activity from extrapituitary tumors in patients with acromegaly. J Clin Invest 65:43–54

12. Rivier J, Spiess J, Thorner M, Vale W (1983) Characterisation of a growth hormone releasing factor from a human pancreatic islet tumour. Nature 300:276–278

13. Guilleman R, Brazeau P, Bohlen PE, Esch F, Ling N, Wehrenberg W (1982) Growth hormone-releasing factor from a human pancreatic tumor that caused acromegaly. Science 218:585–587

14. Thorner MO, Rivier J, Spiess J, Borges JL, Vance ML, Bloom SR, Rogol AD, Cronin MJ, Kaiser DL, Evans WS, Webster JD, MacLeod RM, Vale W (1983) Human pancreatic growth-hormone-releasing factor selectively stimulates growth-hormone secretion in man. Lancet 1:24–28

15. Cowden EA, Ratcliffe WA, Ratcliffe JG, Dobbie JW, Kennedy AC (1978) Hyperprolactinaemia in renal disease. Clin Endocrinol 9:241–248

16. Ijaiya K, Roth B, Schwenk A (1980) Serum prolactin levels in renal insufficiency in children. Acta Paediatr Scand 69:299–304

17. Lim VS, Auletta F, Kathpalia S (1978) Gonadal dysfunction in chronic renal failure. Dial Transplant 7:896–907

18. Swamy AP, Woolf PD, Cestero RVM (1979) Hypothalamic-pituitary-ovarian axis in uremic women. J Lab Clin Med 93:1066–1072

19. Holdsworth S, Atkins RC, De Kretser DM (1977) The pituitary testicular axis in men with chronic renal failure. N Engl J Med 296:1245–1249

20. Hasegawa K, Matsushita Y, Otomo S, Hamada N, Nishizawa Y, Okamoto T, Morii H, Wada M (1975) Abnormal response of thyrotropin and growth hormone to thyrotropin releasing hormone in chronic renal failure. Acta Endocrinol 79:635–643

21. Weissel M, Stummvoll HK, Kolbe H, Hofer R (1979) Basal and TRH stimulated thyroid and pituitary hormones in various degrees of renal insufficiency. Acta Endocrinol 90:23–32

22. Semple CG, Beastall GH, Henderson IS, Thomson JA, Kennedy AC (1982) Thyroid function and continuous ambulatory peritoneal dialysis. Nephron 32:249–252

23. Boero R, Quarello F, Belardi P, Piccoli G (1983) Blunted response to TRH stimulation in CAPD patients. Perit Dial Bull 3:213 (Letter)

24. Borges JLC, Blizzard RM, Gelato MC, Furlanetto R, Rogol AD, Evans WS, Vance ML, Kaiser DL, MacLeod RM, Merriam GR, Lorians DL, Spiess J, Rivier J, Vale W, Thorner MO (1983) Effects of human pancreatic tumour growth hormone releasing factor on growth hormone and somatomedin C levels in patients with idiopathic growth hormone deficiency. Lancet 2:119–124

25. Takano K, Hizuka N, Shizume K, Asakawa K, Miyakawa M, Hirose N, Shibasaki T, Ling NC (1984) Plasma growth hormone (GH) response to GH-releasing factor in normal children with short stature and patients with pituitary dwarfism. J Clin Endocrinol Metab 58:236–241

26. Lim VS, Kathpalia S, Frohman LA (1979) Hyperprolactinemia and impaired pituitary response to suppression and stimulation in chronic renal failure: reversal after renal transplantation. J Clin Endocrinol Metab 48: 101–107
27. Scanlon MF, Smith BR, Hall R (1978) Thyroid-stimulating hormone: neuroregulation and clinical application (part I). Clin Sci Mol Med 55: 1–10
28. Brazeau P, Ling N, Bohlen P, Esch F, Ying S, Guilleman R (1982) Growth hormone releasing factor, somatocrinin releases pituitary growth hormone in vitro. Proc Natl Acad Sci USA 79: 7909–7913
29. Wood SM, Ch'Ng JLC, Adams EF, Webster JD, Joplin GF, Mashiter K, Bloom SR (1983) Abnormalities of growth hormone release in response to human pancreatic growth hormone releasing factor (GRF[1–44]) in acromegaly and hypopituitarism. Br Med J 286: 1687–1691

Thyroid Function in Children on CAPD

N. G. De Santo, C. Carella, R. N. Fine, E. Leumann, S. Fine, G. Amato, G. Capodicasa, F. Nuzzi, V. De Simone, G. Capasso, G. Lama, F. Scoppa, and C. Giordano

Introduction

Thyroid function in uremia has not been studied as extensively in children as it has been in adults. The data available point to a low T_3 and T_4 syndrome, but it is not clear whether these patients are hypothyroid or not [1–5]. In addition, little is known about free hormone concentration with respect to the various dialytic modalities for this age group of patients. This work was designed to study thyroid function in children undergoing CAPD. The data presented indicate that CAPD does not correct the low T_3 and T_4 syndrome. In addition, stunted TSH response to TRH is present.

Patients and Methods

A total of 60 normal children (30 males, 30 females) and 22 uremic children on CAPD (12 males, 10 females) aged 10–17 years were studied. T_3, T_4, rT_3, TSH, TBG, FT_3 and FT_4 were measured in plasma by RIA and hTG by IRMA and, antithyroglobulin antibodies and microsomal antibodies were determined as described elesewhere [5–10]. The lysophase method was used to evaluate FT_4 concentration; this technique is comparable to the equilibrium dialysis method [5]. In addition, we evaluated changes of plasma TRH, T_3, and T_4 following a bolus injection of TRH (7.5 µg/kg BW) i.v. in 30 normal children and nine CAPD patients.

Data are given as mean ± SEM. Statistical analysis was carried out by means of the t test for unpaired observations.

Results

Table 1 shows the basal values of various thyroidal activities and points to the existence of a low T_3 and T_4 syndrome. In fact, T_3 was 161 ± 16.4 µg/dl in normal children and 120 ± 7.1 µg/dl in CAPD children ($P < 0.001$). T_4 concentration was 7.45 ± 1.6 µg/dl in healthy subjects and 6.20 ± 0.30 µg/dl during the CAPD regimen ($P < 0.001$).

There was no significant increase in the mean rT_3 concentration, although six of 22 children showed values above normal. There was a small but significant increase in the mean FT_4 concentration. TSH, hTG, and TBG concentrations did not disclose any significant alterations in the CAPD group.

Table 2 shows the response of plasma TSH to TRH, which was blunted in the CAPD group.

Table 1. Thyroid hormone levels in plasma during CAPD treatment. Data obtained in 60 control subjects and 20 uremic children on CAPD. Data are given as mean ± (SEM). Statistical analysis by the t test of unpaired observations. n.s. = not significant

	Control	CAPD	P
T_3, ng/dl	161.0 ± 16.4	120.7 ± 7.1	0.001
T_4, µg/dl	7.45 ± 1.6	6.20 ± 0.30	0.001
rT_3, ng/dl	24.0 ± 5	28.1 ± 9	n.s.
FT_3, pg/ml	5.70 ± 0.80	6.20 ± 0.41	n.s.
FT_4, pg/ml	11.6 ± 0.95	14.8 ± 0.41	0.05
TBG, µg/ml	25.2 ± 4.7	22.7 ± 4.5	n.s.
hTG, ng/ml	28.1 ± 17.9	27.9 ± 4.1	n.s.
TSH, µU/ml	2.58 ± 0.80	2.89 ± 1.07	n.s.

Table 2. Plasma TSH after a bolus injection of TRH in 30 normal subjects and in nine uremic children on CAPD. Data are means ± SEM; statistical analysis was earried out by the t test for unpaired observations

Time (min)	TSH, µU/ml		P
	Controls	CAPD	
0	2.52 ± 0.83	2.89 ± 1.07	n.s.
20	14.10 ± 2.64	7.10 ± 2.44	0.001
60	12.00 ± 2.43	8.26 ± 2.13	0.05
120	5.74 ± 1.28	6.47 ± 1.75	n.s.

Table 3. Plasma T_3 and T_4 after a bolus injection of TRH in 30 normal children and nine children on CAPD. Data are expressed as percent increase over basal plasma values 120 min after injection. Data are means ± SEM

	Percent increase over basal values		
	Controls	CAPD	P
T_3	50.5 ± 12.7	40.6 ± 15.4	n.s.
T_4	20.7 ± 13.9	15.8 ± 8.8	n.s.

Table 3 depicts the response of T_3 and T_4 plasma concentrations after TRH and indicates that 120 min after stimulation, the percent increase over basal values was normal for both thyroid hormones.

Antithyroglobulin and microsomal antibodies were not detected.

Discussion

The data presented indicate that uremic children on CAPD have a low T_3 and T_4 syndrome usually associated with normal rT_3 concentration, increased FT_4, and blunted TSH response to TRH. In general, these data agree with earlier findings concerning pediatric and adult patients with chronic renal failure [1–23].

The fact that six of 22 patients had increased rT_3 values may reflect impaired peripheral $T_4 - T_3$ conversion due to impaired glucose utilization. This phenomenon deserves further evaluation and is currently being evaluated in our laboratory.

FT_4 concentrations which are crucial to the diagnosis of hypothyroidism in non-thyroidal illnesses were not reduced, a finding similar to the experience of Wassner et al. [2]. The increased amounts of FT_4 may be linked to a reduced KaT_4 for TBG [5] and may indicate a nephrosis-like situation in uremic children on CAPD [5].

No pathology was observed in the FT_3, TBG, and hTG concentrations. The data on hTG are relevant since these are the first reports for uremic children and only the second for uremia [6, 7]. In addition, our control data are similar to the data of Penny et al. [22].

The blunted response of TSH to TRH was associated with a normal percent increase of T_3 and T_4 over basal concentrations and indicates abnormalities of the hypothalamo-pituitary axis.

The present data do not prove or disprove the possibility that uremic children may acquire hypothyroidism, a possibility which has been shown in uremic adults.

Acknowledgments. This work is financed by funds made available by the Italian Ministry of Public Instruction through programs of local and national interest.

References

1. Czernichow P, Dauzet MC, Broyer M, Rappaport R (1976) Abnormal TSH, PRL and GH response to TSH releasing factor in chronic uremia. J Clin Endocrinol Metab 43:630
2. Wassner JJ, Buckingham BA, Kershar AJ, Malekzadeh MH, Pennisi AJ, Fine RN (1977) Thyroid function in children with chronic renal failure. Nephron 19:236
3. Chan JCM, Hung W (1978) Hemodialysis and thyroid function in children. J Dial Transplant 2:387
4. Waters W, Bulla M, Tekook A (1982) Thyroid function in children on regular hemodialysis. In: Bulla M (ed) Renal insufficiency in children. Springer, Berlin Heidelberg New York, p 129
5. De Santo NG, Fine RN, Carella C, Leumann E, Amato G, Fine S, Nuzzi F, Capasso G, Capodicasa G, Lama G, Scoppa F, and Giordano C. Thyroidal status in uremic children. Kidney Int (in press)
6. Giordano C, Carella C, De Santo NG, Mioli V, Bazzato G, Amato G, Tarchini A, Coli U, Landini S (1982) Hormonal status of patients on CAPD and HD. In: La Greca G (ed) Proceedings 1st international course on peritoneal dialysis. Wichtig, Milan, p 330
7. Giordano C, De Santo NG, Carella C, Mioli V, Bazzato G, Di Leo Va, Amato G, Tarchini A, Coli V, Landini S (1982) Thyroid status in uremia, effects of hemodialysis and CAPD. Int J Artif Organs 5:394
8. Giordano C, De Santo NG, Carella C, Mioli V, Bazzato G, Amato G, Tarchini A, Coli V, Capasso G, Landini V, Capodicasa G, Nuzzi F, Esposito A. Thyroidal function during hemodialysis and CAPD. Proceedings 4th ISAO Conference. Artif Organs (in press)
9. Giordano C, De Santo NG, Carella C, Mioli V, Bazzato G, Amato G, Di Leo VA, Tarchini G, Coli U, Capodicasa G, Landini G, Nuzzi F, De Simon V, Esposito A (1984) TSH response to TRH in hemodialysis and CAPD patients. Int J Artif Organs 7:7
10. Giordano C, De Santo NG, Carella C, Capodicasa G, Amato G, Nuzzi F, Mioli V, Bazzato G, De Simone V, Tarchini A, Landini A, Coli U, Bordoni V, Mottola G, Capuano F (1984)

Thyroid status and nephron loss. A study in patients with chronic renal failure, end stage renal disease and/or on hemodialysis. Int J Artif Organs 7:119

11. Ramirez G, Jubitz W, Gutch CF, Bloomer HA, Siegler R, Kolff WJ (1973) Thyroid abnormalities in renal failure. A study on 53 patients on chronic hemodialysis. Ann Intern Med 79:504

12. Carter JN, Eastman CJ, Corcoran P, Lazarus L (1974) Effects of severe illness on thyroid function. Lancet 2:971

13. Spector DA, Davis JP, Helderman JH, Bell B, Utiger RD (1976) Thyroid function and metabolic state in chronic renal failure. Ann Intern Med 85:274

14. Savdie E, Stewart JH, Mahony JF, Hayer JM, Lazarus L, Simons LA (1978) Circulating thyroid hormone levels and adequacy of dialysis. Clin Nephrol 9:68

15. Weissel M, Stummval HK, Wolf A, Fritsche H (1977) Thyroid hormone in chronic renal failure. Ann Intern Med 86:644

16. Kalk WJ, Morley JE, Gold GH, Meyers A (1980) Thyroid function tests in patients on regular hemodialysis. Nephron 25:173

17. Farrington K, Boss AMB, Varghese Z, Kingstone D, Baillod RA, Moorhead JF (1980) Thyroid function tests in dialyzed patients. Dial Transplant 9:846

18. Czekalski S, Malczeva B, Sobieszczyk S, Kozak W, Eder M, Grycynska M, Backzyk K, Kosowicz J (1981) Comparison of some circulating pituitary thyroid and gonadal hormone levels in non dialyzed and dialyzed males with chronic renal failure. Dial Transplant 10:438

19. Nogimori T (1981) A Clinical study on thyroid hormone secretion and metabolism in patients with chronic renal failure on hemodialysis. Folia Endocrinol (Jpn) 57:903

20. Gavin LA, McMahon FA, Castle JN, Cavalier RC (1970) Alteraions in serum thyroid hormones and thyroxin binding globulin in patients with nephrosis. J Clin Endocrinol Metab 49:63

21. Kaptein EM, MacIntyre SS, Weiner SM, Spencer CA, Nicoloff JT (1981) Free thyroxine estimates in non thyroidal illness. Comparison of eight methods. J Clin Endocrinol Metab 52:1073

22. Penny R, Spencer CA, Frasier DS, Nicoloff JT (1983) Thyroid stimulating hormone and thyroglobulin levels decrease with chronological age in children and adolescents. J Clin Endocrinol Metab 56:177

23. De Santo NG, Carella C, Fine RN, Leumann E, Fine S, Amato G, Capodicasa G, Nuzzi F, Capasso G, Lama G, Scoppa F, De Simone V, Giordano C (1984) Data presented at Bari Seminars in nephrology 29–31 March

Somatostatin Secretion in Children on CAPD and CCPD

B. Roth, B. Busch, K. E. Bonzel, R. Drachman, P. Niaudet, and M. Broyer

Introduction

In 1972 a peptide hormone with an inhibitory effect on the release of human growth hormone was isolated and named somatostatin [1]. Further work revealed that somatostatin has a general inhibitory activity on the release of several other hormones from their production sites. Among other hormones, the release of prolactin and thyroid-stimulating hormone can be inhibited by somatostatin in the pituitary gland [2]. Furthermore, the secretion of gastrin from the G cells [3] and possibly of parathormone from the parathyroid glands [2, 4] can be inhibited by somatostatin. The most important organs of synthesis of somatostatin are the hypothalamus and the D cells of the pancreatic islets [5]. The role of somatostatin in clinical medicine has not been defined, and measurement of this substance is primarily of research interest.

In chronic renal failure and during dialysis multiple endocrine disorders are known, especially in children. The pathophysiology of most of these disorders is not weel understood. In this context the role of somatostatin is completely unknown. Therefore, we studied the secretion of somatostatin in children with terminal renal failure undergoing chronic peritoneal dialysis – CAPD and CCPD.

Patients and Methods

Seventeen patients (6 girls, 11 boys) aged 6 months to 13.8 years were studied. Six children were on CCPD, while the remaining 11 had been on CAPD for 1–46 months. Two CCPD patients were dialyzed only during the day, four during the night.

The causes of terminal renal insufficiency in these patients were: dysplastic kidney, four; juvenile nephronophthisis, four; nonimmunological glomerulopathies, four; hemolytic-uremic syndrome, two; postpartum renal failure, two; and cystinosis, one.

Blood was taken at between 8 and 10 a.m. after an overnight fast. During routine investigations 5 ml of venous blood was collected in precooled tubes containing 7.2 mg EDTA and 2500 kIU aprotinin. The blood was centrifuged in the cold as soon as possible, and the plasma was stored at $-30\,°C$. At the same time a 5 ml aliquot of the peritoneal outflow was taken under the same conditions.

Somatostatin in the plasma was determined as somatostatin-like immunoreactivity (SLIR) using a rabbit anti-somatostatin antibody and [Tyr-1]-^{125}J somatostatin tracer (Immuno Nuclear Corporation, Stillwater, Minnesota, USA). Prior to assaying the samples were extracted with cold acetone and petroleum ether.

Growth hormone, gastrin, and C-terminal PTH in plasma and peritoneal dialysate were determined by commercially available radioimmunoassays.

Results

In comparison to the data of 28 healthy infants and children with a mean plasma somatostatin level of 13.4 pg/ml, the children on CAPD and CCPD showed significantly elevated plasma somatostatin levels, with a mean of 56.9 pg/ml (Table 1). The plasma somatostatin concentrations were significantly correlated with the dialysate levels of somatostatin (Fig. 1). Also the elevated levels of plasma gastrin showed a strong positive correlation with the concentrations of plasma somatostatin (Fig. 2).

No correlation could be demonstrated between plasma or dialysate somatostatin and the corresponding values of growth hormone and C-PTH. However, it was interesting to find consistently higher levels of growth hormone in the peritoneal fluid than in the plasma (Table 1).

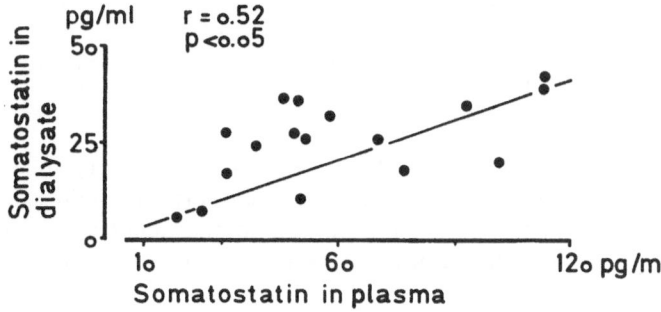

Fig. 1. Correlation between the plasma somatostatin concentrations in children on CAPD and CCPD and the dialysate concentrations of somatostatin

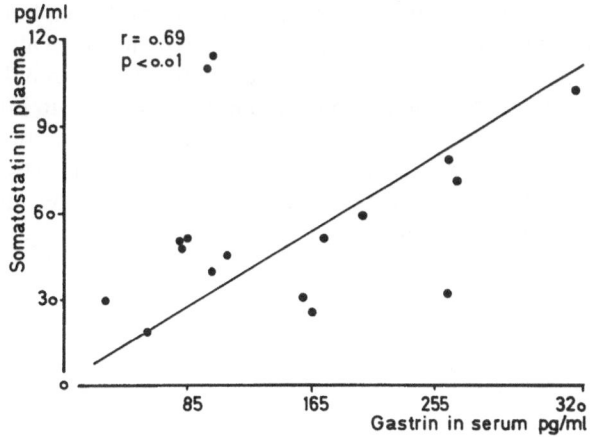

Fig. 2. Correlation between plasma somatostatin concentrations and serum gastrin in children on CAPD and CCPD

Table 1. Somatostatin, gastrin, growth hormone, and C-PTH levels in plasma and peritoneal dialysate[a]

	Somatostatin (pg/ml)	Gastrin (pg/ml)	Growth hormone (ng/ml)	C-PTH (ng/ml)
Normals	13.4[b]	35.0[b]	1.73	0.93[b]
($n=28$)	3.6 – 28.2	22.6 – 170	0.33 – 7.99	0.24 – 1.62
CAPD and				
CCPD ($n=17$)				
Plasma	56.9[b]	153.3[b]	1.34	3.36[b]
	19.5 – 113.5	27.5 – 350.2	0.12 – 4.60	0.58 – 6.02
Dialysate	25.0	19.6	4.47	1.29
	5.0 – 40.7	0.13 – 110.9	2.75 – 7.85	0.20 – 4.34

[a] Figures given are median values and range values.
[b] U-test, $P < 0.01$.

No relationship was found between plasma or dialysate somatostatin levels and sex, underlying disease, duration or mode of peritoneal dialysis, anthropometric data, serum creatinine, and urea, blood glucose, and total protein content of the peritoneal fluid.

Discussion

When discussing these results it is necessary to consider the metabolism of somatostatin. In plasma, somatostatin is very rapidly degraded by plasma proteases. It disappears from the plasma compartment with a mean half-time of elimination ranging between 1 and 3 min [6, 7]. The liver and the kidneys each contribute about one-third of the mean plasma clearance [8, 9]. Recent results showed no changes in the disappearance rate of this peptide hormone in relation to chronic renal failure [9]. Therefore, it seems unlikely that the increased plasma somatostatin levels in the dialyzed patients of the present study can be explained only by the reduced metabolic function of the kidneys. A more plausible explanation is to assume that the somatostatin secretion in children with chronic renal failure on peritoneal dialysis treatment is regulated on a higher level in order to inhibit the exaggerated release of several other hormones in chronic uremia. The most important example supporting this hypothesis is the demonstrated relationship between plasma somatostatin levels and gastrin concentrations in the serum. However, the secretion of gastrin from the G cells and of C-PTH is not sufficiently suppressed, although somatostatin secretion was found to be increased in the patients studied. It is not clear whether or not the somatostatin released is biologically active and/or whether a defect of the somatostatin receptors exists in uremic patients.

In vivo investigations showed that growth hormone levels in plasma were suppressed by somatostatin infusions [2]. Possibly somatostatin can also inhibit the release of growth hormone or of growth hormone releasing factor from production sites in children with chronic renal failure. In future studies it will be necessary to evaluate the biological activity of somatostatin secreted in children with chronic renal failure.

References

1. Brazeau P, Vale H, Burgus R, Ling N, Butcher M, Rivier J, Guillemin R (1973) Hypothalamic polypeptide that inhibits the secretion of immunoreactive pituitary growth hormone. Science 179:77–79
2. Copinschi G, Leclercq-Meyer V, Virasoro E, L'Hermite M (1976) Pituitary and extrapituitary effects of somatostatin in normal man. Horm Metab Res 8:226–231
3. Bloom SR, Mortimer CH, Thorner MO, Besser GM, Hall R, Gomez-Pan A, Roy VM, Russell RCG, Coy DH, Kastin AJ, and Schally AV (1974) Inhibition of gastrin and gastric-acid secretion by growth hormone release-inhibiting hormone. Lancet II:1106–1109
4. Williams GA, Hargis GK, Ensinck JH, Kukreja SC, Bowser EN, Chertow BS, Henderson WJ (1979) Role of endogenous somatostatin in the secretion of parathyroid hormone and calcitonin. Metabolism 28:950–954
5. Schally AV, Meyers CA (1980) Somatostatin, basic and clinical studies. A review. Mater Med Pol 12:28–32
6. Bethge N, Diel F, Roesick M, Holz J (1981) Somatostatin half-life: a case report in one healthy volunteer and a three month follow-up. Horm Metab Res 13:709–710
7. Depraetere Y, Peeters TL, Vantrappen GR, Janssens J (1981) Metabolism of somatostatin in man. Gastroenterology 80:1134
8. Polonsky KS, Jaspan JB, Berelowitz M, Emmanouel DS, Dhorajiwala J, Moossa AR (1981) Hepatic and renal metabolism of somatostatin-like immunoreactivity. J Clin Invest 68:1149–1157
9. Sheppard M, Shapiro B, Pimstone B, Kronheim S, Berelowitz M, Gregory M (1979) Metabolic clearance and plasma half-disappearance time of exogenous somatostatin in man. J Clin Endocrinol Metab 48:50–53
10. Hargis GK, Williams GA, Reynolds HA, Chertow BS, Kukreja SC, Bowser EN, Hendersen WJ (1978) Effect of somatostatin on parathyroid hormone and calcitonin secretion. Endocrinology 102:745–750

Biochemical and Hormonal Abnormalities of Mineral Metabolism in Children on Continuous Ambulatory Peritoneal Dialysis

R. Gusmano, F. Perfumo, R. Oleggini, A. Carrea, G. Basile, and F. Ginevri

Introduction

Renal osteodystrophy is a mosaic of clinical and metabolic abnormalities. In children, it may produce severe abnormalities and is associated with well-known adverse effects on growth [1–3].

In hemodialyzed children, progressive bone lesions have been documented [4, 5]. Data on the effect of continuous ambulatory peritoneal dialysis (CAPD) on renal osteodystrophy in children is controversial [6, 7].

In a previous study of children on CAPD carried out over a period of 12 months [8], we observed an initial improvement of the biochemical and hormonal parameters of renal osteodystrophy. The aim of the present study is to assess the long-term effects of CAPD on mineral metabolism.

Patients and Methods

We studied 18 children (14 boys, 4 girls), aged 0.5–12.3 years, who had been treated with CAPD for a minimum of 6 months. Clinical data is presented in Table 1. Children performed three to four exchanges per day. The dialysate contained 1.5%–2.4% glucose, and the dialysate volume was 35–45 ml/kg. The dialysate calcium was 3.5 mEq/l, and magnesium was 1.5 mEq/l. Children received an unrestricted diet. Calcium was given as carbonate to reach a total intake of 0.5–1.5 g/day, depending on the age and size of the child. Aluminum hydroxide (0.5–15 g/day) was prescribed to ten of 18 children. All children received supplemental vitamin D metabolites: $25(OH)D_3$ (1–3 g/kg/day) or $1,25(OH)_2D_3$ (0.015–0.03 g/kg/day) at dosages related to serum calcium levels.

Biochemical parameters were evaluated every 3 months and hormonal parameters every 6 months. The last observation was made 24 months after the initial one. The assay of vitamin D metabolites was initiated at 6 months. Serum calcium, phosphorus, magnesium, and alkaline phosphatase levels were measured using standard methods. Serum calcium values were corrected using Parfitt's formula. Plasma immunoreactive COOH-PTH and NH_2-PTH were measured by Mallette's method [9]. Serum calcitonin was assayed following a modification of Deftos' method [10].

Serum levels of $25(OH)D_3$ were measured by the method described by Preece et al. [11]; $1,25(OH)_2D_3$ and $24,25(OH)_2D_3$ were assayed by a modified method according to Shepard et al. [12]. Vitamin D binding protein (DBP) was assayed by the technique of Bouillon et al. [13]. All values are expressed as mean ± standard error of mean (SEM).

Table 1. Clinical data of 18 children on CAPD

Patients	Age (years)	Sex	Weight (kg)	Duration of study (months)	Diagnosis
C.L.	5.7	M	16.4	24	GN
M.M.	8.4	M	18.0	24	RN
A.E.	1.0	M	8.0	24	BCN
S.S.	6.1	F	11.0	18	RD
R.G.	4.8	F	19.8	9	FJN
C.D.	11.8	F	16.8	18	Cystinosis
C.C.	4.5	M	12.2	6	RN
P.D.	6.9	M	16.0	24	FJN
S.G.	5.3	M	15.2	24	FGS
A.A.	3.6	M	14.7	12	CNS
Z.F.	11.6	M	31.0	12	HUS
C.N.	1.3	M	10.0	18	DMS
B.G.	12.2	M	24.4	18	RD
M.L.	12.3	M	22.6	12	RN
L.T.	7.7	M	18.7	12	GN
B.L.	1.9	F	8.5	6	RD
D.A.	0.5	M	9.0	12	BCN
B.M.	11.1	M	38.0	6	HUS

GN, glomerulonephritis; RN, reflux nephropathy; RD, renal dysplasia; BCN, bilateral cortical necrosis; FJN, familial juvenile nephronophthisis; FGS, focal glomerulosclerosis; CNS, congenital nephrotic syndrome; HUS, hemolytic uremic syndrome; DMS, diffuse mesangial sclerosis.

Table 2. Changes of serum calcium, phosphorus, and magnesium levels during treatment by CAPD

Months on CAPD		0	3	6	9	12	15	18	21	24
Patients (n)		18	18	18	15	14	9	9	5	5
Calcium	mean	8.62	9.78	9.85	10.39	10.23	10.63	10.48	10.48	11.00
(mg/dl)	SEM	0.28	0.13	0.11	0.26	0.18	0.29	0.15	0.31	0.46
Phosphorus	mean	7.27	5.61	5.34	5.97	6.14	6.11	6.36	6.83	7.03
(md/dl)	SEM	0.39	0.37	0.31	0.27	0.34	0.61	0.49	0.28	0.57
Magnesium	mean	2.31	2.74	2.64	2.63	2.89	2.72	2.87	3.07	3.02
(mg/dl)	SEM	0.09	0.09	0.10	0.13	0.24	0.17	0.17	0.23	0.12

SEM, standard error of mean.

Results

Serum calcium, phosphorus, and magnesium levels are shown in Table 2. Hypocalcemia was present at the beginning and in the early course of dialysis; serum calcium concentration rose from 8.62 ± 0.28 mg/dl to normal levels within 3 months and exceeded 10 mg/dl after 9 months of CAPD. Asymptomatic hy-

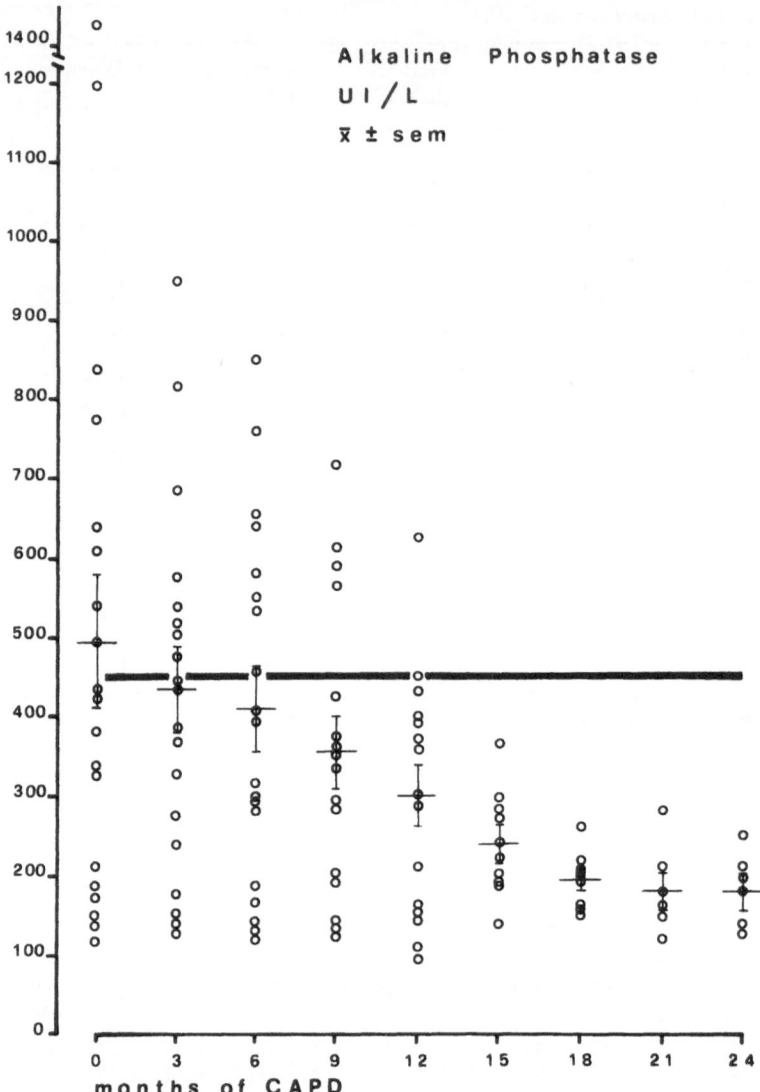

Fig. 1. Serum alkaline phosphatase (AP) values during CAPD treatment. The *horizontal line* indicates the upper limit of normal

percalcemia (> 11 mg/dl) was found seven times in six children; discontinuation of vitamin D metabolite administration resulted in normalization of the serum calcium levels.

Serum phosphate levels showed an initial decrease, but subsequently, an increase above normal values was observed. No patient showed hypophosphatemia. The serum magnesium level remained above normal during the entire period of observation, rising from 2.31 ± 0.09 at the start of CAPD to 3.02 ± 0.12 mg/dl after 24 months.

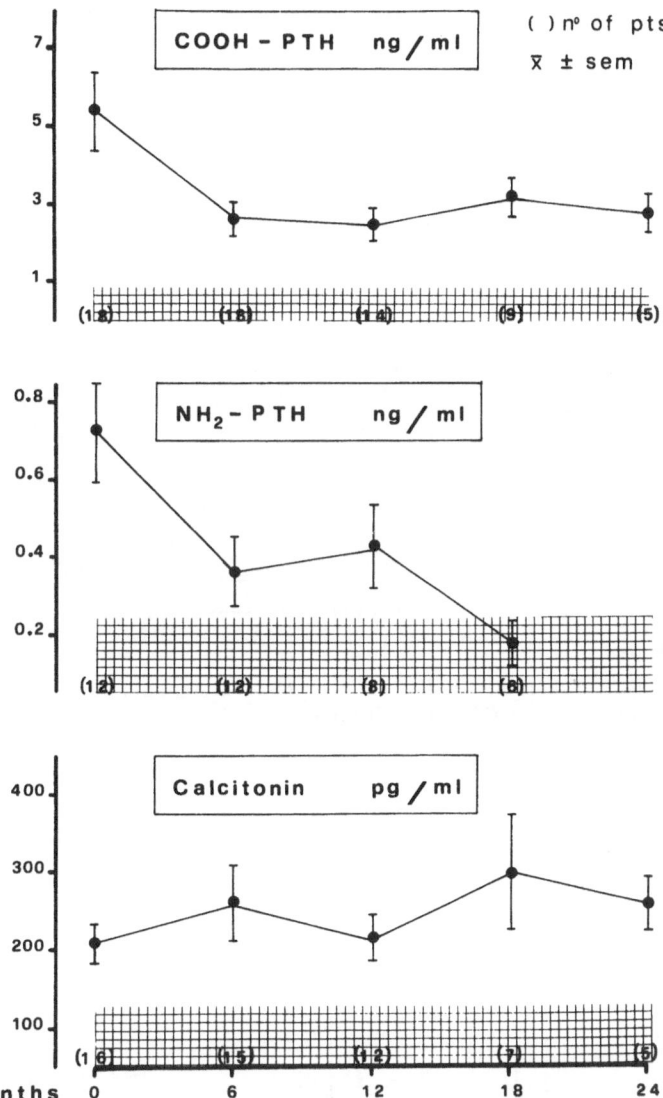

Fig. 2. Calciotropic hormone values during CAPD. *Shaded areas* represent the normal range

Alkaline Phosphatase Levels (AP), (Fig. 1). Total serum AP was elevated in eight of 18 patients at the initiation of CAPD, and in these patients, a steady decline of AP was observed. From the 15th month, normal values were reached in all patients. One child, whose AP values were normal at the start of CAPD, subsequently showed a pathological increase.

Immunoreactive Parathyroid Hormone (iPTH), (Fig. 2). Plasma COOH-PTH initially showed a mean value of 5.4 ng/ml, with great interindividual variation, ranging from 1–16 ng/ml (Fig. 3). A decrease of COOH-PTH values was noted at the 6th

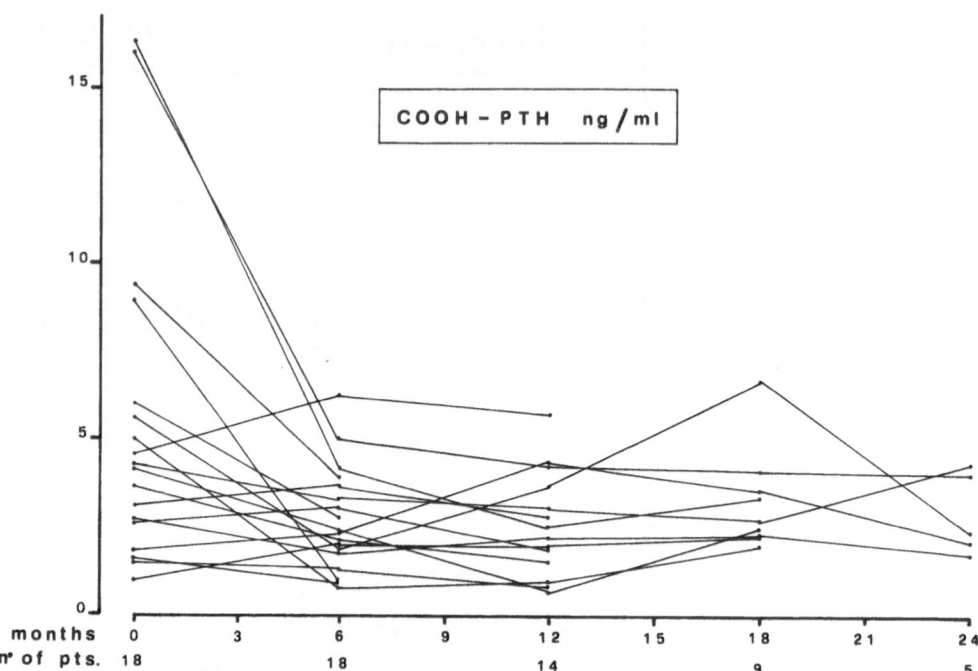

Fig. 3. Values of *COOH-PTH* determined at 6-month intervals. Normal values of our laboratory for *COOH-PTH* are < 0.7 ng/ml

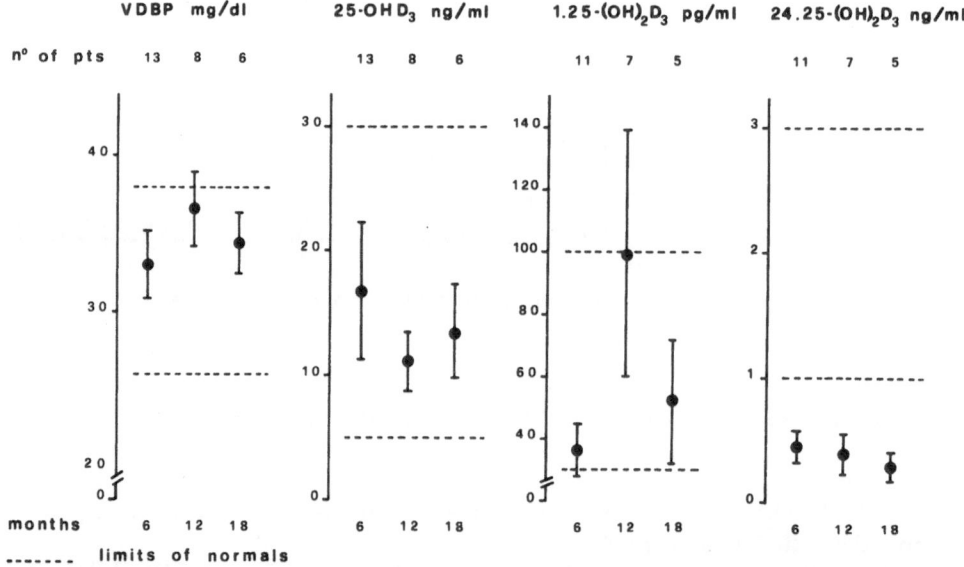

Fig. 4. Serum concentrations of *VDBP* and vitamin D metabolites (mean ± SD). The first values were obtained at the 6th month of CAPD treatment and the last after 18 months of treatment. The *dotted lines* represent the upper and lower limits of control values

and at the 12th month, but COOH-PTH failed to return to the normal range. NH_2-PTH showed the same variation: A fall after 6 months of treatment, with initial value decreasing by 50% and showing a steady decrease thereafter. It should be noted that the NH_2-PTH levels decreased to normal values at 18 months. The study of this fragment was stopped at month 18 for technical reasons.

Calcitonin. The high values of calcitonin remained unchanged during the entire period of the study.

Vitamin D Metabolites and DBP (Fig. 4). Levels of $25(OH)D_3$ and $1,25(OH)_2D_3$ were within normal limits of age-matched controls during the entire period of the study. The same findings were observed for DBP. Values of $24,25(OH)_2D_3$ remained unchanged and were below the lower limit of the control values.

Discussion

Renal osteodystrophy in children is not cured during maintenance hemodialysis and may increase in severity [4, 5]. Few data on bone lesions in children undergoing CAPD have been reported.

Balfe [14] indicated that renal osteodystrophy progresses during CAPD despite therapy with $1,25(OH)_2D_3$ and normalization of serum calcium and phosphorus levels. The same group later [6] reported great variation in bone lesions; hyperparathyroid or rachitic lesions either improved or worsened. Plasma AP also showed great variation, and iPTH remained elevated in all but one patient. Potter et al. [15] reported that hyperparathyroid bone disease appeared or worsened in children not receiving vitamin D therapy. Subsequently, the same authors [7], comparing two groups of patients on hemodialysis and on CAPD, observed that the incidence of bone disease was similar, although AP and PTH were higher (but not significantly so) in children on CAPD.

Parameters of mineral metabolism in the children we treated with CAPD showed an initial improvement. A normalization of calcium was observed, indicating a positive balance as a result of the influx of calcium from the dialysate. Calcium supplements and $1,25(OH)_2D_3$ administration may have contributed to the balance. Lowering serum phosphorus levels were initially observed. In adults on CAPD, a negative mass transfer has been documented [17]. The serum magnesium level remained above the normal range due to a positive balance resulting from the fact that peritoneal dialysis efflux was lower than intestinal absorption. It is possible that intestinal absorption of magnesium increased through the administration of $1,25(OH)_2D_3$ [18]. A lower dialysate magnesium concentration seems desirable.

The serum AP level fell, accompanied by a similar decrease in the iPTH level. Whether the decrease in the iPTH level is due to suppressed secretion of the hormone or to removal by the dialysate is uncertain. The values for clearance of iPTH reported previously in children [19] and those reported in adults [17] support the former hypothesis. In contrast, serum calcitonin levels remained elevated. Values for this hormone did not correlate with the serum calcium level, which was elevated during hypocalcemia and hypercalcemia alike.

The vitamin D metabolites $25(OH)D_3$ and $1,25(OH)_2D_3$ remained within the normal range. High levels of $25(OH)D_3$ and a significant amount of specific DBP were found in the peritoneal dialysis fluid of adults treated with CAPD [20]. In children and adolescents, the loss of 25(OH)D_3 has been demonstrated to represent 10%–38% of the daily oral intake [21]. A significant correlation was found between the peritoneal clearance of 25(OH)D_3 and the DBP level [21].

In our patients, normal blood concentrations of 25(OH)D_3 and 1,25(OH)D_3 demonstrated that the peritoneal losses were compensated for by the oral administration of these metabolites. DBP levels remained in the normal range, notwithstanding the protein losses observed in the dialysate. The low level of 24,25(OH)$_2D_3$, as found in patients with advanced renal failure [22] in the presence of normal concentrations of 25(OH)D_3, is in agreement with clinical and experimental data suggesting that the kidney is the major site of 24-hydroxylation of 25(OH)D_3 [23].

The hormonal values and biochemical parameters of children on CAPD were not stable. After an improvement during the 1st year of treatment, they showed a mild deterioration, manifested as an increase in both serum phosphorus levels and in COOH-PTH. Unfortunately, we have no data on NH$_2$-PTH after the 18th month of CAPD, when values were in the normal range. The behavior of this fragment might have provided a better indication of parathyroid secretory status.

Either the nutritional status or the treatment modality could account for the deterioration with time. Unrestricted diet in our children has been demonstrated to be high in protein [24], causing a high phosphorus intake that is well above the dialysis removal capacity, thus requiring aluminum hydroxide and calcium carbonate administration. A lower protein intake seems to be required in order to obtain a lower serum phosphate level, since compliance with taking phosphate-binding agents is uncertain. Naturally, improved appetite works against reducing protein intake. Hyperphosphatemia could also be caused by enhancement of intestinal phosphorus absorption due to 1,25(OH)D_3 administration [18]. The increase in the serum phosphorus levels paralleled the increase of the serum COOH-PTH values. Normal or slightly elevated serum calcium concentrations did not adequately control PTH secretion. The loss of PTH in the dialysate, although substantial, did not result in an adequate reduction of the elevated serum PTH level. A higher serum calcium concentration might have been an effective method of controlling parathyroid secretion, provided that phosphorus levels normalized first. Nevertheless, even if some alteration of mineral metabolism exists, serum AP remains in the normal range, indicating an alleviation of bone disease.

It appears that CAPD treatment is able to bring mineral metabolism abnormalities under control initially, while for long-term clearance of phosphorus and PTH, regulation of mass transfer is less effective. Calcitonin levels appear unaffected by peritoneal dialysis.

References

1. Fine R, Isaacson AS, Payne V, Grushkin CM (1972) Renal osteodystrophy in children: the effect of hemodialysis and renal homotransplantation. J Pediatr 80:243–249
2. Stickler GB, Bergen BJ (1973) A review. Short stature in renal disease. Pediatr Res 7:978–982

3. Broyer M (1982) Growth in children with renal insufficiency. Pediatr Clin North Am 29:991–1003
4. Mehls O, Krempien B, Ritz E, Schärer K, Schüler HW (1973) Renal osteodystrophy in children on maintenance hemodialysis. Proc Eur Dial Transplant Assoc 10:197–201
5. Potter DE, Wilson CJ, Ozonoff MB (1974) Hyperparathyroid bone disease in children undergoing long-term hemodialysis: treatment with vitamin D. J Pediatr 85:60
6. Hewitt IK, Stefanidis C, Reilly BJ, Kooh SW, Balfe JW (1983) Renal osteodystrophy in children undergoing continuous ambulatory peritoneal dialysis. J Pediatr 103:729–734
7. Baum M, Powell D, Calvin S, McDaid T, McHenry K, Mar H, Potter D (1982) Continuous ambulatory peritoneal dialysis in children: comparison with hemodialysis. N Engl J Med 307:1537–1542
8. Perfumo F, Oleggini R, Basile G, Gusmano R (1982) Biochemical and hormonal parameters of renal osteodystrophy in dialyzed children: comparison between maintenance hemodialysis (MHD) and continuous ambulatory peritoneal dialysis (CAPD). Min Metab Res Italy 3:151–154
9. Mallette LE, Tuma SN, Berger TE, Kirkland JL (1982) Radioimmunoassay for the middle region of human parathyroid hormone using an homologous antiserum with a carboxy-terminal fragment of bovine parathyroid hormone as radioligand. J Clin Endocrinol Metab 34:1017–1024
10. Parthemore JG, Deftos LJ (1978) Calcitonin secretion in normal human subject. J Clin Endocrinol Metab 47:184–188
11. Preece MA, O'Riordan JLH, Lawson DEM, Kodicek E (1974) A competitive protein binding assay for 25-hydroxy-cholecalciferol and 25-hydroxy-ergocalciferol in serum. Clin Chim Acta 54:235–242
12. Shepard RM, Horst RL, Hamstra AJ, De Luca HF (1979) Determination of vitamin D and its metabolites in plasma from normal and anephric man. Biochem J 182:55–69
13. Bouillon R, Van Bealen H, De Moor P (1977) The measurement of the vitamin D binding protein in human serum. J Clin Endocrinol Metab 45:225–231
14. Balfe JW (1983) Metabolic effects of CAPD in the child. Perit Dial Bull 3:S21–S23
15. Potter DE, McDaid TK, McHenry K (1981) Continuous ambulatory peritoneal dialysis (CAPD) in children. Trans Am Soc Artif Intern Organs 27:64–67
16. Chesney RW, Hamstra A, Jax DK, Mazess RB, De Luca HF (1980) Influence of long-term oral 1,25-dihydroxyvitamin D in childhood renal osteodystrophy. Contrib Nephrol 18:51–71
17. Delmez JA, Slatopolsky E, Martin KJ, Gearing BN, Harter HR (1982) Minerals, vitamin D, and parathyroid hormone in continuous ambulatory peritoneal dialysis. Kidney Int 21:862–867
18. Chan JCM, Kodroff MB, Landwehr DM (1981) Effects of 1,25– diyhydroxyvitamin D_3 on renal function, mineral balance, and growth in children with severe chronic renal failure. Pediatrics 68:559–571
19. Oleggini R, Perfumo F, Carrea A, Basile G, Gusmano R (1984) Study of parathyroid hormone behaviour in children in continuous ambulatory peritoneal dialysis. Gaslini (in press)
20. Aloni Y, Shany S, Chaimovitz C (1983) Losses of 25-hydroxyvitamin D in peritoneal fluid: possible mechanism for bone disease in uremic patients treated with chronic ambulatory peritoneal dialysis. Miner Electrolyte Metab 9:82–86
21. Guillot M, Garabedian M, Lavocat C, Guillozo H, Gagnadoux MF, Balsan S, Broyer M (1983) Evaluation of 25-hydroxyvitamin D and vitamin D binding protein losses in thirteen children on continuous ambulatory peritoneal dialysis. Int J Pediatr Nephrol 4:99–102
22. Horst RL, Shepard RM, Jorgensen NA, De Luca HF (1979) The determination of 24,25-dihydroxyvitamin D and 25,26 dihydroxyvitamin D in plasma from normal and nephrectomized man. J Lab Clin Med 93:277–285
23. Knutson JC, De Luca HF (1974) 25-hydroxyvitamin D_3-24-hydroxylase. Subcellular location and properties. Biochemistry 131:1543–1548
24. Gusmano R, Basile G, Ginevri F, Perfumo F (1983) Growth and nutrition in children treated by chronic ambulatory peritoneal dialysis (CAPD). Eur J Pediatr 140:150 (A)

Aluminum-Containing Phosphate Binding Agents and Plasma Aluminum Levels in Children Undergoing CAPD: Preliminary Results with the Use of Calcium Carbonate *

I. B. Salusky, J. W. Coburn, L. Paunier, J. Foley, and R. N. Fine

Introduction

Aluminum-containing phosphate binders are the principal therapy utilized to prevent the development of hyperphosphatemia and secondary hyperparathyroidism in patients with chronic renal failure [1]. Furthermore, the use of vitamin D sterols, which can aid in suppressing hyperparathyroidism, may increase intestinal phosphate absorption, thereby increasing the required dosage of phosphate binders [2–3]. Berlyne et al. [4] first reported that hyperaluminemia can occur after the ingestion of aluminum (Al)-containing anti-acids. Kaehny et al. [5] have confirmed that small amounts of Al can be absorbed after the ingestion of Al hydroxide gels. Initial reports from Europe demonstrated a strong association between the use of Al-contaminated water for preparing dialysate and the prevalence of osteomalacia and encephalopathy in adult dialysis patients [6]. Furthermore, the incidence of osteomalacic bone disease was reduced following the initiation of appropriate water purification [7]. Recently, both encephalopathy and Al-related osteomalacia have been described in infants and adults with advanced chronic renal failure prior to the initiation of dialysis [8–14]. The development of these abnormalities was associated with the ingestion of large quantities of Al-containing phosphate binding agents. Such observations implicate Al absorption from the gastrointestinal tract as the major source of Al accumulation in these patients.

The use of continuous ambulatory peritoneal dialysis (CAPD) as a treatment modality for the management of pediatric patients with end-stage renal disease (ESRD) is increasing; however, this dialytic modality does not adequately control hyperphosphatemia [15–17]. Indeed, Al-containing phosphate binders are usually necessary to reduce the serum phosphorus level in young children who ingest large quantities of formula and milk products, which have a high phosphate content. Thus, infants with ESRD require relatively larger doses of phosphate binders to reduce their serum phosphorus levels.

The aims of this study were (1) to measure serum Al levels and correlate the results with the Al intake in pediatric patients undergoing CAPD and (2) to evaluate the effectiveness of calcium carbonate as a phosphate binder in children with elevated plasma Al levels.

---

* Supported in part by grants AM 28368 and AM 29926 from the National Institute of Health, by the Peter Boxenbaum Fund, and by the Research Fund of the Veterans' Administration.

Patients and Methods

Sixteen patients (seven boys and nine girls) who had undergone CAPD for 16 ± 2.3 (SE) months were studied. At initiation of CAPD the mean age and body weight were 8.9 ± 1.0 (range 1.52–14.2) years and 23.5 ± 2.4 kg, respectively.

The CAPD procedure was performed according to the method described by Oreopoulos et al. [16]. Each patient received four to five daily exchanges of a commercially available dialysate solution (Dianeal, Travenol Laboratories, Deerfield, Ill) with 0.5–2 liters per exchange. The glucose concentration of the dialysate was adjusted to regulate the degree of ultrafiltration required. During the period of the study, three patients received dihydrotachysterol, 0.125–0.250 mg/day and 13 patients received calcitriol, 0.25–2.0 μg/day. Each patient received either Al hydroxide or Al carbonate as a phosphate binder, and the dosage was varied to maintain the serum phosphorus level between 4.5 and 6.0 mg/dl. Serum Al concentration was measured on two occasions, initially after 7.9 ± 2.1 months of CAPD and again after 16.6 ± 2.3 months of CAPD.

The use of calcium carbonate as a phosphate binder was evaluated in five patients, aged 6.0 ± 1.4 years, who initially demonstrated elevated serum Al levels of 60 to 153 μg/l. Each blood Al determination represented the mean of two or more determinations of consecutive months. Three patients had been treated with CAPD for 34 ± 3.9 months and two patients had been undergoing hemodialysis for 14 ± 2.5 months. The dosage of calcium carbonate ranged from 3 to 7 g/day.

Serum Al concentration was determined by flameless atomic absorption spectroscopy with a Perkin-Elmer spectrophotometer and an HGA 500 graphite furnace according to the method previously reported [18]. The normal values in children and adults are < 10 μg/l. The Al intake was estimated from the dosage of Al-containing gels prescribed and recorded for a 3-month period at each clinic visit. The Al concentration in 14 different lots of dialysate inflow was < 5 μg/l.

In two patients with a poor response to calcitriol therapy, a bone biopsy was obtained from the iliac creast with a Bordier needle after double tetracycline labeling [19]. The sample was fixed in 10% buffered formalin, dehydrated in ethanol, embedded in methyl methacrylate, and evaluated as previously described [19]. Data were expressed as mean $\pm$ SD. This study was approved by the UCLA Human Subject Protection Committee, and informed consent was obtained from the patients and/or their parents.

Results

The serum Al levels, measured after 7.9 ± 2.1 and 16.6 ± 2.3 months of CAPD therapy, were 55.2 ± 11.4 and 59.8 ± 10.4 μg/l, respectively (Fig. 1). These values were significantly higher than those of control children (8.2 ± 1.1 μg/l, $P < 0.001$). The mean oral intake of elemental Al at the time of these measurements was 98 ± 20 and 104 ± 32 mg/kg/day, respectively. The serum Al concentration and the estimated oral Al intake were directly related, $r = 0.86$, $P < 0.01$. In addition,

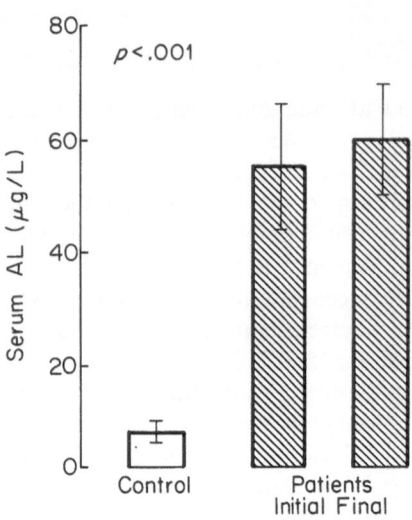

Fig. 1. Serum aluminum levels in children undergoing CAPD

there was an inverse correlation between the serum Al levels and both the patients' body weight ($r = -0.68$, $P < 0.01$) and age ($r = -0.67$, $P < 0.01$).

Bone biopsy showed marked staining for Al on the trabecular surface (3.1 mm/mm^2, normal $P < 0.00$), with an increase in the osteoid surface and no separation of the tetracycline labels. These findings are characteristic of low turnover, Al-related osteomalacia.

In the patients with elevated serum Al levels treated with calcium carbonate, the mean serum calcium and phosphorus levels were $10.3 + 0.8$ and $5.5 + 0.7$ mg/day, respectively, after 9.4 ± 2.4 months of treatment. The plasma Al level decreased significantly ($P < 0.02$) following calcium carbonate therapy (Table 1).

Discussion

The present study demonstrates that patients undergoing CAPD have elevated serum Al levels while receiving Al-containing phosphate binders. Furthermore, the serum Al levels are directly related to the oral intake of Al expressed per kg body weight, and are indirectly related to the patients' age and body weight.

The reason for the elevated serum Al levels in the younger patients could be related to the high Al intake expressed per kg body weight, or to a greater intestinal absorption of Al in patients of this age.

Vitamin D-resistant osteomalacia and/or encephalopathy secondary to Al accumulation resulting from oral Al compounds have been described in infants and adults prior to the initiation of dialysis [8–14]. Furthermore, reports from Europe have shown a strong association between the use of Al-containing water used for the preparation of dialysate and the prevalence of osteomalacia and encephalopathy in adult hemodialysis patients. On the other hand, osteomalacic bone disease was less

Table 1. Blood calcium, phosphorus, carbon dioxide, and aluminum levels in pediatric patients treated with oral calcium carbonate

Pt	Age (years)	Serum[a]			P-Al[b] (μg/l)		Duration on $CaCO_3$ (months)	Side-effects
		Ca (mg/dl)	P (mg/dl)	CO_2 (mEq/l)	Initial determinations	Final determinations		
1	1.5	8.8 ± 0.8	6.2 ± 2.3	21 ± 3	140	45	12	None
2	4.9	11.5 ± 1.4	6.4 ± 1.6	26 ± 3	153	78	8	Ca[c]
3	5.4	10.5 ± 0.7	5.3 ± 0.6	20 ± 4	60	39	5	None
4	8.7	9.9 ± 1.7	5.1 ± 1.5	19 ± 2	84	58	10	None
5	9.3	10.4 ± 0.8	6.0 ± 1.4	22 ± 2	153	82	9	None
Mean $\pm$ SD		10.3 ± 0.8	5.5 ± 0.7	22 ± 3	118 ± 43	60 ± 19[d]	9 ± 2	

[a] These values represent the mean levels of serum *Ca, P,* and CO_2 while the patients received calcium carbonate as the only phosphate binder.
[b] These values represent the plasma Al levels while the patients received only calcium carbonate.
[c] This patient had two episodes of asymptomatic hypercalcemia (Ca = 12.6 mg/dl).
[d] Paired *t*-test, final vs initial P-Al level $P < 0.02$.

common following the initiation of water purification used for the preparation of dialysate. The prevalence of Al-related bone disease is at present unknown. However, data from Oklahoma [20] and Australia [21] in asymptomatic adults on dialysis who were randomly biopsied suggest that it may be at least 20%–25%. The incidence is probably greater in patients with a longer duration of dialysis therapy, and preliminary data suggest that nearly 40% of adults on hemodialysis for more than 8 years with have eivdence of Al-related bone disease despite the use of water that is free of Al [22]. These epidemologic observations indicate an association between osteomalacia and the accumulation of Al from the oral Al intake contained in the phosphate binding agents.

Baluarte et al. described the development of encephalopathy in uremic infants receiving Al hydroxide, and recommended that the dose of Al hydroxide should not exceed 100 mg/kg/day [23]. The Al intake in many of the children included in the present report greatly exceeded this recommended level. Our findings suggest that the use of Al-containing phosphate binders should be minimized, especially in young children.

Clinical studies with the use of calcium carbonate as an alternative phosphate binder in patients undergoing maintenance dialysis have demonstrated effective control of hyperphosphatemia with this agent [24–25]. However, diarrhea and hypercalcemia can occur with large doses of calcium carbonate [25]. In addition, the concomitant use of vitamin D sterols and calcium carbonate can enhance the potential of hypercalcemia. Our preliminary results, in a small number of patients who were followed for at least 10 months, have shown that calcium carbonate can control serum phosphorus levels with a concomitant reduction in the serum Al levels. Long-term studies with calcium carbonate as the primary phosphate binding agent are needed to evaluate the efficiency and side-effects of this agent. Until such studies are available, calcium carbonate should be the primary agent used to control the serum phosphorus level in younger children with chronic renal failure.

Acknowledgments. We thank William van Buren, Korneil Gerzi, and Norma Maloni, Ph. D. for excellent technical assistance, and Ms. Amy Landsberg for secretarial assistance in preparing the manuscript.

References

1. Slatopolsky E, Caglar S, Gradowska L, Canterbury JM, Reiss E, Bricker NS (1972) On the prevention of secondary hyperparathyroidism in experimental chronic renal disease using "proportional reduction" of dietary phosphorus intake. Kidney Int 2:147–151
2. Brickman AS, Hartenbower DL, Norman AW, Coburn JW (1977) Actions of 1 α-dihydroxyvitamin D_3 and 1,25 dihydroxyvitamin D_3 on mineral metabolism in man. Effect on net absorption of phosphorus. Am J Clin Nutr 30:1064–1069
3. Chesney RW, Hamstra A, Jax DK, Mazess RB, DeLuca HF (1980) Influence of long-term oral 1,25 dihydroxyvitamin D in childhood renal osteodystrophy. Contrib Nephrol 18:55–71
4. Berlyne GM, Ben-Ari J, Pest D, Winberger J, Stern M, Gilmore GR, Levine R (1970) Hyperaluminaemia form aluminum resins in renal failure. Lancet 2:494–496
5. Kaehny ND, Hegg AP, Alfrey AC (1977) Gastrointestinal absorption of aluminum from aluminum-containing antacids. N Engl J Med 296:1389–1390
6. Cournot-Witmer G, Zingraff J, Piachot JJ, Escaig F, Lefevre R, Boumati P, Bourdean A, Garabedian M, Galle P, Bourdon R, Druecke T, Balsan S (1981) Aluminum localization in bone from hemodialyzed patients: Relationship to matrix mineralization. Kidney Int 20:376–385
7. Pierides AM, Eduards WG Jr, Cullum VX Jr, McCall JT, Ellis HA (1980) Hemodialysis encephalopathy with osteomalacic fractures and muscle weakness. Kidney Int 18:115–124
8. Nathan E, Pedersen SE (1980) Dialysis encephalopathy in a non-dialyzed uremic boy treated with aluminum hydroxide orally. Acta Paediatr Scand 69:793–796
9. Felsenfeld AJ, Gutman RA, Llach F, Harrelson JM (1982) Osteomalacia in chronic renal failure: a syndrome previously reported only with maintenance dialysis. Am J Nephrol 2:147–154
10. Griswold WR, Reznik V, Mendoza SA, Tauner D, Alfrey AC (1983) Accumulation of aluminum in a nondialyzed uremic child receiving aluminum hydroxide. Pediatrics 71:56–58
11. Randall ME (1983) Aluminum toxicity in an infant not on dialysis. Lancet 1:1327–1328
12. Kaye M (1983) Oral toxicity in a non-dialyzed patient with renal failure. Clin Nephrol 20:208–211
13. Andreoli SP, Bergstein JM, Sherrard DJ (1984) Aluminum intoxication from aluminum-containing phosphate binders in children with azotemia not undergoing dialysis. N Engl J Med 310:1079–1084
14. Salusky IB, Coburn JW, Paunier L, Sherrard DJ, Fine RN (1984) Role of aluminum hydroxide in raising serum aluminum levels in children undergoing continuous ambulatory peritoneal dialysis. J Pediatr 105, 717–720
15. Balfe JW, Vigneux A, Willumsen J, Hardy BE (1981) The use of CAPD in the treatment of children with end-stage renal disease. Perit Dial Bull 1:35–38
16. Salusky IB, Lucullo L, Nelson P, Fine RN (1982) Continuous ambulatory peritoneal dialysis in children. Pediatr Clin North Am 29:1005–1012
17. Baum M, Powell D, Calvin S, McDaid T, McHenry K, Mar H, Potter D (1982) Continuous ambulatory peritoneal dialysis in children. Comparison with hemodialysis. N Engl J Med 307:1537–1542

18. Legendre GR, Alfrey AC (1976) Measuring picogram amounts of aluminum in biological tissue by flameless atomic absorption analysis of a chelate. Clin Chem 22:53–56
19. Ott SM, Maloney NA, Coburn JW, Alfrey AC, Sherrard DJ (1982) The prevalence of bone aluminum deposition in renal osteodystrophy and its relation to the response to calcitriol therapy. N Engl J Med 307:709–713
20. Llach F, Felsenfeld AJ, Coleman MD, Pederson JA, Rosen R (1984) Renal osteodystrophy in unselected hemodialysis patients. In: Coburn JW (ed) Calcitriol. A clinical update. Excerpta Medica, Princeton, New Jersey, p 11
21. Buchanan MRC, Ihle BV, Dunn CM (1981) Hemodialysis related osteomalacia: a staining method to demonstrate aluminum. J Clin Pathol 34:1352–1354
22. Andress DL, Ott SM, Endress DB, Maloney NA, Milliner DS, Coburn JW, Sherrard DJ, Aluminum bone disease in chronic renal failure: high prevalence in a long-term dialysis population. (submitted for publication)
23. Baluarte HJ, Gruskin AB, Himer LB, Foley CM, Grover WD (1977) Encephalopathy in children with chronic renal failure. Proc Dial Transplant Forum 7:95–98
24. Meyrier A, Marsac J, Richet G (1973) The influence of a high calcium carbonate intake on bone disease in patients undergoing hemodialysis. Kidney Int 4:146–153
25. Morniere PH, Roussel A, Tahiri Y, de Fremont JF, Maurel G, Jaudon MC, Gueris I, Fournier A (1982) Substitution of aluminum hydroxide by high doses of calcium carbonate in patients in chronic hemodialysis: Disappearances of hyperaluminemia and equal control of hyperparathyroidism. Proc Eur Dial Transplant Assoc 19:784–787

Evolution of Renal Osteodystrophy and the Effect of High-Dose Calcitriol in Children Undergoing CAPD *

I. B. Salusky, L. Paunier, J. W. Coburn, H. Kangarloo, E. Slatopolsky, and R. N. Fine

Introduction

The presence of bone disease has been recognized in patients with renal failure for many years. Since dialysis and transplantation are available for the management of end-stage renal disease (ESRD) in children, the management of bone disease has become extremely important in this patient population. While CAPD is an effective dialytic modality for children with ESRD [1–3], it has been previously shown that hemodialysis per se does not prevent the development of secondary hyperparathyroidism in children [4]. Furthermore, the persistence or worsening of the bone disease has been observed in adult and pediatric patients treated with CAPD [3–8]. In addition, in a retrospective study of children undergoing CAPD, we demonstrated that low doses of calcitriol or dihydrotachysterol did not prevent the progression of renal osteodystrophy in 65% of the patients. We therefore undertook a prospective study to evaluate the clinical consequences and the effect on serum immunoreactive parathormone (iPTH) when the dose of calcitriol is progressively increased to raise the serum calcium level [9].

This article reviews the results we derived from two studies, a retrospective one [8] and a prospective one [9], on the management of renal osteodystrophy in pediatric patients treated with CAPD.

Methods

In the retrospective study (phase I), we evaluated 14 patients who received treatment with CAPD for 12 ± 5.6 months. Of this group, 11 patients received calcitriol (Rocaltrol, Hoffman LaRoche), 0.25–0.5 µg/day, and three patients received dihydrotachysterol, 0.125–0.25 mg/day.

In the prospective study (phase II), 17 pediatric patients who had undergone CAPD for a mean of 24.0 ± 9.5 months were studied, including ten patients evaluated in phase I. The mean duration of follow-up was 14.7 ± 3.0 months.

All patients were dialyzed through an in-dwelling Tenckhoff catheter, according to the method we have previously described [2]. Serum calcium, phosphorus, alka-

* Supported in part by grants AM 28368 and AM 29926 from the National Institutes of Health, the Peter Boxenbaum Research Fund, and the Research Fund of the Veterans' Administration.

line phosphatase, and iPTH levels were measured monthly. The iPTH levels were determined with the Ch 9 antibody, which recognizes the midregion of the carboxy fragment of the PTH molecule [10]. Skeletal roentgenographs obtained at the onset of the study and every 6 months thereafter were evaluated by an independent observer. The methods used to quantitate the X-ray scores have been published elsewhere [8].

During phase II, the dose of calcitriol was increased each month by 0.25 µg/day if the serum calcium level was below 10.5–11.0 mg/dl or if the serum alkaline phosphatase activity was increasing. All the patients received aluminum-containing phosphate-binding agents to maintain serum phosphorus level below 6 mg/dl.

These studies were approved by the UCLA Human Subject Protection Committee, and informed consent was obtained from the patients and/or their parents. All values are expressed as mean ± SD, and the Student's paired or unpaired *t* tests were used to compare results.

Results

In the phase I study, the patients were grouped according to serum alkaline phosphatase levels into a group with increasing levels and a subgroup with stable or decreasing levels (Fig. 1). The group with the increasing serum alkaline phosphatase levels had a mean serum calcium and iPTH levels of 9.7 ± 0.8 mg/dl and 208 ± 108 µlEq/ml respectively. On the other hand, the group with stable or decreasing serum alkaline phosphatase levels had serum calcium and iPTH levels of 10.6 ± 0.9 mg/dl and 75 ± 49 µlEq/ml respectively. The radiological score of hyperparathyroidism was significantly more abnormal in the group with increasing serum alkaline phosphatase levels (4.1 ± 1.2 compared with 2.3 ± 1.1, $P < 0.05$) [8].

Serial serum levels of calcium, phosphorus, and alkaline phosphatase during the phase II of the study are shown in Table 1. Serum calcium level increased from 10.1 ± 0.9 mg/dl at the initiation of the study to 10.8 ± 0.7 mg/dl at the end of the

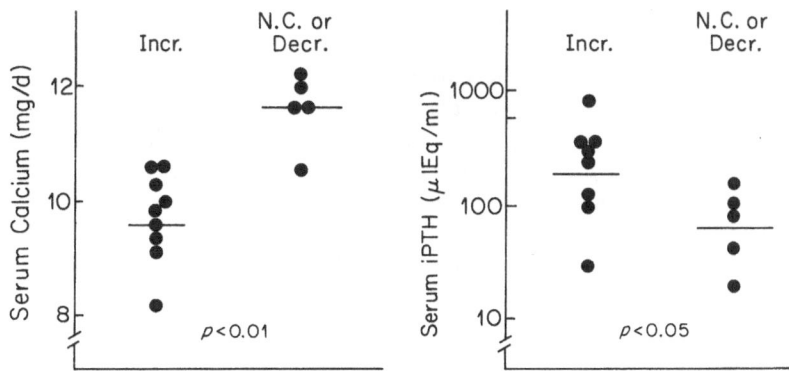

Fig. 1. Mean serum calcium and iPTH levels of patients grouped according to serum alkaline phosphatase levels in phase I study (Incr., increase; N.C., no change; Decr., decrease)

Table 1. Serial serum levels of calcium and phosphorus and alkaline phosphatase activity in 17 pediatric patients during treatment with calcitriol (From Salusky et al. [9] with permission)

	Measurement[a]		
	Initial	Final	P[a]
Calcium (mg/dl)	10.1± 0.9	10.8± 0.7	<0.01
Phosphorus (mg/dl)	5.1± 1.0	5.7± 0.7	NS
Alkaline phosphatase (IU/l)	433.0±300	210.0±60	<0.01

[a] In each patient, the initial and final measurements were the means of three consecutive measurements. Thus, the means (±SD) presented in this table are averages based on mean values in 17 patients.

period of observation ($P < 0.01$). The mean initial and final serum phosphorus levels were 5.1 ± 1.0 and 5.7 ± 0.7 mg/dl respectively. Serum alkaline phosphatase levels decreased from 433 ± 300 IU/l to 210 ± 60 IU/l ($P < 0.01$) [9]. Serum iPTH levels decreased by 56% from initial values in 11 patients ($P < 0.01$). In four patients, the serum iPTH levels either increased or were persistently elevated. Two of these patients were subsequently found to have aluminum-related bone disease. Skeletal roentgenographs showed improvement in 16 of the 17 patients.

The average daily dosage of calcitriol was 0.60 ± 0.40 µg/day with a range from 0.25 to 2.25 µg/day during phase II. The only side effect of calcitriol therapy was the occurrence of hypercalcemia. In 11 patients, 13 episodes of hypercalcemia occurred. When hypercalcemia occurred, the dosage of calcitriol was discontinued or decreased. Serum calcium levels returned to within normal limits within 20 days after discontinuing or decreasing the dose in all patients except one. In this patient, the hypercalcemia persisted for 15 weeks, and a bone biopsy showed aluminum– related osteomalacia. The hypercalcemia was asymptomatic in all instances except for two patients who had acute conjunctival erythema.

Discussion

In phase I of the study, the patients exhibited one or two divergent courses: 36% showed either stabilization or lack of progression of bone disease, and the other 64% showed evidence of progression or worsening of secondary hyperparathyroidism. The latter group had significantly lower serum calcium levels and higher iPTH levels than the group who did not show progression of the bone disease. Thus, the serum calcium level may need to reach values above normal to achieve parathyroid suppression in children with uremia. This is consistent with the in vitro observation that there may be alterations in the calcium-regulated inhibition of PTH released by the parathyroid cells from uremic patients with secondary hyperparathyroidism [11]. It has been shown that the "set point," or calcium concentration at which iPTH secretion by parathyroid cells is half maximally inhibited by an increase in ambient calcium concentration, is higher in cells from patients with secondary hyperparathyroidism than in normal parathyroid cells [11]. Whether the serum iPTH level could have been suppressed in the group with progressive hyperparathyroidism if the serum calcium level had been increased was not established by our initial observations in phase I [8].

On the basis of this hypothesis, we now consider the results of phase II, in which increased doses of calcitriol were used to raise the serum calcium level and suppress iPTH secretion [9].

Our observations in phase II indicate that "high" doses of calcitriol can heal and/or prevent the development of hyperparathyroidism in children undergoing CAPD [9]. The serum calcium levels increased significantly, serum alkaline phosphatase levels returned to normal values, and the serum phosphorus level remained unchanged. Serum iPTH levels fell significantly in 76% of the patients. In 24% of the patients, elevated serum iPTH levels persisted. Two of these patients were found to have aluminum-related bone disease. The radiographical features of secondary hyperparathyroidism improved in all the patients except in a patient with aluminum-related osteomalacia.

Aluminum-related osteomalacia has been typically described in adult patients on maintenance hemodialysis [12]. The syndrome can arise from aluminum contamination of the dialysate [13], or aluminum-containing phosphate binders can be another source for aluminum intoxication [15–20]. The pathogenesis is uncertain, but aluminum may inhibit bone matrix synthesis, the mineralization process, or both. The biochemical characteristics include the finding of normal to elevated serum calcium levels [21]; normal plasma alkaline phosphatase levels in patients reported from the United Kingdom, with elevated levels of plasma alkaline phosphatase found by others; and serum iPTH levels that are usually lower than those noted in dialysis patients [21]. There are few reports of this syndrome among pediatric patients [14, 16, 20]. The finding of high iPTH levels in patients with aluminum-related bone disease is unusual in adult patients. The characteristics of this syndrome requires further study in children.

Calcitriol has been shown to increase intestinal absorption of phosphorus [22], and its use could aggravate the hyperphosphatemia in children with renal failure, as has been previously suggested [23]. During phase II of this study, the amount of phosphate binders required did not increase as patients received high doses of calcitriol. On the other hand, as described earlier [20], the patients receiving higher doses of aluminum-containing phosphate binder agents had the highest serum aluminum levels. Moreover, the two patients with the highest aluminum intake and the highest serum aluminum levels had findings of aluminum-related osteomalacia.

The optimal dose of calcitriol for pediatric patients with ESRD is not clearly delineated. Chan et al. recommended initial daily dosages of calcitriol of 0.25 µg for those weighing less than 10 kg, 0.50 µg for those weighing 10–20 kg, and 1.0 µg for those with body weight greater than 20 kg undergoing hemodialysis [24]. Furthermore, in most patients studied by Hewitt et al. [7], who used a daily dosage of calcitriol ranging from 0.25 to 1.5 µg in children undergoing CAPD, the features of secondary hyperparathyroidism persisted after 1 year of treatment.

During phase II of our study, the dosage of calcitriol varied widely, with a maximal dosage range of 0.25 to 2.25 µg/day [9]. From the present observations, we would recommend a dynamic approach to the use of calcitriol adjusted for each individual patient, with the maintenance of serum calcium at a level between 10.5 to 11.0 mg/dl to achieve optimal suppression of iPTH.

We previously demonstrated that CAPD patients who have received high doses of aluminum-containing phosphate binder agents have high serum aluminum levels [20]. The use of calcium carbonate as the only phosphate binder has been suggested. Our own preliminary experience has shown adequate control of serum phosphorus levels and a decrease in plasma aluminum levels. Under these conditions, vitamin D sterols should be given only with great caution.

The only side effect of calcitriol therapy was the development of hypercalcemia in 65% of the patients; most were asymptomatic, but two patients developed acute conjunctivitis.

During phase II of the study, there was a substantial improvement in the radiological findings of renal osteodystrophy; no patient developed extraskeletal calcifications.

In conclusion, the use of "high" doses of calcitriol in children on CAPD corrected hyperparathyroidism, as demonstrated by radiographical findings, serum iPTH levels, alkaline phosphatase, and calcium levels. In most instances, these effects did not occur until the serum calcium level increased to 10.5 to 11.0 mg/dl. These findings are consistent with the in vitro data showing an abnormal "set point" for the parathyroid glands in patients with ESRD [11].

References

1. Balfe JW, Vigneux A, Williumsen J, Hardy BE (1981) The use of CAPD in the treatment of children with end-stage renal disease. Perit Dial Bull 1:35–38
2. Salusky IB, Lucullo L, Nelson P, Fine RN (1982) Continuous ambulatory peritoneal dialysis in children. Pediatr Clin North Am 29:1005–1012
3. Baum M, Powell D, Calvin S, McDaid T, McHenry K, Mar H, Potter D (1982) Continuous ambulatory peritoneal dialysis in children. Comparison with hemodialysis. N Engl J Med 307:1537–1542
4. Fine RN, Isaacson AS, Payne V, Grushkin CM (1972) Renal osteodystrophy in children. The effect of hemodialysis and renal homotransplantation. J Pediatr 80:243–249
5. Tielemans C, Aubry C, Dratwa M (1981) The effects of continuous ambulatory peritoneal dialysis (CAPD) on renal osteodystrophy. In: Gahl GM, Kessel M, Nolph KD (eds) Advances in peritoneal dialysis. Excerpta Medica, Amsterdam, p 455
6. Digenis G, Khanna R, Pierratos A, Mena HE, Rabinovich S, Petit J, Oreopoulos DG (1983) Renal osteodystrophy in patients maintained on CAPD for more than three years. Perit Dial Bull 2:81–86
7. Hewit IK, Stefanidis C, Reilly BJ, Kooh SW, Balfe JW (1983) Renal osteodystrophy in children undergoing continuous ambulatory dialysis. J Pediatr 103:729–734
8. Paunier L, Salusky IB, Slatopolsky E, Kangarloo H, Kopple JD, Horst RL, Coburn JW, Fine RN (1984) Renal osteodystrophy in children undergoing continuous ambulatory peritoneal dialysis. Pediatr Res 18:742–747
9. Salusky IB, Fine RN, Paunier L, Slatopolsky E, Kangarloo H, Coburn JW (1984) Use of high-dose calcitriol in pediatric patients undergoing CAPD. In: Coburn JW (ed) Calcitriol. A clinical update. Excerpta Medica, Princeton, New Jersey, p 36
10. Hruska KA, Kopelman R, Rutherford WE, Klahr S, Slatopolsky E (1975) Metabolism of immunoreactive parathyroid hormone in the dog. The role of the kidney and the effects of chronic renal disease. J Clin Invest 56:39–48

11. Brown EM, Wilson RE, Eastman RC, Pallota J, Marynick SP (1982) Abnormal regulation of parathyroid hormone release by calcium in secondary hyperparathyroidism due to chronic renal failure. J Clin Endocrinol Metab 54:172–179
12. Hodsman AB, Sherrard DJ, Alfrey AC, Ott SM, Brickman AS, Miller NL, Maloney NA, Coburn JW (1982) Bone aluminum and histomorphometric feature of renal osteodystrophy. J Clin Endocrinol Metab 54:539–546
13. Platt MM, Goode GC, Hislop JS (1977) Comparison of the domestic water supply and the incidence of features of fractures and encephalopathy in patients on home dialysis. Br Med J 2:657–660
14. Nathan E, Pedersen SE (1980) Dialysis encephalopathy in a non-dialyzed uremic boy treated with aluminum hydroxide orally. Acta Paediatr Scand 69:793–796
15. Felsenfeld AJ, Gutman RA, Llach F, Harrelson JM (1982) Osteomalacia in chronic renal failure: a syndrome previously reported only with maintenance dialysis. Am J Nephrol 2:147–154
16. Griswold WR, Reznik V, Mendoza SA, Trauner D, Alfrey AC (1983) Accumulation of aluminum in a non-dialyzed uremic child receiving aluminum hydroxide. Pediatrics 71:56–58
17. Randall ME (1983) Aluminum toxicity in an infant not on dialysis. Lancet 1:1327–1328
18. Kaye M (1983) Oral toxicity in a non-dialyzed patient with renal failure. Clin Nephrol 20:208–211
19. Andreoli SP, Bergstein JM, Sherard DJ (1984) Aluminum intoxication from aluminum-containing phosphate binders in children with azotemia not undergoing dialysis. N Engl J Med 310:1079–1084
20. Salusky IB, Coburn JW, Paunier L, Sherrard DJ, Fine RN (1984) Role of aluminum hydroxide in raising serum aluminum levels in children undergoing continuous ambulatory peritoneal dialysis. J Pediatr 105:717–720
21. Ott SM, Maloney NA, Coburn JW, Alfrey AC, Sherrard DJ (1982) The prevalence of bone aluminum deposition in renal osteodystrophy and its relation to the response to calcitriol therapy. N Engl J Med 307:709–713
22. Brickman AS, Hartenbower DL, Norman AW, Coburn JW (1977) Actions of 1-hydroxyvitamin D_3 and 1,25-dihydroxyvitamin D_3 on mineral metabolism in man. Effects on net absorption of phosphorus. Am J Clin Nutr 30:1064–1069
23. Chesney RW, Hamstra A, Jax DK, Mazess RB, DeLuca HF (1980) Influence of long term oral 1,25-dihydroxyvitamin D in childhood renal osteodystrophy. Contrib Nephrol 8:55–71
24. Chan JCM, DeLuca HR (1979) Calcium and parathyroid disorders in children. J Am Med Assoc 241:1242–1244
25. Meyrier A, Marsac J, Richet G (1973) The influence of a high calcium carbonate intake on bone disease in patients undergoing hemodialysis. Kidney Int 4:146–149
26. Moriniere PH, Roussel A, Tahiri Y, Fremont JF de, Maurel G, Jaudon MC, Gueris I, Fournier A (1982) Substitution of aluminum hydroxide by high doses of calcium carbonate in patients in chronic hemodialysis: Disappearances of hyperaluminemia and equal control of hyperparathyroidism. Proc Eur Dial Transplant Assoc 19:784–787

Renal Anemia in Children on CAPD

D. E. Müller-Wiefel, K. E. Bonzel, R. Wartha, O. Mehls, and K. Schärer

Introduction

In patients with end-stage renal disease (ESRD), uremic intoxication leads to increased blood loss, especially in the gastrointestinal tract, to reduced erythropoiesis, and to exaggerated hemolysis [1]. The resulting anemia cannot be eliminated by regular hemodialysis (HD) but is almost completely reversed by renal transplantation [2]. The aim of this study is to investigate whether CAPD is better able to counteract renal anemia (RA) than·HD – a question that has received conflicting answers in the literature to date.

Patients

The data of eight children older than 1 year of age at initiation of CAPD, which was performed for at least 6 months, were analyzed (Table 1). Two patients had previously been treated by HD, and one child was treated for acute renal failure by continuous peritoneal dialysis. At the start of treatment, the mean age of the children was 7 years and 8 months. None of the children suffered from hepatitis or poly-

Table 1. Clinical data of eight patients

No.	Previous treatment	Age at start of treatment (years)	Time on CAPD (months)	Outcome of treatment
1	Conservative	11	6	still on CAPD
2	Conservative	12 10/12	6	still on CAPD
3	Hemodialysis	6 2/12	10	transplantation
4	Conservative	1 8/12	11	transplantation
5	Hemodialysis	9 3/12	12	transplantation
6	Conservative	3 9/12	16	transplantation
7	Continuous peritoneal dialysis	5 7/12	18	death
8	Conservative	11 7/12	23	transplantation
	Mean	7 7/12	13	

cystic kidneys, and none had been transfused for immunological reasons or had received iron supplementation. All the patients were orally supplemented with 2 mg folate per m² body surface area per day. One patient underwent bilateral nephrectomy within the observation period. Five children received transplants, one child died, two are currently on CAPD. A total of 100 CAPD treatment months were analyzed.

Methods

The concentrations of whole blood hemoglobin (Hb), mean erythrocyte corpuscular hemoglobin (MCH), and mean corpuscular volume (MCV) were measured in a total of 300 peripheral venous blood samples using the Coulter Counter S. The reticulocyte count (R) was determined in 55 peripheral blood smears after coloration with brillant cresyl blue and corrected for the degree of anemia by calculating the production index

$$\frac{\text{Hb(g/l)} \times \text{R(\%)}}{150}.$$

In addition, serum ferritin, folate, and vitamin B_{12} levels were measured by radioimmunoassay [1]. The values were combined to give a mean value for a 3-month period. After blood transfusion (BT), a period of at least 2 weeks was required before further measurements were made. If possible, data were compared with those obtained for 17 children on home hemodialysis (HHD) [1].

Results

In the 3-month period prior to the start of treatment, patients on CAPD and HHD had nearly the same Hb level (Fig. 1). For the group on CAPD, we observed a sig-

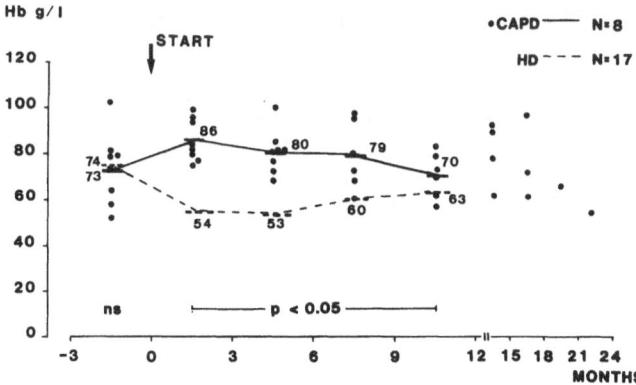

Fig. 1. Mean values (3 months periods) of blood hemoglobin concentration in eight children on CAPD, compared to data in 17 children on HHD (– – – –, from [1])

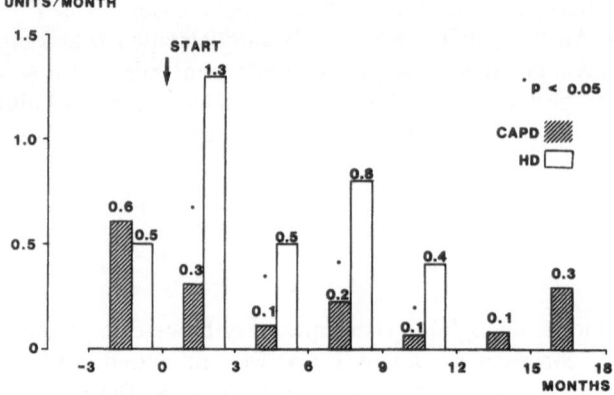

Fig. 2. Mean number of erythrocyte transfusions (3 months) expressed in units (250 ml/m² body surface area) per month before and after start of CAPD (▨) and HHD (□, from [1])

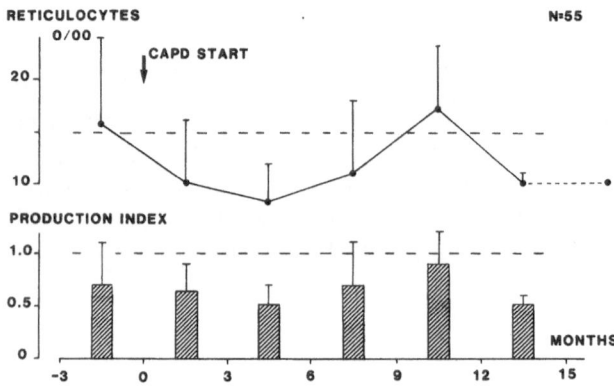

Fig. 3. Mean values ± SD (3 months) of reticulocyte counts and production indices (see this chapter, Methods) with their standard deviations for patients on CAPD. The *broken lines* are the mean normal values

nificant initial increase from 73 to 86 g/l in the Hb levels for the first 3-month period. At the same time the mean Hb values in the HHD group fell significantly from 74 to 54 g/l. Subsequently, the Hb levels varied in the two treatment groups: in the patients on CAPD, a gradual decrease was observed, while regular HHD was associated with a slow increase. After 9–12 months of dialysis treatment, the mean Hb concentration was 70 g/l for the CAPD group and 63 for the patients on HHD.

With the start of CAPD, the need for blood transfusions (BT) decreased, ranging from 0.1 to 0.3 units per month (1 unit = 250 ml erythrocytes per m² body surface area) (Fig. 2). However, in the course of HHD, the frequency of BT sharply increased to 1.3 units per months and remained two to four times higher than for CAPD. CAPD did not lead to an increase of R. Values usually remained below 1.5% with a nadir seen between 3 and 6 months (Fig. 3). The mean production index never achieved the normal value of 1. MCH and MCV did not change significantly during the observation period and neither increased nor decreased (Fig. 4). At the onset of CAPD, serum ferritin (SF) levels were slightly increased, with a further rise observable during the first 6 months of treatment (Fig. 5). Over 1 year of treatment,

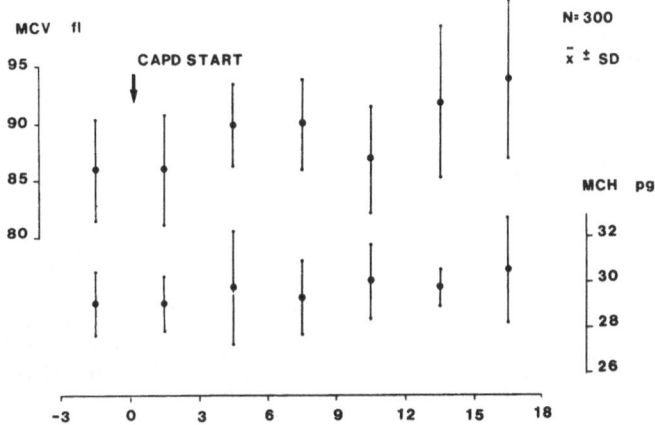

Fig. 4. Mean values (3 months) and standard deviation of mean corpuscular erythrocyte volume (MCV) and mean corpuscular erythrocyte hemoglobin (MCH) in CAPD patients

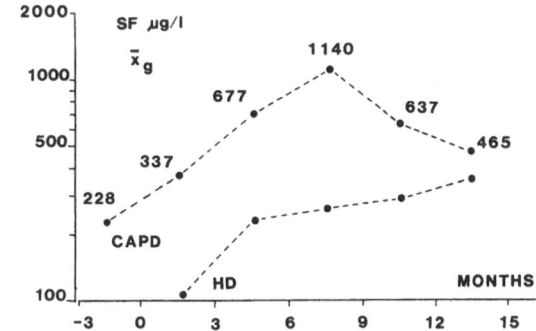

Fig. 5. Changes in 3-month values of serum ferritin concentration in children on CAPD compared with those on home hemodialysis (HHD, from [1])

the SF levels for the children on CAPD were higher than for those on HHD in spite of the lower incidence of BT on CAPD. In both groups, the number of BT per patient significantly correlated with SF levels. The correlation curve was, however, at a higher level for the CAPD group (Fig. 6). No deficiency of serum folate of vitamin B_{12} was noted during CAPD, all values being within or above the normal range (Fig. 7).

Discussion

At present, RA remains a major clinical problem in ESRD, especially in children [2]. It is a primary factor limiting physical fitness and well-being [3]. Unfortunately, RA is neither sufficiently compensated for hematologically [4, 5] nor ameliorated by a single therapeutic regimen because of its heterogenous nature, which stems from the unfavorable interaction of reduced erythropoiesis, increased hemolysis, and exag-

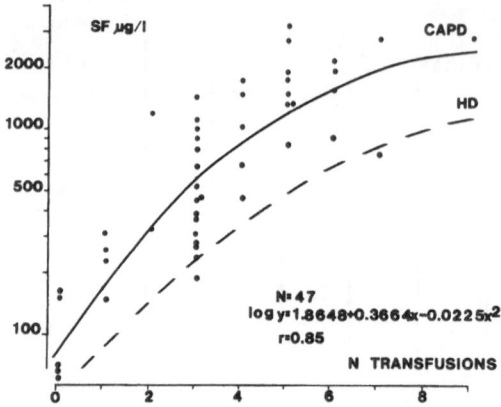

Fig. 6. Correlation of serum ferritin (SF) concentration with the number of erythrocyte units transfused. The correlation curve (—) is compared with that calculated in children on HD (– – –, from [1])

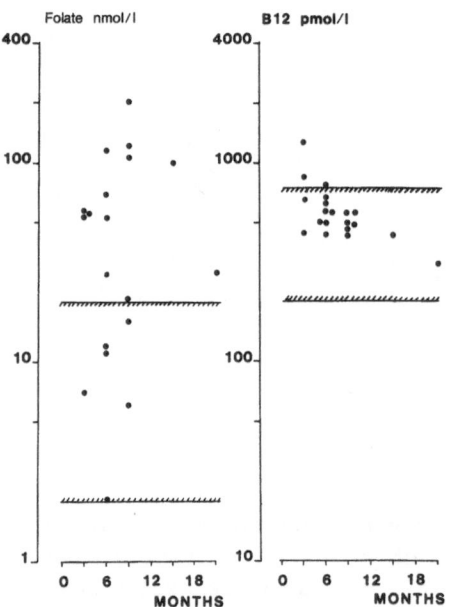

Fig. 7. Concentration of serum folate and vitamin B_{12} in children on CAPD. The upper and lower limits of normal are indicated by the *horizontal lines*

gerated blood loss [1]. Even different methods of extracorporeal blood purification, including the elimination of low and high molecular weight compounds or toxins have failed to cure RA [3].

However, there have been enthusiastic reports of improvement of RA after the initiation of CAPD [6, 7]. Currently, most authors confirm a favorable effect of CAPD on Hb concentration or hematocrit and/or BT rate in contrast to hemodialysis, becoming apparent over the course of treatment [8–22]. The latter observation has been denied by others [23–26]. The controversy might easily be explained by differences in patient selection that include parameters having an influence on Hb levels, such as age, residual renal function, uremic state, degree of hyperparathyroidism, primary renal disease, bilateral nephrectomy, persistent renal graft [27] or hepatitis. Moreover, divergent interpretations might result from different investigation times during the course of treatment [28] or from discrepancies in therapeutic schedules, especially where blood transfusions are involved. Valid statements about the influence of CAPD on RA should only be made in comparison with a control group and/or a period, conditions which are usually, however, very difficult to achieve. By comparing under identical conditions and at different stages of treatment the degree of RA in children on CAPD with that of children on HHD, we have tried to minimize the variables mentioned above.

During the 1-year period analyzed, the Hb concentration in children on CAPD was higher than in those on HHD, but during the same period of observation, a gradual decrease in Hb occurred – again in contrast to HHD. Investigations including the measurements of both total red cell mass and plasma volume have demonstrated a real increase of erythrocyte volume, together with plasma volume constriction in CAPD patients [14, 20], a finding which was, however, not reproducible in another study [24]. Because of unchanged erythrocyte indices (MCH and MCV) during the course of treatment, it is rather unlikely that the increase in Hb concentration noted in our patients is due to dehydration. Therefore, we assume an increase of total red cell mass, the origin of which is neither sufficiently clarified by the data in this study nor by the literature.

From our investigation, the higher Hb values observed for patients on CAPD compared with those on HHD cannot be attributed to increased erythropoiesis because of low reticulocyte counts observable for both forms of dialysis. This observation is in accordance with the study of Summerfield et al. [20]. On the other hand, a progressive increase in the reticulocyte count during CAPD has been noted by other investigators [11]. The insufficient erythropoiesis as indicated by the low erythrocyte production index was demonstrated in our children by the level of reticulocytosis corrected for the degree of anemia. The insufficient erythropoiesis in patients on dialysis – whether CAPD or HD – has been proven by ferrokinetic studies [24] as well as by bone marrow cell culture techniques [18]. These results are in line with the lack of any difference between the serum erythropoietin concentration of patients on CAPD and on HD [18, 20]. For both treatment modalities, moderate elevations of the serum erythropoietin concentration were found to be counteracted to the same extent by plasma inhibitors of erythropoiesis; however, a higher peak 7cl clearance for CAPD has been pointed out by others [17]. Only rarely, such as in patients with polycystic kidney disease, does bone marrow inhibition appear to be overcome by erythropoietic activity, even during CAPD [22]. On the whole, increased red cell mass during CAPD is probably not the consequence of a significant amelioration of erythropoiesis.

Correspondingly, increased hemolysis, as measured by decreased erythrocyte life span, is not eliminated by CAPD [23, 29], and these data parallel those of children and adults on regular HD [30]. In this context, it might be noted that levels of the enzymes of the hexose monophosphate shunt and the glycolytic pathway are normal and comparable to those of HD patients [29]. Although Summerfield et al. [20] and Salahudeen et al. [24] demonstrated an increased erythrocyte life span during the course of CAPD treatment, both studies were unable to show a relationship between these findings and the degree of anemia. Therefore, it remains questionable whether reduced hemolysis contributes toward alleviating RA in patients on CAPD at all.

Blood loss – the third major component of RA – is considerably lower for patients on CAPD than for those on HD because there is no extracorporeal circuit. In previous investigations, we calculated a blood loss of 2.5 1/1.73 m²/year into the extracorporeal dialysis system and an additional loss of 6.7 1/1.73 m²/year into the gastrointestinal tract due to uremic enteropathy and heparinization [1, 30]. Although the significance of this factor has not been accurately assessed, it is likely that the smaller quantities of blood lost during CAPD as compared with HD contribute toward alleviating RA in patients on CAPD, an explanation that has been proposed by other investigators [23, 28]. Accordingly, iron deficiency as measured by erythrocyte indices and SF levels did not develop in our CAPD patients, in spite of the fact that this group had a lower BT rate than the HHD patients. The SF level has been shown to correlate as well with bone marrow iron stores in CAPD patients [31] as it does in HD patients [32]. To detect iron deficiency in patients on CAPD, one has to take into consideration that SF levels are usually higher in this group than in patients on HD, despite the same number of blood transfusions given (Fig. 6). The inappropriately high SF levels for CAPD patients could be a consequence of inflammation, a notion which has recently been proposed by others [21]. From our data, we recommend oral iron supplementation when SF levels are below 100 µg/l (immunoradiometric assay, heterologous antibody system).

The normal serum levels of folate and vitamin B_{12} are in accordance with the normal erythrocyte indices, with no evidence of a megaloblastic component of RA for CAPD patients. However, without the daily oral supplementation of 2 mg folate our children were given, they could have developed folate deficiency, as has recently been reported for adults [33].

In summary, RA in CAPD patients is normocytic and normochromic and, in contrast to HD, shows improvement during the first year of treatment, probably as a result of smaller blood losses. It is characterized by elevated SF levels, which are possibly the result of inflammation.

References

1. Müller-Wiefel DE (1982) Renale Anämie im Kindesalter. Thieme, Stuttgart
2. Schärer K, Müller-Wiefel DE (1982) Renal anemia in children. A review. Int J Pediatr Nephrol 3:193–198
3. Schärer K, Müller-Wiefel DE (in press) Hematological and cardiovascular problems in renal insufficiency. In: Holliday MA, Barratt TM, Vernier R (eds) Pediatric Nephrology. Williams and Wilkins, Baltimore
4. Müller-Wiefel DE, Schärer K, Fischer W, Michalk D (1978) Erythrocyte organic phosphates in anemia of renal failure in childhood. Eur J Pediatr 128:103–111
5. Müller-Wiefel DE, Schärer K (1983) Serum erythropoietin in children with chronic renal failure. Kidney Int 24 Suppl 15:70–76
6. Oreopoulos GD (1979) Introductory remarks: Selection criteria and clinical results of continuous ambulatory peritoneal dialysis. In: Legrain M (ed) Continuous Ambulatory Peritoneal Dialysis. Excerpta Medica, Amsterdam, p 101
7. Popovich RP, Moncrief JW, Nolph K, Ghods AJ, Twardowski ZJ, Pyle WK (1978) Continuous ambulatory peritoneal dialysis. Ann Intern Med 88:449–456
8. Amair P, Khanna R, Leibele B (1982) Continuous ambulatory peritoneal dialysis in diabetics with end-stage renal disease. N Engl J Med 306:625–630

9. Baum M, Powell D, Calvin S, McDaid T, McHenry K, Mar H, Potter D (1982) Continuous ambulatory peritoneal dialysis in children. N Engl J Med 307: 1537–1542
10. Buoncristiani U, Brugnano R, DiPaolo N, Cozzari M, Carobi C (1984) Steadiness of anemia correction in long-term CAPD patients. Perit Dial Bull 4 Suppl 2: 9
11. Burgess WP, Diaz-Buxo JA, Chandler JT, Farmer CD, Walker PJ (1984) Increased erythropoiesis accounts for long-term improved anemia in patients undergoing peritoneal dialysis (PD). Perit Dial Bull 4 Suppl 2: 10
12. Cantaluppi A, Scalamogha A, Castelnovo C, Graziani G, Ponticelli C (1983) Anemia in CAPD and hemodialysis. Lancet 2: 1489
13. Colombi A, Wyss R, Pfister G, Stoll B, Bussmann HU, Rosenthal CH, Müller G, Brodhage H, Schneider A (1982) Kontinuierliche ambulante Peritonealdialyse (CAPD). Ther Umsch 39: 396–401
14. De Paepe MB, Schelstraete KH, Ringoir SM, Lameire NH (1983) Influence of continuous ambulatory peritoneal dialysis on the anemia of end-stage renal disease. Kidney Int 23: 744–748
15. Fenell RS, Orak JK, Garin EH, Iravani A, Richard G, St. John M (1983) Continuous ambulatory peritoneal dialysis in a pediatric population. Am J Dis Child 137: 388–392
16. Lacke C, Senekjian HO, Knight TF (1981) Twelve months' experience with continuous ambulatory and intermittent peritoneal dialysis. Arch Intern Med 141: 187–190
17. Lamperi S, Carrozzi S, Icardi A (1983) Improvement of erythropoiesis in uremic patients on CAPD. Int J Artif Organs 6: 191–194
18. Mc Gonigle RJS, Husserl F, Wallin JD, Fisher JW (1984) Hemodialysis and continuous ambulatory peritoneal dialysis effects on erythropoiesis in renal failure. Kidney Int 25: 430–436
19. Nolph K, Sorkin M, Rubin J (1980) Continuous ambulatory peritoneal dialysis: three-year experience at one center. Ann Intern Med 92: 609–613
20. Summerfield GP, Gyde OHB, Forbes AMW, Goldsmith HJ, Bellingham AJ (1983) Hemoglobin concentration and serum erythropoietin in renal dialysis and transplant patients. Scand J Haematol 30: 389–400
21. Winearls CG, Sovage COS, Oliviera DBG, Midgley K (1983) Anemia in CAPD and haemodialysis. Lancet 2: 1488
22. Zappacosta AR, Caro J, Erslev A (1982) Normalization of hematocrit in patients with end-stage renal disease on continuous ambulatory peritoneal dialysis. Am J Med 72: 53–57
23. Marcovici P, Boner G, Rosenfeld JB (1983) Effect of continuous ambulatory peritoneal dialysis on anemia in uremic patients. Isr J Med Sci 19: 604–607
24. Salahudeen AK, Keavey PM, Hawkins T, Wilkinson R (1983) Is anemia during continuous ambulatory peritoneal dialysis really better than during hemodialysis? Lancet 2: 1046–1049
25. Spinowitz BS, Sherwood J, Galler M, Charytan C (1982) Anemia and oxygen affinity in patients on continuous ambulatory peritoneal dialysis. Dial Transplant 12: 33–35
26. Wilkinson R, Salahudeen AK, Keavey P, Hawkins T (1984) Anemia and dialysis. Lancet 1: 112–113
27. Chandra M, Garcia JF, Miller ME, Waldbaum RS, Bluestone PA, McVicar M (1983) Normalization of hematocrit in a uremic patient receiving hemodialysis: role of erythropoietin. J Pediatr 103: 80–83
28. Summerfield GP, Bellingham AJ, Goldsmith HJ (1983) Anemia in CAPD and hemodialysis. Lancet 2: 1489
29. Hefti JE, Blumberg A, Marti HR (1983) Red cell survival and red cell enzymes in patients on continuous peritoneal dialysis (CAPD). Clin Nephrol 19: 232–235
30. Müller-Wiefel DE, Sinn H, Gilli G, Schärer K (1977) Hemolysis and blood loss in children with chronic renal failure Clin Nephrol 8: 581–586
31. Blumberg AB, Marti HR, Graber CG (1983) Serum ferritin and bone marrow iron in patients undergoing continuous ambulatory peritoneal dialysis. JAMA 250: 3317–3319
32. Müller-Wiefel DE, Waldherr R, Feist D, van Kaick G (1984) The assessment of iron stores in children on regular dialysis treatment. Contrib Nephrol 38: 141–152
33. Blumberg A, Hanck A, Sander G (1983) Vitamin nutrition in patients on continuous ambulatory peritoneal dialysis (CAPD). Clin Nephrol 20: 244–250

Loss of Ultrafiltration and Peritoneal Membrane Alterations in Children on CAPD

P. Niaudet, R. Drachman, M.-C. Gubler, and M. Broyer

Introduction

Continuous ambulatory peritoneal dialysis (CAPD) is widely used as maintenance therapy in patients with end-stage renal disease (ESRD). CAPD was introduced as a treatment for children in 1978, and the use of CAPD has increased steadily since then [1–4]. Although this technique is a valuable short-term therapeutic approach, little information is available concerning the long-term side effects of this mode of treatment in children. Several reports in adults have described a permanent loss of ultrafiltration associated with increased glucose absorption from the dialysate [5–8]. Several factors are probably responsible for this complication; for example, prolonged exposure of the peritoneum to acetate-containing dialysate has been incriminated [6, 7]. The histologic changes of the peritoneal membrane associated with isolated loss of ultrafiltration have not been documented. Some patients develop an encapsulating sclerosing peritonitis, in which a thick, fibrous membrane surrounds and compresses the bowel [9]. Most patients with sclerosing peritonitis suffer loss of ultrafiltration. However, it is not known if isolated loss of ultrafiltration and encapsulating peritonitis represent two extremes of the same disease process.

In this report, we present our experience with several ultrafiltration studies performed on 11 children as well as the results of peritoneal biopsies performed in five children treated with CAPD.

Patients and Methods

The study involved 13 children, nine girls and four boys, who were treated with CAPD for 6 to 31 months. Peritoneal dialysis was performed through a permanent Tenckhoff catheter. The age at initiation of CAPD ranged from 2.5 to 17.6 years. Intermittent peritoneal dialysis (IPD) was introduced in four children after 14 to 31 months of CAPD. Two patients (No. 7, 8) were switched to intermittent cycling peritoneal dialysis (ICPD) using an automatic cycler system (AMP 80/2) during the night after 21 and 31 months of CAPD respectively. The daytime dwell was discontinued by eliminating the instillation of fluid in the peritoneum during this period. Two other children (No. 6 + 9) were switched to intermittent ambulatory peritoneal dialysis (IAPD) using standard bags during the day and instilling no fluid during the night period after 14 and 23 months of CAPD respectively. The solutions used were commercially available dialysis solutions containing lactate. Dialysate volumes were 35–50 ml/kg BW/cycle with three to five exchanges performed daily.

Peritoneal effluent was measured daily, and ultrafiltration was calculated from the difference between the peritoneal dialysate inflow and the peritoneal dialysate outflow. Ultrafiltration is expressed as ml/kg BW/day. Negative ultrafiltration indicates net fluid transfer of fluid from dialysate to blood. Ultrafiltration was studied in 11 patients (Table 1), of which nine patients used Fresenius solution (No. 1–9) and two used a Travenol solution (No. 9 and 10). The glucose, urea, and creatinine content of the dialysate effluent during a 24-hour period was measured monthly.

Peritoneal biopsy specimens were obtained from seven children: at the time of catheter removal in six of these patients and during laparotomy for bowel obstruction 9 months after transfer to hemodialysis in one patient. Formaldehyde fixation was used. Samples were embedded in paraffin and 4 μm sections were examined after staining with hematoxylin-eosin, Masson's trichromic stain, PAS, and Orcein.

Results

Ultrafiltration Data

Table 1 summarizes the ultrafiltration characteristics of the 11 patients. The peritoneal ultrafiltration capacity (PFUC) of each patient decreased progressively with time. The mean initial PFUC using a 1.5% glucose dialysate solution was 15.5 ml/kg BW/day (range, 26.3 to 6 ml/kg BW/day). The PFUC dropped to a mean of −2.4 ml/kg BW/day (range, 7.8 to −14.5 ml/kg BW/day).

Five children had negative ultrafiltration which varied from −4.3 to −14.5 ml/kg BW/day. The duration of peritoneal dialysis at the time of negative ultrafiltration was 1.5–25 months. As shown on Table 1, there was no significant correlation between the loss of ultrafiltration, the age at initiation of CAPD, the duration of CAPD, the occurrence of peritonitis, and the use of 4.25% glucose dialysate solutions. Only one of the five patients with negative ultrafiltration had had a peritonitis episode and in four patients, glucose dialysate solutions with a concentration of 1.5% were used.

The glucose concentration in the dialysate effluent accumulated for the 24-hour period decreased from 24.9 mmol/l to 11.8 mmol/l within 6–23 months of CAPD for these six children. The increased glucose absorption from dialysate was correlated with the loss of ultrafiltration.

Despite the loss of ultrafiltration, there was no significant reduction in the creatinine clearance (mean 4.55 ml/min/1.73 m²; range, 2.4–6.2 ml/min/1.73 m²) or the urea clearance (mean 4.94 ml/min/1.73 m²; range, 2.4–7.7 ml/min/1.73 m²).

In four children (No. 6–9), the PFUC increased following initiation of IAPD or ICPD (Table 2). The mean PFUC rose from −3.75 ml/kg BW/day to + 5 ml/kg BW/day within 1 month. In these patients, the mean peritoneal dialysate dwell time per exchange was reduced from a mean of 7 hours to a mean of 3.8 hours. The glucose concentration in the effluent increased from 11.8 mmol/l to 19.6 mmol/l. IAPD and ICPD were continued for 6–14 months, and the PFUC remained stable after the initial increase (Figs. 1 and 2).

Table 1. Ultrafiltration data

Patients	Age at initiation of CAPD (years)	Duration of peritoneal dialysis (months)	PFUC. (ml/kg BW/day)		Duration of PD before negative ultrafiltration (months)	Use of hyperosmolar solutions	Peritonitis episodes
			maximum	minimum			
1	13	14	18.5	2.5		+	+
2	5	11	14.5	2.5		+	–
3	3	15	26.3	7.8		+	+
4	6	9	14.5	1.8		+	–
5	2.5	31	23	–14.5	19	+	–
6	10	20	11.5	–13	3	–	–
7	16	34	18.5	1.5		–	–
8	13	39	9.2	–8.5	25	–	–
9	17	26	17	5		–	–
10	13.5	6	6	–7.6	1.5	–	–
11	17	6	17	–4.3	4.5	–	+
Mean		19	15.5	–2.4			

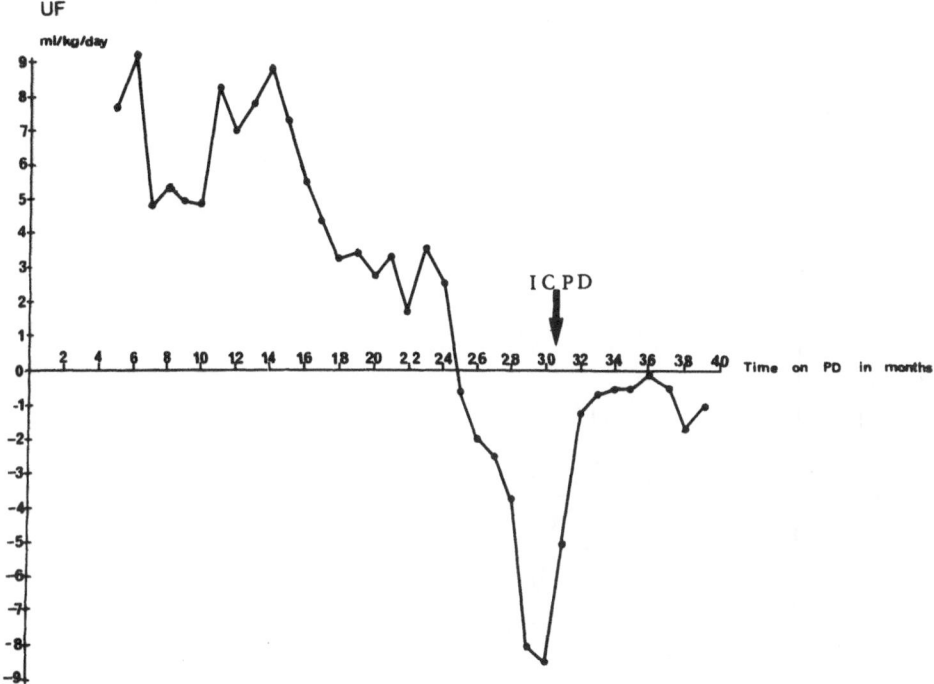

Fig. 1. Evolution of peritoneal ultrafiltration capacity *UF* during CAPD and effects of *ICPD* in patient 8

Table 2. Effects of IAPD or ICPD on ultrafiltration

Patients	Mean dwell time (hours)		PFUC ml/kg BW/day	
	CAPD	IAPD/ICPD	CAPD before onset of IAPD/ICPD	IAPD/ICPD
6	8.0	5.0	−13.0	−2.0
7	6.25	2.75	1.5	12.5
8	5.85	2.5	−8.5	0
9	8.15	5.0	5.0	10
Mean	7.0	3.8	−3.75	5.0

Peritoneal Biopsies

Peritoneal biopsy specimens were obtained in seven children after 12–34 months of peritoneal dialysis. Samples were obtained from the parietal peritoneum in seven patients, from the omentum in one, from the hepatic capsule in one, and from the appendix, the Meckel's diverticulum, and the mesenteric peritoneum in one patient who had undergone laparotomy for bowel obstruction.

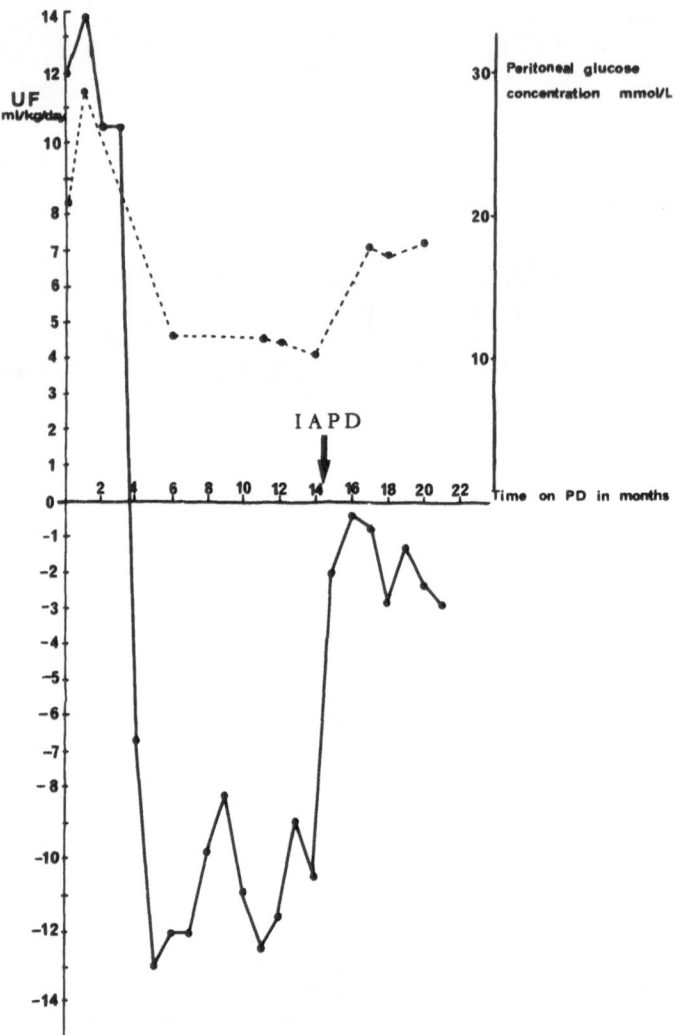

Fig. 2. Evolution of PFUC and glucose concentration in the effluent on CAPD and effects of *IAPD* in patient 6. The *solid line* indicates ultrafiltration (*UF*); the *broken line* indicates peritoneal glucose concentration

In three patients, microscopic examination showed focal mesothelial denudation with marked infiltration of inflammatory cells which included neutrophils. These inflammatory cells predominanted around blood vessels and the submesothelial area. Fibrin exsudates were also seen. The peritoneum was thickened due to the presence of fibroconnective tissue. Moderate hyaline and sclerotic thickening of arteriocapillary walls was observed in vessels located in the submesothelial fibrous tissue in two patients.

In three patients, no inflammatory cells were present, and the main findings were fibrous peritoneal thickening, severe vascular changes, and focal mesothelial denudation. In two patients, histologic examination showed progressive fibrous organization of fibrin exsudates. In all four patients, the vascular changes involved arteries and capillaries in the submucosal area, which consisted of marked thickening of the vascular walls with fibrosis and hyaline deposits leading at times to complete obstruction of the vascular lumen.

One patient had signs of bowel obstruction 6 months after catheter removal. At laparotomy, the mesentery was retracted, and the peritoneal surface was opaque and markedly thickened. The fibrous tissue was lysed and the bowel liberated. The appendix and the Meckel's diverticulum were removed. On light microscopy, the submesothelial tissue was strikingly thickened and sclerotic. Irregular sclerotic involvement of the intestinal muscular layers was observed, with patchy disappearance of the external and, less frequently, of the intestinal layers of the muscular coat. Severe vascular lesions were present in the serosa, but the vessels in the lamina propria and the submucosal region were normal.

Discussion

Several reports have described a loss of ultrafiltration in patients undergoing CAPD [5–8, 10]. In early reports, loss of ultrafiltration was defined as the inability to reach dry weight despite the use of hypertonic dialysate solutions [8]. Recently, an international cooperative study [7] was undertaken in order to determine the incidence of reduced ultrafiltration. The protocol consisted of a 2-liter hypertonic (4.25% glucose) exchange. The effluent was weighed and the glucose concentration measured. The study concluded that patients using acetate had significantly lower ultrafiltration values when compared with those using lactate. In patients using lactate only, ultrafiltration remained stable with time. There was no significant correlation between the loss of ultrafiltration and the rate of peritonitis or the duration of CAPD.

In our study, the definition of loss of ultrafiltration was different. UF was calculated from the difference between peritoneal inflow and peritoneal outflow values using 1.5% glucose solution. We observed a loss of ultrafiltration in all patients undergoing CAPD. The age of the patients at initiation of CAPD, the duration of treatment, the number of episodes of peritonitis, or the use of hypertonic dialysate solutions were not related to the loss of ultrafiltration. In all patients, we observed a decrease in glucose concentration in the effluent dialysate. Rapid glucose absorption reduces the osmolality in the dialysate and thus decreases the period of time during which an adequate osmotic gradient exists to promote transfer of water. The use of hypertonic solutions allowed adequate ultrafiltration in one patient, but only for a short period of time (Fig. 3). It is of interest that all our patients were treated with lactate-containing solutions. However, it should be noted that at the initiation of CAPD, all patients were treated with acetate-buffered solutions during machine dialysis for 6–10 days. Other factors which may be responsible for the loss of ultrafiltration include the pH or buffer capacity of the solutions, the presence of particulate matter, or the sterilizing substances used [11].

Peritoneal biopsies were performed in seven children. The submesothelial area was moderately thickened in three patients, and was characterized by the presence

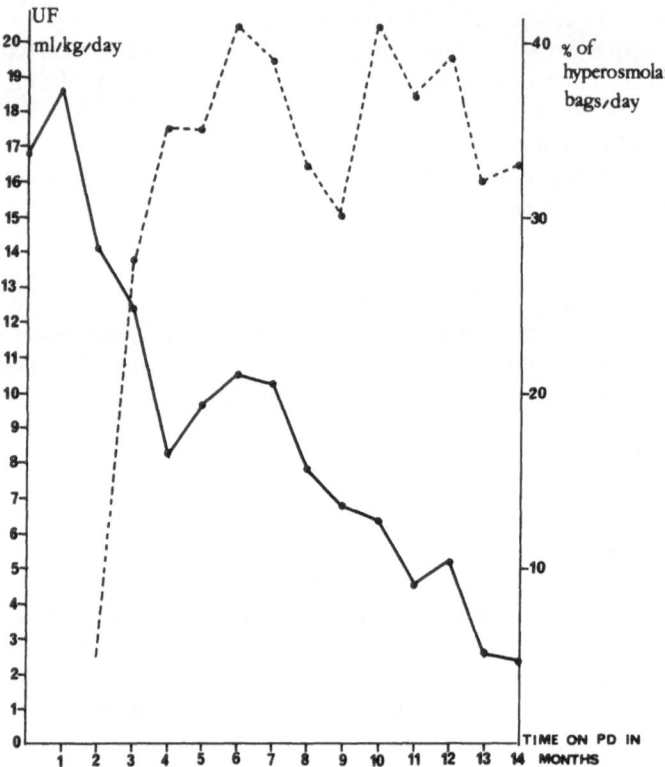

Fig. 3. Evolution of PFUC with the use of 4.25% glucose solutions in patient. 1. The *solid line* indicates ultrafiltration (*UF*); the *broken line* indicates percentage of hyperosmolar used bags per day

of inflammatory cells. In four patients, the peritoneum was markedly thickened with a proliferation of fibroconnective tissue. The vessels in the submesothelial area showed lesions of hyalinosis, sclerosis, and sometimes obstruction. The etiology of these membrane changes is unknown [12]. During acute peritonitis, mesothelial denudation and numerous leukocytes on the peritoneal surface are present [13]. Prolonged peritonitis may result in fibrosis of the submesothelial area. However, in our study, peritoneal changes were present even in the absence of peritonitis epidoses.

Two major questions are whether the minor histologic alterations detected by systematic peritoneal biopsies can progress to encapsulating peritoneal sclerosis and whether these alterations are reversible upon cessation of peritoneal dialysis. There are no definite answers to these questions. However, one of our patients developed intestinal obstruction 6 months after cessation of CAPD, and the macroscopic and histologic findings were compatible with encapsulating peritoneal sclerosis. Several factors may be responsible for structural alterations of the peritoneum. Peritonitis episodes have been incriminated, but several of our patients did not experience this complication. The deposit of foreign material from plastic bags or the use of hy-

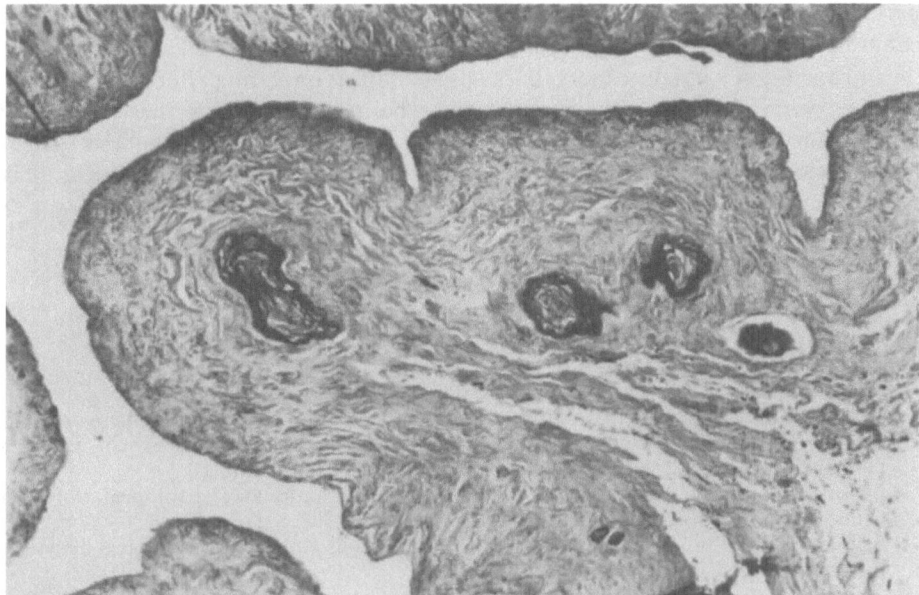

Fig. 4. Section of the omentum in patient 8. Thickening of the peritoneum by a dense connective tissue without any cell infiltrate. Severe hyalinosis leading to obstruction of vessels (PAS, × 160)

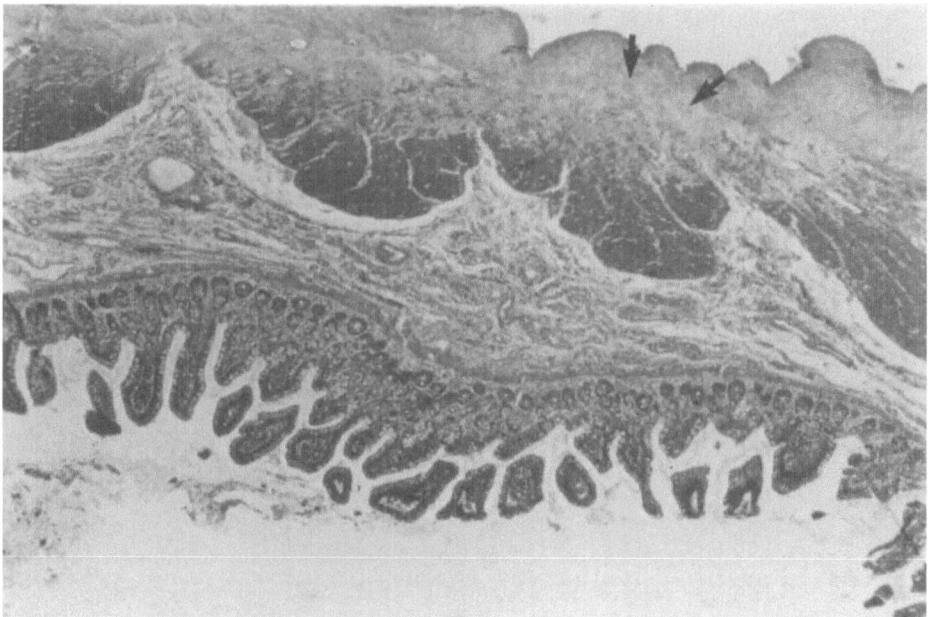

Fig. 5. Section of Meckel's diverticulum in patient 1. Thickening and sclerosis of the visceral peritoneum. Sclerosis of the outer layer of the muscular wall. Arrows indicate thickening of blood vessels in the serosa. Normal blood vessels in the submucosa and in the lamina propria (Trichrom high green, × 60)

pertonic solutions may be involved. It is not likely that the catheter plays a significant role since the peritoneal lesions are diffuse.

In conclusion we have observed loss of ultrafiltration in all children treated with CAPD. Peritoneal histologic changes may be responsible for the reduced ultrafiltration. The long-term evolution of these alterations is unknown, and patients may develop encapsulating peritonitis months after discontaining peritoneal dialysis.

References

1. Alexander SR (1983) Pediatric CAPD update 1983. Perit Dial Bull 3:15–22
2. Balfe JW, Irwin MA (1980) Continuous ambulatory peritoneal dialysis in pediatrics. In: Legrain M (ed) Continuous ambulatory peritoneal dialysis: proceedings of an international symposium, 2–3 Nov 1980. Excerpta Medica, Amsterdam
3. Baum M, Powell D, Calvin S et al. (1982) Continuous ambulatory peritoneal dialysis in children: Comparison with hemodialysis. N Engl J Med 307:1537–1542
4. Salusky IB, Lucullo L, Nelson P et al. (1982) Continuous ambulatory peritoneal dialysis in children Pediatr Clin North Am 29:1005–1012
5. Ariefie M (1983) Failure of ultrafiltration in patients on CAPD. Perit Dial Bull 3:38–40
6. Faller B (1984) Loss of ultrafiltration in continuous ambulatory peritoneal dialysis: a role for acetate Perit Dial Bull 4:10–13
7. First report of an international cooperative study (1984) Factors affecting ultrafiltration in continuous ambulatory peritoneal dialysis. Perit Dial Bull 4:14–19
8. Slingeneyer A, Canaud B, Mion C (1983) Permanent loss of ultrafiltration capacity of the peritoneum in long term peritoneal dialysis: An epidemiological study. Nephron 33:133–138
9. Gandhi VC, Humayum HM, Ing TS et al. (1980) Sclerotic thickening of the peritoneal membrane in maintenance peritoneal dialysis patients. Arch Intern Med 140:1201–1203
10. Wolfish NM (1983) Loss of ultrafiltration capacity in children. Nephron 35:277–278
11. Oreopoulos DG (1983) Peritoneal membrane: Handle with care Perit Dial Bull 3:111–113
12. Verger C, Brunschvicg O, Le Charpentier Y, Lavergne A, Vantelon J (1981) Structural and ultrastructural peritoneal membrane changes and permeability alterations during CAPD. Proc Eur Dial Transplant Assoc 18:199–203
13. Verger C, Luger A, Moore H, Nolph KD (1983) Acute changes in peritoneal morphology and transport properties with infectious peritonitis and mechanical injury. Kidney Int 23:823–831

Sclerosing Peritonitis in Patients Treated by CAPD

J. Rottembourg, B. Issad, P. Langlois, P. Y. Cossette, A. Boudjemaa, H. Mehamha, U. Assogba, and G. M. Gahl

Introduction

Since 1977, continuous ambulatory peritoneal dialysis (CAPD) has been proposed as an effective maintenance therapy for patients with end-stage renal disease. Despite encouraging results [1], recurrent peritonitis represents a major cause of treatment failure [2] and a limitation to the expansion of the technique [1]. Among severe abdominal complications observed in patients on CAPD [3, 4], sclerosing peritonitis (SP) is a major problem. This report deals with 12 patients observed over a 5-year period and concentrates on the analysis of the risk factors involved in the genesis of this syndrome which have emerged from the literature and our own personal data.

Patients and Methods

The Population at Risk

Between August 1978 and October 1983, 163 patients (104 males and 59 females) were trained to perform CAPD in a specialized unit of the Department of Nephrology. The mean age was 61.7 ± 16.6 years, with a range of 17–83 years. At start of treatment, 65 patients were older than 65 years, and 41 were insulin-dependent diabetic patients.

Cumulative duration of treatment was 237 patient-years, with a mean period on CAPD of 1.5 years (range, 1–56 months). In October 1983, 59 patients were still on CAPD, 39 had been transferred to hemodialysis, 3 had received a kidney transplant, 3 had recovered renal function, and 59 had died while still on CAPD or within 3 months after transfer to hemodialysis (HD).

Technical Procedure

CAPD was conducted through a double-cuff Tenckhoff catheter, with a preference for the curled type. Most patients performed four exchanges a day; the usual sequence involved three 2-liter bags with a dialysate solution of 1.5% dextrose concentration during the day and one 2-liter bag containing a solution of 4–4.5% dextrose concentration overnight. Most diabetics used intraperitoneal insulin injected into the line four times a day when the bag was changed. Heparin injection (2500 units) was preferred to prevent fibrin formation.

Dialysate from four different sources was used. A total of 65 patients were treated over a period of 1430 patient months with a dialysate from Assistance Publique de Paris; 36 patients were treated during 450 patient months with a dialysate from Aguettant Laboratories, Lyon; 38 patients used a dialysate from Travenol Lab, Deerfield, USA, for 650 patient months; and eight patients were treated for 120 patient months with a dialysate from Fresenius Lab, West Germany. Another 16 patients were successively dialyzed with fluids from different sources. Polyvinyl chloride (PVC) was used to prepare the bags by means of various techniques. The different dialysates were almost identical in composition, except for the buffer: sodium acetate was used in the dialysates from Assistance Publique and Aguettant, and sodium lactate was used in the dialysate from Travenol and Fresenius. The buffer concentration was uniform: 35 mmol/l.

All peritonitis episodes were treated by intrapertioneal administration of antibiotics. Continuous lavage was the preferred treatment until May 1981, with continuation of CAPD procedure since October 1981.

Results

Patients with Sclerosing Peritonitis (SP)

On the patients observed, 12 patients (six males and six females) developed SP, meaning there was an incidence of one case per 16.6 patient years (Table 1). The mean age of the patients at the start of CAPD was 57 ± 12 years. Primary renal disease was caused by glomerulonephritis in seven cases and diabetic nephropathy in two cases, with one case each of interstitial nephropathy, polycystic kidney disease, and nephropathy of unknown origin.

The diagnosis of SP was made in nine patients while they were still undergoing CAPD, and in three patients, the diagnosis was made 9, 12, and 15 months after transfer to HD because of recurrent peritonitis and malnutrition (cases 4, 7, and 10 respectively). The clinical symptoms observed before anatomical confirmation of SP included a decrease in ultrafiltration for seven patients and recurrent abdominal pain with anorexia, nausea and vomiting in nine patients, which led to severe malnutrition in seven of these patients. Intermittent subocclusive episodes were observed in eight patients. Delay between the first clinical symptom and anatomical confirmation varied from 1 to 15 months. Major signs following a barium x-ray study were haustration of the ileum and fixed and rigid bowel loops with ineffective peristaltic contractions. Diagnosis was anatomically confirmed in all cases. In six cases, the lesions were observed during an attempt to replace a catheter. Space for cleavage was not found, and the catheter was not replaced. In five cases, the diagnosis was confirmed during a surgical procedure for acute bowel obstruction. In the last case, the diagnosis was an autopsy finding; death was attributable to an acute bowel obstruction.

Anatomical Lesions

The macroscopic findings observed were similar for all cases: the peritoneum was opaque, thickened, and sclerotic; the small bowel was either partly or entirely en-

Table 1. Patient characteristics and course of sclerosing peritonitis

Patient	Sex	Age	Renal disease	CAPD (months)	Buffer dialysate	Episodes of peritonitis (n)	Mode of diagnosis	Treatment on HD (months)	outcome
1	F	32	PN	22	Acetate	3	Catheter replacement	36	Alive on HD
2	F	64	GN	42	Acetate	6	Catheter replacement	1	Dead on HD
3	M	49	DN	37	Acetate Lactate	9	Catheter replacement	15	Alive on HD
4	F	58	GN	16	Acetate	3	Surgery for bowel obstruction	15	Dead on HD
5	F	70	PKD	7	Acetate	3	Surgery for bowel obstruction	6	Dead on HD
6	M	44	GN	14	Acetate	1	Catheter replacement	12	Alive on HD
7	M	72	GN	13	Lactate Acetate	2	Surgery for bowel obstruction	1	Dead on HD
8	M	60	DN	31	Acetate	5	Catheter replacement	11	Alive on HD
9	F	50	unknown	10	Acetate	2	Autopsy	–	Dead on CAPD
10	M	74	GN	17	Acetate	7	Surgery for bowel obstruction	17	Dead on HD
11	F	57	GN	36	Acetate	2	Surgery for bowel obstruction	3	Dead on HD
12	M	54	GN	27	Acetate	3	Catheter replacement	4	Alive on HD

F, female; M, male; HD, hemodialysis; GN, glomerulonephritis; DN, diabetic nephropathy; PKD, polycystic kidney disease; PN, pyelonephritis closed in a bag made of a thickened peritoneum. In four cases, the colon was free, but the root of the mesentery was sclerotic and retracted. In six cases, numerous fibrous adhesions were encountered.

Histologic examination showed a marked and diffuse thickening of the peritoneum due to the proliferation of the connective tissue and an infiltration with mostly mononuclear inflammatory cells. The mesothelial layer was disrupted or absent.

Clinical Course after Diagnosis

All patients except case 9, who died while on CAPD, were transfered to HD. Six patients died, 1 to 17 months after transfer to HD. All deaths were attributable to the sclerosing process. Four patients required recurrent laparotomies for bowel obstruction. Five patients are still alive after 5 to 33 months on HD, three without any clinical symptoms, two with minor abdominal problems.

Potential Risk Factors

The following risk factors were analyzed: time on dialysis, dialysate composition, peritonitis episodes and treatment, drug administration, and composition of the dialysate bags.

Dialysate Buffer

Ten patients with SP were exclusively dialysed with fluid containing acetate buffer. Two other patients received successively dialysate containing both acetate and lactate buffer. Until now, SP has never been observed in patients dialysed exclusively with lactate-buffered dialysate.

Duration of Treatment by Dialysis

The mean duration of CAPD treatment for the 12 patients with SP was 22.6 ± 11.6 months. Five patients were dialyzed for more than 2 years, of whom three continued CAPD treatment for more than 3 years, while only two patients were dialyzed for less than 1 year. The incidence of SP appears to increase with time and may reach a rate of 20%, if the three out of 15 patients dialyzed for at least 3 years are considered.

Peritonitis: Rate, Etiology, and Treatment

A total of 46 episodes were observed in the 12 cases during the period of observation. The rate was more frequent in the group with SP: one every 6 patient months.

In the entire population, the incidence was one every 10 patient months. The organisms grown from the peritoneal fluid were Gram-positive in 34 episodes, Gram-negative in eight episodes, and in one case proved to be a fungus. Cultures were negative in three episodes. In 8 patients, 20 episodes were treated by means of intraperitoneal administration of co-trimoxazole for an average of 9 days. Another 14 episodes were treated with a combination of Cephalothin and Tobramycin. Other antibiotics were required to treat 12 other episodes. In ten patients, 21 episodes were treated by lavage with 24–36 liters of acetate-buffered dialysate using a cycler. The mean duration of lavage was 3.8 ± 1.2 days. A prolonged lavage was performed in three cases (cases 3, 7, and 8). Another 18 episodes of peritonitis occurring in seven patients were not treated by lavage.

The PVC Bags

Bags furnished by Assistance Publique and Fresenius were manufactured by the same firm in tubular form. Travenol and Aguettant provided bags they had manufactured themselves. Substances added to the PVC used in the different types of bags varied, as did the sterilization process.

Drugs

Routine treatment of the patients with SP included the prolonged intraperitoneal administration of heparin, which the addition of insulin for the diabetic patients. The patients also received oral Furosemide, Clonidine, α-methyldopa, dihydralazine, antiangorous drugs, digitalis, thyroxine, calcium salts, vitamin D derivates, and aluminium-containing phosphate binders. Eight patients with SP received acebutolol for an extended period of time. Propanolol was given to some patients for a short period of time. Four patients received no betablockers. In the control group, 122 out of 151 patients (81%) were treated with betablockers.

Discussion

The peritoneal membrane is a delicate structure composed of capillary interstitial tissue and a simple layer of mesothelial cells which is definitely not designed for peritoneal dialysis [5, 6]. Sclerosing encapsulating peritonitis is a distressing abdominal complication that can occur as a result of either intermittent peritoneal dialysis [3, 7] or CAPD [9, 10]. The disease can progress slowly or remain asymtomatic for a long period of time. The first symptoms may occur several months or even years after transfer of the patient to HD or transplantation [3].

Clinical symptoms are directly related to abnormalities of gastrointestinal transit. The most common complaints are abdominal pain, nausea, vomiting, and partial or intermittent bowel obstruction. Acute episodes of more or less complete intestinal obstruction may require emergency surgery. The modification of the peritoneal membrane can induce a decrease in the ultrafiltration rate, while peritoneal clearances remain unchanged. The severity of SP should be emphasized: out of 34 cases reported in the literature [3, 4, 9–12], 17 died rapidly, mostly of sepsis and malnutrition after a surgical procedure indicated because of bowel obstruction.

The factors involved in the genesis of SP are not clearly defined. *Infection* should be considered as a major risk factor, and thickening of the peritoneum may develop secondary to recurrent inflammation of the peritoneum [3]. Patients with SP suffer more episodes of peritonitis than other patients, but SP may develop despite a very low rate of peritoneal infection. After comparing the various modes of treatment for peritonitis, we were unable to detect any connection between the development of SP and the intraperitoneal administration of antibiotics. Peritoneal lavage using a cycler and a dialysate with an acetate buffer had been used in all cases of SP. These risk factors should be avoided.

The origin and the composition of the dialysis fluid may play a major role. All the patients with SP we studied had been treated with dialysate containing an acetate buffer. No similar complication was observed when lactate solutions were used. However, new cases of SP have recently been reported with the use of dialysate containing a lactate buffer prepared by Fresenius.

Further research should look for factors related to the composition of *dialysate* and the *containers.* The rare cases reported in which lactate-buffered solutions were used have occurred in patients using plastic bags from Fresenius. This company and Assistance Publique receive the plastizer used to make the bags from the same company.

SP has been reported among patients receiving various *betablockers,* including practolol, propanolol, oxprenolol, atenolol, and metoprolol [3]. Treatment with betablockers was routinely prescribed among our patients during the early phase of dialysis. However, the proportion of patients who subsequently developed SP remained the same in our population.

SP is a dramatic complication which can jeopardize the long-term efficacy of maintenance CAPD. The large discrepancy in the number of cases observed in different countries suggests that various risk factors are involved in the genesis of SP. Careful retrospective and prospective analysis should facilitate detection and permit delineation of the cause of the disease. Preventive measures can then be devised. At present, a reasonable approach is to avoid the use of acetate solution and to reduce as much as possible the indications of peritoneal lavage. More precise knowledge about containers is imperative.

References

1. Williams CC and the University of Toronto Collaborative Dialysis group (1983) CAPD – an overview. Perit Dial Bull 3 (suppl):6–8
2. Rottembourg J, Jacq D, Singlas E et al. (1980) Medical management of peritonitis in continuous ambulatory peritoneal dialysis. In: Legrain M (ed) Continuous ambulatory peritoneal dialysis, Proceedings of an international symposium, Paris. Excerpta Medica, Amsterdam, pp 248–257

3. Slingeneyer A, Canaud B, Mourad G et al. (1983) Progressive sclerosing peritonitis: a late and severe complication of maintenance peritoneal dialysis. Trans Am Soc Artif Intern Organs 29:633–640
4. Rottembourg J, Gahl GM, Poignet JL et al. (1983) Severe abdominal complications in patients undergoing continuous ambulatory peritoneal dialysis. Proc Eur Dial Transplant Assoc 20:236–242
5. Verger C, Brunschvig O, Le Charpentier Y et al. (1981) Structural and ultrastructural peritoneal membrane changes and permeability alterations during CAPD. Proc Eur Dial Transplant Assoc 18:199–203
6. Oreopoulos DG (1983) Peritoneal membrane: handle with care. Perit Dial Bull 3:111–112
7. Gandhi VC, Humayun HM, Inig TS et al. (1980) Sclerotic thickening of the peritoneal membrane in maintenance peritoneal dialysis patients. Arch Intern Med 140:1201–1203
8. Bradley JA, MacWhinnie DL, Hamilton et al. (1983) Sclerosing obstructive peritonitis after continuous ambulatory peritoneal dialysis. Lancet 2:113–114
9. Oreopoulos DG, Khanna R, Wu G (1983) Sclerosing obstructive peritonitis after CAPD. Lancet 2:409
10. Denis J, Paineau J, Potel G et al. (1980) Continuous ambulatory peritoneal dialysis. Ann Intern Med 93:508
11. Hauglustaine D, Monballyu J, Van Meerbeek J et al. (1983) Sclerosing obstructive peritonitis, betablockers and continuous ambulatory peritoneal dialysis. Lancet 2:734
12. Marigold JH, Pounder RE, Pemberton J et al. (1982) Propanolol, oxprenolol and sclerosing peritonitis. Br Med J 284:870

Five Years' Experience with CAPD/CCPD Catheters in Infants and Children

S. R. Alexander, E. S. Tank, and A. T. Corneil

Introduction

A reliable catheter is the cornerstone of successful chronic peritoneal dialysis. As continuous ambulatory peritoneal dialysis (CAPD), and more recently, continuous cycler peritoneal dialysis (CCPD), have evolved as effective treatments for infants and children with irreversible renal failure, so have techniques for peritoneal catheter placement in these young patients. In this report, we review our experience with 50 consecutive peritoneal dialysis catheters placed in 27 pediatric CAPD/CCPD patients during the first 5 years of our program.

Patients and Methods

Patient Population

Between February 8, 1979 and February 10, 1984, we surgically placed 50 peritoneal dialysis catheters in 27 pediatric CAPD/CCPD patients whose ages ranged from 12 days to 17 years (mean, 8.5 ± 5.3 SD years) and whose weights at the onset of peritoneal dialysis ranged from 2.5–60 kg. There were eight girls and 19 boys. One child who received a renal transplant and then returned to CAPD when the graft was rejected 1 year later was considered in this report as two different patients. As of June 20, 1984, uninterrupted time on peritoneal dialysis for these children ranged from 4 to 61 months (mean, 24.9 ± 16.7 SD months). Patients in our program whose catheters had been placed at other centers were not included in this study.

During the study period, which continued for 5 years and 4 months, two patients died, four were transferred to hemodialysis, one of whom died shortly thereafter, one was transferred to another center, and six underwent successful renal transplantation.

Catheters

Table 1 lists the catheters used during the study period by catheter type. Choice of catheter type was not made randomly, but occurred longitudinally as our experience evolved. Initially, we used adult-sized, straight, 2-cuff Tenckhoff catheters (T-2) [1], gluing the cuffs ourselves 12–24 h prior to catheter placement and trimming the intraperitoneal portion of the catheter intraoperatively to fit the individual child. A to-

Table 1. Pediatric CAPD/CCPD catheters

Catheter type	Catheters used (n)	Patients (n)	Dates of placement	Total experience[a] (months)
T-2	19	11	2/79 – 6/81	296.1
T-1	7	7	7/81 – 3/82	123.1
C-1	24	24	4/82 – 2/84	252.5
	50			671.7

T-2, Tenckhoff, straight, 2-cuffs; T-1, Tenckhoff, straight, 1-cuff; C-1, curled, 1-cuff
[a] 8 Feb 1979 – 20 June 1984.

tal of 19 such catheters were placed in 11 patients during the first 2.3 years of our program. Early experience with these catheters has been reported previously [2].

After observing the development of tunnel infections requiring catheter replacement in six of the 11 patients with T-2 catheters, we became concerned that the superficial cuff might be playing a role in the acquisition of these infections, as a result of trauma to the skin overlying the cuff and/or erosion of the cuff through the skin at the exit site. Several early T-2 catheters were placed with only 0.5 cm separating the superficial cuff from the exit site, thus predisposing them to cuff erosion.

Because of these concerns, in 1981 we began using adult-sized, straight, 1-cuff, Tenckhoff catheters (T-1), the cuff placed at the peritoneum, with a short (4–6 cm) subcutaneous tunnel. The cuff was glued by the manufacturer at a point 3.0 cm away from the first catheter fenestrations. Seven T-1 catheters were placed in seven patients during 1981 and 1982.

Early in our experience with straight Tenckhoff catheters, we noted that some children complained of localized pelvic pain during infusion of dialysate through their recently placed T-1 or T-2 catheters. This pain usually decreased when the infusion rate was slowed, and the pain gradually resolved over the first few weeks of CAPD. We presumed that infusion pain was caused by a forceful jet of dialysate repeatedly striking the same peritoneal surface, perhaps because the intraperitoneal catheter segment was too long. In one child who was experiencing localized infusion pain, the T-1 catheter became obstructed after migration under the liver. These problems prompted us to abandon the T-1 catheter in April, 1982 in favor of a modified, adult-sized, curled, 1-cuff Tenckhoff (or "Palmer") catheter (C-1) [3] for all subsequent patients weighing more than 5 kg. The use of this catheter configuration in adult CAPD patients has been described recently [4].

The location of the single cuff on the curled catheter posed a problem when attempting to use it in children of different sizes. We chose to have the cuff glued by the manufacturer at a point either 5.0 or 8.5 cm away from the onset of fenestrations in the curled intraperitoneal portion of the C-1 catheter (Fig. 1a). These relatively short cuff-to-fenestration distances resulted in a catheter which began curling almost immediately upon entry into the peritoneal cavity and which then lay flat in a very superficial position in the center of the abdomen, anterior to the peritoneal contents

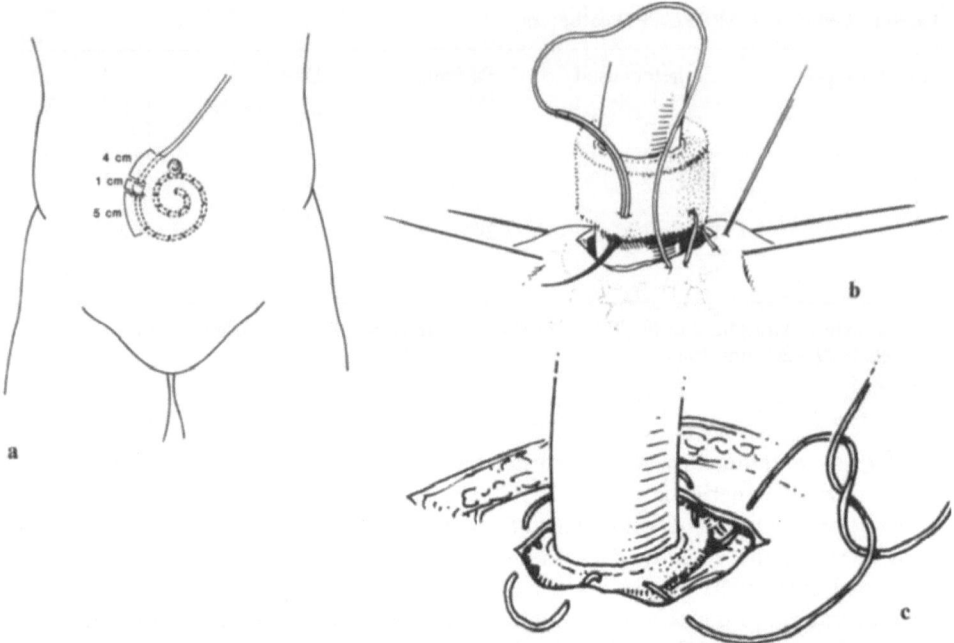

Fig. 1. a Technique for placement of the curled Tenckhoff catheter in a young child. A 4-cm subcutaneous tunnel is shown directed medially. Lateral direction of the tunnel is also acceptable (see *Fig. 2a*). The 1-cm cuff is depicted sutured at the point of entry into the peritoneal cavity. Catheter fenestrations begin 5-cm below the cuff. **b** Attachment of the base of the cuff to the peritoneum with a nonabsorbable purse string suture. **c** Closure of the anterior rectus sheath incorporating the top of the cuff. Details of surgical technique are outlined in text

(Fig. 2a, b). During the period of this study, 24 C-1 catheters were placed in 17 patients (Table 1).

All 50 catheters were constructed of silastic rubber which had been made either totally or partially radiopaque by impregnation with barium sulfate. Only dacron felt cuffs were used. All catheters were supplied by a single manufacturer (Quinton Instrument Company, Seattle, Washington 98121).

Surgical Technique

All catheters were placed by open technique in the operating room by a team of different surgical residents who on all but four occasions were directed by one of the authors (EST). Variations in surgical technique and approach were minimal. When the first two catheters in this series developed persistent leakage at the peritoneal entry site, the placement technique was modified to include incorporation of the deep cuff in a permanent peritoneal purse-string suture. Early catheters had a midline, subumbilical, peritoneal entry site; this was later changed to a position beneath the body of the rectus muscle. In all other important aspects, the surgical technique used in this series was essentially the same as our current approach to catheter placement, of which a description follows:

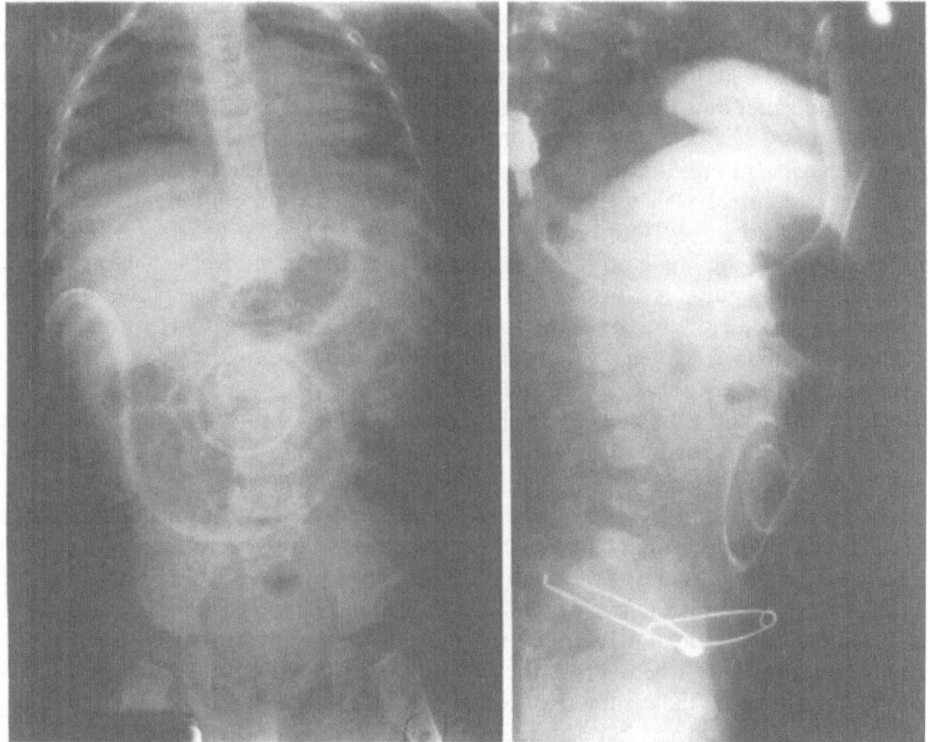

a   b

Fig. 2. a Supine abdominal radiograph showing a curled Tenckhoff catheter in place in an 8-kg infant. The intraperitoneal catheter curl rides higher in the abdomen as a result of the lateral direction of the subcutaneous tunnel. **b** Lateral abdominal radiograph of the same infant showing the desired anterior position of the curled catheter, superficial to the peritoneal contents

The catheter, catheter entry site, and course of the subcutaneous tunnel are chosen preoperatively, avoiding old surgical scars as much as possible and attempting to keep the proposed tunnel either completely above or completely below the level at which the older child wears his/her belt.

We currently use the C-1 catheter with the shorter (5.0 cm) cuff-to-fenestration distance for patients weighing from 5 kg to about 12 kg, and the slightly more distal cuff placement (8.5 cm) in larger patients, but this difference is probably unimportant. Infants weighing less than 5 kg are too small for the only size curled catheter available (our smallest C-1 patient weighed 6 kg); for infants weighing less than about 5 kg, we recommend a trimmed T-1 catheter (our smallest T-1 CAPD patient weighed 2.5 kg). For acute dialysis in even smaller premature infants, we have used a pediatric-sized, straight, 1-cuff Tenckhoff catheter, the cuff of which is only 0.6 cm wide and glued at a point 2.5 cm away from the onset of catheter fenestrations [5]; we would recommend this catheter also for chronic dialysis in these tiny infants.

The operative procedure begins with a 2–4 cm-incision made horizontally over the midportion of the rectus muscle near the level of the umbilicus. This incision may be made somewhat lower in older children and adolescents, depending on the child's belt line. The anterior rectus sheath is incised, and the rectus muscle is separated bluntly. The peritoneum is exposed, fixed by two temporary sutures, and then incised. Digital examination assures that no bowel is adherent to the peritoneum. The small patch of omental tissue which is readily available through the incision is then excised, thus clearing the path of the catheter. The curled catheter is threaded over a long, lubricated catheter guide and then inserted just beneath the anterior abdominal wall to a point in the midline, several centimeters below the level of the entry site. Holding the catheter guide in this position, the catheter is gently eased off the guide until the catheter cuff reaches the level of the incision, at which point the guide is removed. As the catheter slides off of the guide, it will assume the coiled configuration it had prior to placement; care is taken to ensure that the coil lies flat on a plane anterior to the abdominal contents (Fig. 2b), thereby avoiding entanglement with omentum or loops of bowel.

The peritoneum is now closed. A purse string of nonabsorbable suture is placed in the peritoneum surrounding the catheter with the suture being passed through the substance of the cuff at its lowest point in several places (Fig. 1b). When secured, this suture pulls a collar of peritoneum around the base of the cuff, creating a near watertight seal and anchoring the catheter in position. A similar purse string suture is then used to close the anterior rectus sheath and fix it to the upper aspect of the cuff in the same manner (Fig. 1c). At this point, about 15 cc/kg of dialysate is infused and then immediately drained. If the closure is tight and the dialysate leaves the peritoneal cavity freely, the catheter is felt to be in good functional position. If outflow is not brisk, the catheter is flushed, and if drainage is still not improved, the catheter is removed and repositioned. In our experience, catheters which drain poorly in the operating room rarely improve with subsequent use. Acceptance of anything less than excellent outflow at the time of catheter placement places successful initial dialysis management at risk and invites a second procedure.

When the catheter has been shown to infuse and drain freely, a short subcutaneous tunnel is created, with care taken that the skin exit aperture is small and fits tightly onto the catheter. A small skin biopsy punch can be useful in the creation of the smallest practical skin exit aperture. The direction of the tunnel may be either toward or away from the midline (Fig. 1a).

New patients are then placed in a reverse Trendelenberg position, and peritoneography [6, 2] is performed by infusing 8 cc/kg of contrast material mixed with an equal volume of dialysate. An abdominal radiograph (which includes the inguinal areas) confirms correct position of the catheter and defines any actual inguinal hernias or patent *processus vaginalis* which might be present. If a hernia or a patent *processus vaginalis* is demonstrated, the inguinal area on that side is explored, the peritoneal protrusion excised, and the internal ring closed as tightly as possible. Our recent experience suggests that high ligation is not enough to prevent development of a clinical hernia when the high intraperitoneal hydraulic pressures generated by CAPD occur in the presence of even a seemingly insignificant patent *processus vaginalis;* tight closure of the internal inguinal ring is necessary to prevent hernias [7]. Umbilical and incisional defects are also closed at the time of catheter placement.

Following catheter placement, dialysis is continued without interruption, beginning with frequent low-volume (15 cc/kg) exchanges. Gradual increases in exchange volume and dwell period are used to stabilize patients on a maintenance regimen ideally achieved by 5–10 days after catheter placement [8]. The dialysate currently used postoperatively for the first 12–24 h contains 500 units of sodium heparin per liter and 125 mg of cephapirin per liter. Subsequent use of heparin is limited to those patients with obvious fibrin or blood in their dialysate and during episodes of peritonitis.

Catheters are routinely left in place for approximately 3 months following successful renal transplantation [9, 10].

Management of Catheter Complications

Exit Site and Tunnel Infections

We generally followed the descriptive definitions and management guidelines regarding exit site and tunnel infections outlined by Vas [11]. Exit site care varied widely throughout the study period, and no generally successful preventive maintenance technique was discovered. Patients took showers and avoided occlusive dressings for the most part, although some nonocclusive coverage of the exit site with sterile gauze pads was used in younger children. When an exit side became infected, we used hydrogen peroxide and povidone iodine solution for local care and administered oral antibiotics, usually dicloxacillin or erythromycin. Topical antibiotics were not used.

The presence of a tunnel infection was usually signaled by pain, tenderness, enduration, edema and/or erythema of the tissue overlying the subcutaneous course of the tunnel and extending more than 1 cm from the exit site; purulent drainage was also often present at the exit site. When *staph epidermidis* was cultured from this purulent drainage, we attempted to treat the tunnel infection with appropriate antibiotics for up to 6 weeks before replacing the catheter, so long as the peritoneal fluid remained sterile. Management of *staph aureus* tunnel infections varied from prompt replacement of the catheter to treatment with oral and/or intraperitoneal antibiotics for up to 3 weeks prior to catheter replacement. Medical management of *staph aureus* tunnel infections was uniformly unsuccessful. Recurrent peritonitis, defined as recurrence of peritoneal infection with the same pathogen within 2 weeks of discontinuing appropriate antibiotics [12], prompted catheter replacement in one child following the second recurrence despite an entirely negative tunnel examination. The pathogen (a *staph epidermidis*) was cultured from the cuff of the removed catheter.

In the absence of peritonitis, catheters removed for tunnel infections were replaced during the same operative procedure, with great care taken to minimize contamination of the new catheter, positioning the new tunnel as far as possible from the old. On one occasion we successfully resected and removed the infected superficial cuff of a T-2 catheter [13], leaving the catheter in place with a very short subcutaneous tunnel. This procedure was unsuccessful on two other occasions and was abandoned with the conversion to single cuff catheters.

Complex Peritonitis

Catheters were removed as a part of the treatment of candidal and tuberculous peritonitis and replaced after a period off peritoneal dialysis lasting from 1 to 4 weeks.

In one case of bacterial peritonitis involving a highly resistant pathogen, we were required to replace the catheter as a part of therapy with what was then an investigational third-generation cephalosporin. During the study period, 91 episodes of bacterial peritonitis were successfully treated without catheter replacement.

One-Way or Complete Obstruction

When a catheter developed one-way or complete obstruction, we injected contrast material under fluoroscopy in an attempt to determine the source of obstruction [14]. Occasionally, the rapid flushing of contrast material into the catheter was followed by improved drainage. In one case, an obstructed catheter was successfully repositioned in the operating room through a separate incision without disturbing the tunnel and peritoneal entry site. On three other occasions of obstruction due to omental encasement, including one in which the catheter had migrated beneath the liver, the catheter was surgically exchanged without attempting in situ revision.

Trauma and Spontaneous Cracking

Spontaneous catheter cracking and breakage was a common problem among catheters which had been in place for more than 1 year. Usually these breaks occurred at or near the titanium adapter and were managed by removing a portion of the catheter and inserting a new adapter. When this procedure would have resulted in an unacceptably short external catheter, additional silastic catheter tubing was added using a splicing kit (Peripatch, Quinton Instruments Company, Seattle, Washington 98121). Splicing was also used to extend the life spans of catheters traumatized by scissors, zippers, and animal bites. Splicing was used successfully in 12 of the study catheters, and no catheter was lost as a result of trauma or spontaneous breakage.

Data Analysis

Life table analysis was used to assess catheter survival. We defined "terminal events" to include only catheter replacement occasioned by any mechanical complication (leakage, obstruction, etc.) or by tunnel infection or complex peritonitis. When a complication-free catheter was removed following successful renal transplantation or transfer to hemodialysis, and when patients died or were transferred to another center, these catheters were considered "lost to follow-up."

Statistical analysis was performed using the statistical package for the social sciences as most recently updated [15]. Catheter survival curves were compared using the Lee-Desu test for significance independently applied at 6-month intervals [16, 15]. For all other tests of statistical significance we used the students's t test.

Results

The catheter requirements of the 27 study patients can be summarized as follows: six catheters in one, five catheters in one, four catheters in two, three catheters in

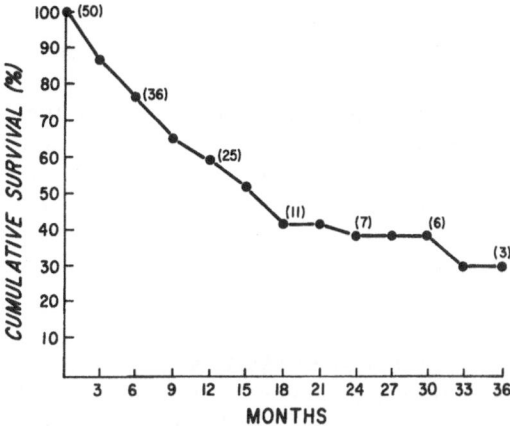

Fig. 3. Cumulative survival of 50 pediatric CAPD/CCPD catheters by life table analysis. Catheter replacement due to mechanical complication, tunnel infection or complex peritonitis was considered as catheter "death". Numbers in *parentheses*: number of catheters entering each six-month observation period

Table 2. Fate of catheters by type

Catheter type	(n)	Technical failure (n)	Omental obstruction (n)	Complex peritonitis[c] (n)	Tunnel infection (n)	No problems (n)	Total experience (months)
T-2	19	3[a]	2	5	7	2	296.1
T-1	7	0	1	1	0	5	123.1
C-1	24	1[b]	0	1	8	14	252.5
	50	4	3	7	15	21	671.7

T-2, Tenckhoff, straight, 2-cuff; T-1, Tenckhoff, straight, 1-cuff; C-1, curved, 1-cuff.
[a] Leakage, 2; cuff slippage, 1.
[b] Preperitoneal position.
[c] Bacterial, 1; tuberculous, 1; candidal, 5.

two, two catheters in four, and one catheter in 17 patients. At the time of study, 22 of 27 children had received CAPD and/or CCPD for more than 1 year and only two children had been treated for less than 6 months (4.5 and 4.0 months, respectively).

Overall actuarial catheter survival observed among the 50 study catheters is presented in Fig. 3. Cumulative survival at 6, 12, 18, and 24 months was 76%, 58%, 43%, and 37% respectively.

A total of 29 catheters were removed as a result of either mechanical (seven) or infectious (22) complications, as listed in Table 2. Mean catheter age at the time of replacement for mechanical complications was 1.4 ± 1.0 (mean $\pm$ SD) months; mean catheter age at removal for infectious complications was 13.7 ± 11.2 months ($P < 0.0005$).

Tunnel infections forced removal of 15 catheters, including early removal of two of five catheters left in place following successful renal transplantation. Primary pathogens were identified in 13 of 15 tunnel infections as follows: *staph aureus*, 8; *staph epidermidis*, 2; mixed *staph aureus* and *staph epidermidis*, 1; *pseudomonas aeruginosa*, 1; *serratia marcescens*, 1. All but the two posttransplant staphylococcal tunnel infections were preceded by chronic exit site infections unresponsive to local care and oral antibiotics. Mean catheter age at the time of removal for tunnel infection was 12.8 ± 10.3 SD months ($P < 0.0005$, compared to age at removal for mechanical complications). Catheter removal and replacement were accomplished in the same operative procedure in ten patients who had sterile peritoneal fluid and were on appropriate antibiotics at the time of surgery; peritoneal fluid remained sterile postoperatively in all ten patients, and tunnel infection did not recur.

Mechanical complications accounted for the loss of seven catheters, three due to obstruction from omental encasement and four due to technical failures. Of the technical failures, the first two of these catheters were implanted with a peritoneal purse string suture placed just below, but unattached to the cuff. Persistent dialysate leakage forced replacement of both of these catheters. Following introduction of the peritoneum-to-cuff purse-string suturing technique, no catheter was replaced because of dialysate leakage. Minor leakage did occur in two children, both of whom were receiving prednisone at the time of catheter placement. Leakage resolved in 24 and 72 h respectively with reduction in exchange volume and bed rest during dwell periods.

One catheter failed because the cuffs were glued at the time of catheter implantation; 7 weeks later, the child simply pulled out her catheter, leaving the cuffs behind. Cuffs were glued at least 12 h preoperatively in all other instances, and cuff slippage did not occur.

The last technical failure in this series occurred in 1982, when a less experienced surgical team improperly positioned an early C-1 catheter in a large extraperitoneal potential space.

Table 2 also summarizes the fate of the 50 study catheters according to catheter type. No catheter type was without "fatal" complications, although "fatalities" among T-1 (29%) and C-1 catheters (42%) were less common than among T-2 catheters (89%).

During the study period, 100 episodes of peritonitis occurred representing an incidence of one episode every 6.7 patient months. These data are compiled in Table 3 according to catheter type. Incidence of peritonitis was greater in patients with 2-cuff catheters (one episode every 5.7 patient months) than 1-cuff catheters (one episode every 8.7 patient months). This difference may be misleading because 2-cuff catheters were used exclusively during the early years of our program when the incidence of peritonitis was very high. Since 1980, the annual peritonitis rate in our program has improved from 4.1 to 9.3 patient months per episode.

Table 3. Peritonitis in pediatric CAPD/CCPD patients by catheter type

Catheter type	Peritonitis episodes (n)	Total experience (months)	Incidence[a] (months/episode)
T-2	57	296.1	5.7
T-1	15	123.1	8.2
C-1	28	252.5	9.0

T-2, Tenckhoff, straight, 2-cuff; T-1, Tenckhoff, straight, 1-cuff; C-1, curled, 1-cuff.
[a] Difference between 1-cuff (T-1 plus C-1) and 2-cuff (T-2) catheters not significant.

Table 4. Actuarial survival of 1-Cuff[a] and 2-Cuff[b] catheters

Months	1-Cuff		2-Cuff		P[d]
	%	n[c]	%	n[c]	
Survival at:					
6	80%	27	76%	15	NS
12	65%	19	53%	11	NS
18	61%	10	28%	8	NS

[a] T-1 plus C-1 catheters.
[b] Catheters, excluding first two, which were placed without cuff-to peritoneum purse string suture (see text).
[c] Number of catheters entering interval for analysis.
[d] Lee-Desu test.

Actuarial survival of the 31 1-cuff catheters (C-1 plus T-1) is compared to that of 17 of 19 2-cuff (T-2) catheters in Table 4. For this analysis, the first two T-2 catheters were excluded because they were the only catheters in the series placed without benefit of the cuff-to-peritoneum purse string suture. At 6, 12, and 18 months, the intervals at which there were enough catheters at risk to make comparisons meaningful, there was no significant difference in survival of 1-cuff and 2-cuff catheters, although a trend in favor of 1-cuff catheters was present (Table 4).

Tunnel infections forced removal of eight of 31 1-cuff catheters (26%) and seven of 19 2-cuff catheters (37%). In order to compare the occurrence of tunnel infections in 1-cuff and 2-cuff catheters, we used life table analysis to calculate actuarial survival rates for each catheter configuration, considering tunnel infection as the only "terminal event" and all other reasons for catheter removal as yielding catheters "lost to follow-up." In this way, we could correct for the fact that tunnel infections were relatively late complications in this study. Simple comparison of incidence figures would have ignored the fact that some catheters in each group had not been in place long enough to be properly considered equally "at risk" for a tunnel infection. Considered in this manner, there was no significant difference in the occurrence of catheter loss due to tunnel infection in 1-cuff as compared with 2-cuff catheters.

We then compared survival of 24 straight (T-2 plus T-1) and 24 curled (C-1) catheters, again excluding the first two T-2 catheters. As shown in Table 5, there was no significant difference in survival of straight as compared with curled catheters at 6, 12, and 18 months after catheter placement.

Finally, after excluding the first two catheters, we compared the incidence of mechanical complications in straight catheters (four of 24, or 16.7%) and in curled catheters (one of 24, or 4.2%). Direct comparison of incidence was reasonable in this case first of all because time on dialysis for all study patients exceeded the mean catheter age at time of loss due to mechanical complications by more than two standard deviations and secondly because loss due to infectious complications occurred at a much greater mean catheter age. All 48 catheters could thus be considered equally at risk for loss due to mechanical complications. Despite an obvious trend in favor of curled catheters, the small sample size prevented this difference from achieving statistical significance.

Table 5. Actuarial survival of straight[a] and curled[b] catheters

Months	Straight		Curled		P[d]
	%	n[c]	%	n[c]	
Survival at:					
6	79%	21	78%	21	NS
12	58%	16	64%	14	NS
18	38%	11	57%	7	NS

[a] T-2 plus T-1, excluding first two T-2 catheters (see text).
[b] C-1 catheters.
[c] Number of catheters entering interval for analysis.
[d] Lee-Desu test.

Discussion

In the 6 years since the successful adaptation of CAPD for use in infants and children [8, 17], the choice of a chronic peritoneal dialysis catheter and catheter placement technique have become increasingly important to a growing number of pediatric dialysis centers around the world. Early experience with various catheter configurations and placement techniques suitable for use in children on CAPD has been reported by several investigators [2, 18–21]. The straight Tenckhoff catheter has been almost universally preferred by pediatric dialysis centers, although the use of the Toronto Western Hospital catheter [22] and the curled Tenckhoff catheter [23] in a few children has been described. Pediatric programs have differed in their choice of 1-cuff or 2-cuff Tenckhoff catheters, with the preference in recent years swinging toward the 1-cuff configuration [24, 25].

Catheter placement techniques have also varied. Most centers rely on surgical placement under general anesthesia, although a technique for percutaneous placement by the pediatric nephrologist has been devised (Lum GM, personal communication). Partial omentectomy is included in most surgical techniques; the resection of larger portions of omentum has also been recommended [20]. In some placement techniques, the intraperitoneal tip of the straight Tenckhoff catheter is sutured either deep in the pelvis [26] or above the liver [27]. When 1-cuff catheters are used, the cuff is usually located at the peritoneal entry site, held in place by a nonabsorbable purse string suture. The technique chosen for placement of this purse string suture has differed widely, reflecting the preferences of individual surgeons.

The relative merits of the various catheters and placement techniques currently used in children are difficult to assess because published data on catheter outcome have been largely anecdotal, describing relatively short-term observations. Some early reports discussed catheter survival in terms of average life span (i.e., patient months per catheter) [19, 28, 29]. Other reports have compared the incidence of various complications among different catheters. Such an approach is valid only if all of the catheters considered are more or less equally at risk in developing the complication in question. For example, early in our use of the 1-cuff catheter, we were encouraged by an apparently low incidence of tunnel infections as compared with our previous experience with 2-cuff catheters [25]. Longer experience with the 1-cuff catheters dispelled this impression (see below). The longitudinal use of different catheter configurations rather than random use in a prospective manner also introduces variables which are difficult to control. However, even prospective, randomized trials can yield misleading results when the study period is not long enough and patient characteristics are different among the study groups [30, 31].

In the present study, we have used life table analysis to assess our experience. Life table analysis has recently been shown to be a simple and reliable statistical method with which to evaluate catheter experience [31, 32]. To determine catheter survival in this manner, one must identify those situations leading to catheter removal which are to be considered terminal events (i.e., catheter "deaths"), and those situations in which catheter removal is tantamount to withdrawal from the study (i.e., catheters "lost to follow-up"). Terminal events criteria should be chosen such that catheter "deaths" occur only when removal is largely (but not necessarily exclusively) the result of complications related to the catheter itself and/or the implantation technique.

Terminal events criteria have differed in previous reports. Gloor and associates [33] defined terminal events in two ways: (a) all reasons for catheter removal, including successful renal transplantation, and return of renal function; and (b) only mechanical catheter failures, excluding tunnel infections or any other complication in which the removed catheter remained functional. We believe that these methods would result in either underestimation (method a) or overestimation (method b) of catheter-related survival.

In the present study, we defined terminal events to include all mechanical complications as well as those tunnel infections and complex peritonitis episodes which resulted in catheter removal. Complication-free catheters removed from patients who died, transferred to another center, transferred to hemodialysis, or underwent successful renal transplantation were considered lost to follow-up. Our terminal events criteria are similar to those used by others [13, 32, 34]. They differ from those proposed by Ponce and associates [31] only in that Ponce and associates do not consider recurrent or intractable peritonitis to be a terminal event. We believe that recurrent peritonitis is very likely to be catheter-related, as was seen in one of our patients in whom an occult tunnel infection presented in this manner. The role played by the catheter in the development and maintenance of complex peritonitis is less clear; recent studies describing infected catheter biofilms [35] and questioning the biocompatibility of various catheter materials [36] have suggested that catheter-related factors may indeed be important in the etiology of peritonitis. We were also influenced to include candidal and tuberculous peritonitis as catheter-related terminal events by the fact that catheter removal is considered to be of such vital importance to the successful treatment of these infections [37].

Actuarial survival observed in our series of 50 catheters was 58% at 1 year and 37% at 2 years. There was no significant difference in survival of similarly implanted 1-cuff and 2-cuff catheters, although there was a trend in favor of 1-cuff catheters.

Tunnel infection was the most common terminal event, accounting for over 50% of catheter "deaths." There was no difference in the likelihood of tunnel infections when 1-cuff and 2-cuff catheters were compared. In the absence of peritonitis, it was

Table 6. Actuarial catheter survival and complications seen in four long-term studies of Tenckhoff catheters

	Present study		Slingenayer et al. (1981) [13]		Ponce et al. (1982) [31]		Gloor et al. (1983) [33]	
	n	%	n	%	n	%	n	%
Patients	27 (children)		247 (adults)		NR (adults)		50 (adults)	
Catheters	50[a]		315[b]		57[b]		85[b]	
Study period (years)	5.3		7		7		7	
Catheter Survival:								
at 1 year:		58[c]		80[c]		76[d]		63[e]
at 2 years:		37		70		67		55
Complications:								
Leakace								
Total:	4	(8)[f]	NR		10	(17.5)[f]	NR	
Requiring catheter removal:	2	(4)[f]	11	(3)[f]	NR		12	(14)[f]
Obstruction[g]	3	(6)[f]	12	(4)[f]	10[h]	(17.5)[f]	14	(16)[f]
Exit site tunnel infection								
Total:	16	(32)[f]	40	(13)[f]	1	(1.7)[f]	23	(27)[f]
Requiring catheter removal:	15	(30)[f]	37	(12)[f]	NR		20	(24)[f]
Complex recurrent peritonitis:	7	(14)[f]	1	(<1)[f]	None		10	(12)[f]

[a] See text for details of catheter configurations used.
[b] All were straight, 2-cuff Tenckhoff catheters surgically implanted.
[c] Actuarial survival; terminal events criteria included all mechanical and infectious complications causing catheter removal (see text).
[d] Terminal events criteria exclude complex/recurrent peritonitis; otherwise as in footnote c.
[e] Terminal events criteria limited to mechanical catheters failures (see text).
[f] Numbers in parentheses indicate percentage of total catheters studied.
[g] One-way or complete obstruction requiring catheter removal.
[h] Does not include ten catheters with poor drainage whose fate was not reported.
NR = not recorded

possible to remove safely and replace at the same operative procedure catheters with infected tunnels. Curled catheters had fewer mechanical complications than straight catheters, but this difference did not achieve statistical significance.

Similarly derived data on catheter survival from other pediatric dialysis programs are not available. Three large adult series involving surgically placed Tenckhoff catheters were recently published [13, 31, 33]. Table 6 summarizes data on catheter survival and complications from these adult series and compares them with our results.

Comparison of actuarial survival data is possible only with the report by Slingenayer and associates (1981) because the other investigators used different terminal events criteria. In their review of 315 2-cuff Tenckhoff catheters implanted in 247 adult patients over a 7-year period, Slingenayer et al. observed a 1-year actuarial catheter survival of 79.7%, which only fell at 2 years to 69.6%. These results were substantially better than our experience with 50 pediatric catheters.

The better survival seen among the catheters reported by Slingenayer et al. [13] may be in part related to the aggressive approach taken by these investigators to in situ revision. Successful surgical revision was accomplished by Slingenayer in 18 of 39 attempts, which reduced the number of catheters suffering terminal events in their series by over 20%. We successfully revised only two catheters in four attempts, thereby reducing terminal catheter events in our series by only 6%.

The catheter placement technique used by Slingenayer is similar to our approach in that partial omentectomy is performed and the deep cuff is sutured directly to the peritoneum. This may account for the similarly lower incidence of leakage seen in our series and that of Slingenayer when compared to the two other adult series (Table 6). The combined incidence of all infectious complications was more than three times greater in our series than in those of Slingenayer et al. [13] and Ponce et al. [31] but was similar to that reported by Gloor et al. [33].

In summary, our experience has shown that catheter failure due to mechanical complications can be minimized by using a surgical placement technique which includes partial omentectomy and creation of a near watertight seal at the peritoneal entry site. The use of a curled catheter with the peritoneal cuff placed close to the curl may further reduce the likelihood of mechanical catheter failures.

Our data also revealed that when the study period is adequate, tunnel infections are as likely to occur in 1-cuff as in 2-cuff catheters. Peritonitis was seen in our patients no more frequently in patients with 1-cuff than in those with 2-cuff catheters. In view of the longitudinal nature of our series, conclusions should be drawn with caution; however, based on our experience, there seems to be little reason to favor either the 1-cuff or the 2-cuff configuration. In fact, the frequency of chronic exit site and tunnel infections among patients with either catheter type suggests that basic changes may be needed in the materials used and/or the design of the peritoneal catheter at its interface with the abdominal wall [38–40].

During the 5 years of this study, we were encouraged by the virtual disappearance of mechanical complications as a cause of catheter failure. Unfortunately, catheter "death" in our center due to infectious complications remains as serious a problem today as it was 5 years ago. Until this problem is resolved, the truly permanent pediatric peritoneal dialysis catheter will remain an elusive goal.

References

1. Tenckhoff H, Schechter H (1968) A bacteriologically safe peritoneal access device. Trans Am Soc Artif Intern Organs 14: 181–187
2. Alexander SR, Tank ES (1982) Surgical aspects of continuous ambulatory peritoneal dialysis in infants, children and adolescents. J Urol 127: 501–504
3. Palmer RA, Quinton WE, Gray J-F (1964) Prolonged peritoneal dialysis for chronic renal failure. Lancet 1: 700–702
4. Rottembourg J, Jacq D, Vonlanthen M, Issad B, Ed Shaliat Y (1981) Straight or curled Tenckhoff peritoneal catheter for continuous ambulatory peritoneal dialysis (CAPD). Perit Dial Bull 1: 123–124

5. Alexander SR (1984) Peritoneal dialysis in infants and children. In: Nolph KD (ed) Peritoneal dialysis, 2nd edn. Nijhoff, Amsterdam, pp 525–560
6. Maxwell MH, Rockney RB, Kleeman CR (1959) Peritoneal dialysis I. Technique and applications. JAMA 170:917
7. Tank ES, Hatch DA (1984) Hernias complicating chronic ambulatory peritoneal dialysis in children. J Urol (in press)
8. Alexander SR, Tseng CH, Maksym KA, Campbell RA, Talwalkar YB, Kohaut EC (1981) Clinical parameters in continuous ambulatory peritoneal dialysis for infants and children. In: Moncrief JW, Popovich RP (eds) CAPD update: continuous ambulatory peritoneal dialysis. Masson, New York, pp 195–209
9. Stefanidis CJ, Balfe JW, Arbus GS, Hardy BE, Churchill BM, Rance CP (1983) Renal transplantation in children treated with CAPD. Perit Dial Bull 3:5–8
10. Patel S, Rosenthal JT, Hakala TR (1983) Management of the peritoneal dialysis catheter after transplantation. Transplantation 36:589–590
11. Vas SI (1981) What are the indications for removal of the permanent peritoneal catheter? Perit Dial Bull 1:145–146
12. Pierratos A (1984) Peritoneal dialysis glossary. Perit Dial Bull 4:2–3
13. Slingenayer A, Mion C, Charpiat A, Balmes M (1981) Is an alternative to the Tenckhoff catheter necessary? In: Gahl GM, Kessel M, Nolph KD (eds) Advances in peritoneal dialysis: proceedings of the second international symposium on peritoneal dialysis, 16–19 June 1981. Excerpta Medica, Amsterdam, pp 179–184
14. Hemmeloff-Anderson KE, Damgaard-Morch P (1981) Catheterography in the diagnosis of catheter failure in peritoneal dialysis. Clin Nephrol 16:142–145
15. Hull CH, Nie NH (1981) Statistical package for the social sciences: update 7–9. McGraw Hill, New York
16. Lee E, Desu M (1972) A computer program for comparing K samples with rightcensored data. Comput Programs Biomed 2:315–321
17. Balfe JW, Vigneux A, Willumsen J, Hardy BE (1981) The use of CAPD in the treatment of children with end-stage renal disease. Perit Dial Bull 1:35–38
18. Balfe JW, Irwin MA, Oreopoulos DG (1981) An assessment of continuous ambulatory peritoneal dialysis (CAPD) in children. In: Moncrief JW, Popovich RP (eds) CAPD update: continuous ambulatory peritoneal dialysis. Masson, New York, pp 211–220
19. Potter DE, McDaid TK, Ramirez JA (1981) Peritoneal dialysis in children. In: Atkins RC, Thomson NM, Farrell PD (eds) Peritoneal dialysis. Churchill Livingstone, New York, pp 356–367
20. Guillot M, Clermont MJ, Gagnadoux MF, Broyer M (1982) Continuous ambulatory peritoneal dialysis in pediatrics: preliminary results on 18 months experience. In: Bulla M (ed) Renal insufficiency in children. Springer, Berlin Heidelberg New York, pp 197–203
21. Salusky IB, Lucullo L, Nelson P, Fine RN (1982) Continuous ambulatory peritoneal dialysis in children. Pediatr Clin North Am 29:1005–1012
22. Hogg RJ, Coln D, Chang J, Arant BS Jr, Houser M (1983) The Toronto Western Hospital catheter in a pediatric dialysis program. Am J Kidney Dis 3:219–223
23. Alexander SR (1983) Pediatric CAPD update – 1983. Perit Dial Bull [Suppl]3:S15–S22
24. Vigneux A, Hardy BE, Balfe JW (1981) Chronic peritoneal catheter in children-one or two dacron cuffs? Perit Dial Bull 1:151
25. Alexander SR, Tank ES (1982) Technical considerations in the implantation of Tenckhoff catheters for continuous ambulatory peritoneal dialysis in children. Nefrologia [Suppl] 11:49–52
26. Bay WH, Gerilli GJ, Perrine V, Powell S, Erlich L (1983) Analysis of a new technique to stabilize the chronic peritoneal dialysis catheter. Am J Kidney Dis 3:133–135
27. Sherman NJ, Atkinson JB (1984) Vascular and peritoneal access: technical considerations. In: Fine RN, Gruskin AB (eds) End-stage renal disease in children. Saunders, Philadelphia, pp 85–87
28. Hickman R (1978) Nine years' experience with chronic peritoneal dialysis in childhood. Dial Transplant 7:803
29. Brouhard BH, Berger M, Cunningham RJ, Petrusick T, Allen W, Lynch RE, Travis LB (1979) Home peritoneal dialysis in children. Trans Am Soc Artif Intern Organs 25:90–94

30. Oreopoulos DG, Izatt S, Zellerman G, Karanicolas S, Mathews RE (1976) A prospective study of the effectiveness of three permanent peritoneal catheters. Proc Dial Transplant Forum 1976:96–100
31. Ponce SP, Pierratos A, Izatt S, Mathews R, Khanna R, Zellerman G, Oreopoulos DG (1982) Comparison of the survival and complications of three permanent peritoneal dialysis catheters. Perit Dial Bull 2:82–86
32. Ash SR, Struewing JD (1983) Clinical trials of the column disc peritoneal catheter (Lifecath ™). Perit Dial Bull 3:77–80
33. Gloor HJ, Nichols WK, Sorkin MI, Prowant BF, Kennedy JM, Baker P, Nolph KD (1983) Peritoneal access and related complications in continuous ambulatory peritoneal dialysis. Am J Med 74:593–598
34. Khanna R, Izatt S, Burke D, Mathews R, Vas S, Oreopoulos DG (1984) Experience with the Toronto Western Hospital permanent peritoneal catheter. Perit Dial Bull 4:95–98
35. Reed WP, Light PD, Newman KA (1984) Biofilm on Tenckhoff catheters: a possible source for peritonitis (Abstract). Perit Dial Bull [Suppl] 4:S53
36. Amair P, DeCamejo OC, Dominguez O, Boissiere M (1984) Skin reaction against the catheter: an explanation for exit site infection in CAPD (Abstract). Perit Dial Bull [Suppl] 4:S2
37. Hogg RG, Arant BS Jr, Houser MT (1982) Candida peritonitis in children on continuous ambulatory peritoneal dialysis. Int J Ped Nephrol 3:287–292
38. Bay WH, Powell SL (1984) Long-term clinical trial of the Gore-tex ™ peritoneal catheter (Abstract). Kidney Int 25:255
39. Poirier VL, Daly BDT, Dasse KA (1984) Elimination of tunnel infection (Abstract). Perit Dial Bull [Suppl] 4:S51
40. Trooskin SZ, Harvey RA, Donetz AP, Greco RS (1984) Application of antibiotic bonding to CAPD catheters (Abstract). Perit Dial Bull [Suppl] 4:S66

Peritonitis in Children Undergoing CAPD Versus CCPD*

H. E. Leichter, I. B. Salusky, D. Davidson, M. Wilson, T. Hall, and R. N. Fine

Introduction

Continuous ambulatory peritoneal dialysis (CAPD) has been shown to be an effective and well-tolerated dialysis technique for pediatric patients with end-stage renal disease (ESRD) [1, 2] awaiting renal transplantation [3–8]. The major advantages of CAPD are the appropriate control of the clinical manifestations of uremia, improved control of hypertension, and decreased severity of anemia. Furthermore, increased freedom and mobility, less frequent hospital visits, and minimal dietary restriction contribute to better rehabilitation. However, repetitive performance of the exchange procedure, frequent episodes of peritonitis, and catheter problems contribute to the burnout of the patients and their families. In order to reduce the peritonitis incidence caused by contamination while performing the exchange procedure and to prevent potential burn-out, continuous cyclic peritoneal dialysis (CCPD) was introduced [9]. CCPD utilizes an automated cycler to deliver frequent exchanges at night and a single daytime dwell. We undertook a retrospective evaluation of the incidence of peritonitis in children undergoing CAPD and CCPD.

Patients and Methods

In the 3 1/2 years since the initiation of the CAPD/CCPD program at UCLA in August 1980, 68 patients (35 males, 33 females) with a mean age of 11.1 ± 7 (SE) years (range, 3 months – 21 years) have been trained for CAPD and/or CCPD. The initial dialysis modality was CAPD in 63 patients (93%) and CCPD in 5 patients (7%). Of the 63 patients initially trained for CAPD, 24 (38%) were switched to CCPD after 12.7 ± 2.0 months. Only one patient (3%) returned to CAPD. Four patients (6%) were transferred to hemodialysis because of peritoneal membrane failure secondary to peritonitis. This represents a total experience of 654 patient months of CAPD and 251 patient months of CCPD.

Dialysis Technique and Peritoneal Access

CAPD was performed with four or five daily exchanges and a volume ranging from 30–50 ml/kg body weight per exchange, depending upon commercially available dialysate solutions (Dianeal, Travenol Laboratories, Deerfield, Ill.). CCPD was ac-

* Heinz Leichter is sponsored by a grant from the *Deutsche Forschungsgemeinschaft*. This work is supported in part by the Peter Boxenbaum Research Fund.

complished with five 2-hour, nighttime exchanges performed with an AMP 80/2 cycler (American Medical Products Corporation, Freehold, N.J.), followed by a single diurnal dwell at one-half the nocturnal volume, or no daytime dwell. The dialysate glucose concentration was adjusted to the desired degree of ultrafiltration, which depended upon the patient's blood pressure and body weight. According to the degree of acidosis, either PD 1 or PD 2 (Dianeal, Travenol Laboratories, Deerfield, Ill.) was used to maintain the serum bicarbonate level within normal limits.

All patients were dialyzed through a permanent indwelling catheter. Partial omentectomy was performed at the time of catheter placement. Single-cuff and double-cuff Tenckhoff catheters, as well as column disc (Life cath) catheters were used.

For the first 48–72 hours following catheter insertion, automated peritoneal dialysis with low volumes and frequent exchanges was initiated. Antibiotics (cefazolin 250 mg/l) and heparin (250 u/l) were added to the dialysate for the first 48 hours following surgery. If uremic symptoms did not necessitate the immediate initiation of CAPD, the patients or their parents were trained in ten training sessions to perform CAPD and/or CCPD. Patients who required immediate dialysis to relieve symptomatology had intermittent peritoneal dialysis (IPD) for 8 hours three times a week until appropriate training was initiated.

Diagnosis and Initial Management of Peritonitis

During the training period, each patient and/or parent was taught to recognize the signs and symptoms of peritonitis, which were cloudy dialysate fluid, abdominal pain, and fever. If any of these symptoms occurred, the patient and/or parent was told to call the CAPD nurse, who was available 24 hours a day, 7 days a week. The nurse instructed patients to drain the dialysate solution from the abdominal cavity, save the bag in the refrigerator, and proceed with three rapid exchanges with the usual volumes, followed by 6-hour exchanges with dialysate containing heparin (250 u/l) and cefazolin (250 mg/l). The first and fourth bag were saved and brought to the hospital. The decision to hospitalize the patient and to start parenteral antibiotic therapy depended on the severity of the clinical symptoms.

A sample of 10 ml of peritoneal dialysis fluid was obtained from each bag and analyzed for cell count, Gram stain, and culture. The diagnosis of peritonitis was based upon clinical findings and an increased cell count (> 100 cells/mm^3) in the dialysate fluid. CAPD patients continued their regular exchanges. CCPD patients were switched to CAPD for at least 4–6 days. Recurrent peritonitis was defined as the presence of the same organism within 2 weeks of stopping antibiotic therapy. Persistent infection was defined as the persistence of positive dialysate cultures with the same organism despite appropriate antibiotic treatment.

Treatment of Peritonitis

Initially, all patients were placed on cefazolin (250 µg/l) and heparin (250 µg/l) intraperitoneally (IP). In the presence of "no growth" or gram-positive infections, this treatment was continued for 12 days. Repeated cultures were taken at day 5 and 10, and if the last culture (day 10) was negative after 48 hours, therapy was discontinued. If tunnel infections coincided with the peritonitis, additional parenteral oxacillin was given for 3–5 days, followed by oral therapy according to the clinical situation. The following findings were indications for additional intraperitoneal treatment with tobramycin (8 mg/l): (a) gram-negative bacteria on the gram stain, (b) gram-negative organisms in the first culture at 48 hours, and (c) persistence of cloudy bags following 48 hours of standard treatment. Gram-negative peritonitis episodes were treated for 21 days with intraperitoneal antibiotics. In some instances, depending upon the clinical situation and/or different sensitivities of the bacteria, other antibiotics were added.

Indications for catheter removal were recurrent or persistent peritonitis and tunnel infections resistent to therapy.

Data are expressed as mean ± SE. Life table analysis was used to describe the interval to the first episode of peritonitis.

Results

There were 94 episodes of peritonitis in the 68 patients undergoing CAPD/CCPD over a period of 910 patient months. During 654 patient months of CAPD, 63 episodes of peritonitis occurred (1 every 10.4 patient months). During 256 patient months of CCPD 31 episodes of peritonitis occurred (1 every 8.3 patient months). The first peritonitis episode for 31 children on CAPD occurred after 6.0 ± 1.0 months, while 15 children on CCPD suffered the first episode after 6.3 ± 1.4 months. According to life table analysis, 46% of the patients were peritonitis free after 12 months of CAPD/CCPD, and 33% after 24 months. The predominant symptoms of peritonitis were cloudy dialysate fluid, abdominal discomfort, vomiting, and fever, although in nine episodes (9.6%), only one of these symptoms was present. The etiology of the infections occurring during both CAPD and CCPD are shown in Table 1. Nearly half of the 94 cultures (44%) showed no growth, while 27 (28%) yielded a gram-positive organism. Gram-negative bacteria accounted for 20 (22%) of the infections. *Candida albicans* was present in 2 patients (2%).

In 15 patients (22%) representing 16 episodes (17%) these were associated with recurrent or persistent infection. Two patients with *pseudomonas aeruginosa* peritonitis were temporarily switched to hemodialysis for 4 weeks. One pseudomonas infection responded to intraperitoneal antibiotic therapy, and two children with residual renal function had the catheter removed and were off dialysis for 10 days before reinsertion of a new catheter. Fungal infections (*candida albicans*) occurred in two patients who had not had any previously treated bacterial peritonitis. In both cases, the catheter was removed.

Membrane loss occurred in three children. Two of them experienced significant damage to the peritoneum after *candida albicans* peritonitis. The remaining patient had a second *staphylococcus aureus* peritonitis episode within 1 year, making continuing peritoneal dialysis impossible. All patients had a loss of ultrafiltration and

Table 1. Etiology of peritonitis in patients undergoing CAPD and CCPD

Organism	Episodes on CAPD (n)	%	Episodes on CCPD (n)	%	Total (n)	%
No growth	30	47	11	37	41	44
Gram-positive:						
Staph. aureus	9		4			
Coag. neg. staph.	7	31	3	23	27	28
Strep. viridans	3		–			
Beta strep.	1		–			
Gram-negative:						
Pseudomonas aerug.	2		3			
Enterobacteria	1		3			
Klebsiella pneum.	1		2			
Serratia marc.	2	14	1	37	20	22
E. coli	–		2			
Hemophilus infl.	1		–			
Acinetobacter	2		–			
Anaerobe	1	2	–	–		
Fungi (Candida)	2	3	–	–	6	6
More than one organism:						
2 gram-neg.	1	3	1	3		
2 gram-pos.	1		–			
Total	64	100	30	100	94	100

were switched to hemodialysis. Death occurred in two of the 68 patients (3%), but neither death was related to either peritonitis or the dialysis procedure.

Discussion

Since the use of peritoneal dialysis for treatment of patients with ESRD, peritonitis has been a major complication. The initially high peritonitis rates associated with CAPD when glass bottles were used [10] were reduced with the introduction of plastic bags [11]. Following the instillation of the dialysate solution into the peritoneal cavity, it was possible to attach the plastic bag to the body and utilize it for efflux of the dialysate several hours later. Through this modification, the number of disconnections were reduced by 50%, thereby decreasing the incidence of peritonitis [11]. There are only a few reports detailing the incidence of peritonitis in children undergoing CAPD [12–15]. Potter, et al. [12] and Alexander [13], reported one episode every 3.3 and 4.1 patient months, respectively. However, these reports represent their experience prior to the availability in the United States of bags of an appropriate size for children. On the other hand, in subsequent studies from Balfe et al. [14] and our Center [15], one episode every 13.1 patient months and one every 12.5 patient months, respectively, were reported. The present report indicates a peritonitis rate of one episode every 9.7 patient months when CAPD and CCPD are taken into account together. Despite the use of CCPD, the infection rate did not improve (1/8.3 months on CCPD, 1/10.4 months on CAPD), as was the case in other studies [9], indicating that fewer connections do not necessarily decrease the risk of peritonitis. However, our data does not represent a prospective, controlled study comparing CAPD with CCPD. Some of our patients were switched to CCPD because they had suffered frequent episodes of peritonitis while on CAPD. These patients represent a high-risk group which can falsely influence the peritonitis rate with CCPD. Furthermore, other factors such as the status of the cellular and humoral defense system may play an important role in the detection of high-risk patients.

Keane et al. [16] have shown that reduced bacterial opsonization, which is critical to the effective defense of the peritoneal cavity by phagocytic cells, may predispose patients to develop peritonitis. The peritonitis rate with *staphylococcus epidermidis* in patients with a "high" rate of opsonic activity against this bacteria species in the peritoneal dialysis effluent was lower than in patients with "low" peritoneal dialysis opsonic activity.

In the present study, we found a relatively high percentage of cultures (44%) with no growth, which might be related to the method of culture. No attempt was made to concentrate the dialysate in order to increase the yield as previously described [17, 18]. Another factor contributing to the low yield may be the lag time between the initiation of the symptoms and the time of culturing. Because of long distances from the hospital, the "infected" dialysate was frequently refrigerated overnight prior to culturing. A look at the different organisms causing peritonitis in patients on CAPD or CCPD shows a significantly higher percentage (37%) of gram-negative infections in patients on CCPD than in patients on CAPD. No other significant differences in the spectrum of peritonitis were observable when the two dialysis modalities were compared.

Gram-positive infections responded to cefazolin treatment; however, seven of the 16 recurrent or persistent peritonitis episodes were caused by Staphylococci and Streptococci and required catheter removal. Gram-negative infections were present in seven recurrent episodes of peritonitis. It is interesting to note that no patient with a gram-negative infection had to be transferred to hemodialysis.

Fungal infections are the most serious cause of peritonitis. They do not respond to antifungal therapy, and catheter removal with subsequent switching to hemodialysis is necessary for at least 2–3 weeks. There is no doubt that fungal infections are a strong indication for prompt catheter removal [19]. This is consistent with our finding that peritoneal damage consequent to fungal peritonitis led to discontinuation of peritoneal dialysis in two patients.

Therapy for peritonitis in patients on CAPD and CCPD has not been standardized. With patients on CCPD, there is the additional question of whether patients should be transiently switched to CAPD or whether CCPD with daytime dwells are adequate treatment. Our regimen for uncomplicated peritonitis episodes seems to be effective. In complicated peritoneal infections (i.e., gram-negative peritonitis), even a prolonged course of intraperitoneal and parenteral treatment could not prevent early catheter removal. As indicated in another study [20], catheter removal is the treatment of choice in some patients.

Although the peritonitis rates can be kept reasonable, peritonitis in addition to catheter-related problems continues to be a significant problem in treating children with continuous peritoneal dialysis. The long-term efficiency of the peritoneum as a dialyzing membrane, especially after several peritonitis episodes, is a factor that may ultimately limit the long-term use of peritoneal dialysis.

In our population, the introduction of CCPD did not decrease the incidence of peritonitis, indicating that factors other than contamination caused by connecting and disconnecting may be responsible. Because of the multifactorial etiology of peritonitis (contamination, exit site infection, immunological status of the patient), further efforts should be made to reduce the incidence of peritonitis.

Acknowledgement. We thank Ms. Amy Landsberg for excellent secretarial assistance.

References

1. Oreopoulos DG, Katirtzoglou A, Arbus G et al. (1979) Dialysis and transplantation in young children. Br Med J 1:1628
2. Balfe JW, Irwin MA (1980) Continuous ambulatory peritoneal dialysis in pediatrics. In: Legrain M (ed) Continuous ambulatory peritoneal dialysis. Excerpta Medica, Amsterdam, p 131
3. Alexander SR, Tseng CH, Maksym KA et al. (1981) Clinical parameters in CAPD for infants and children. In: Moncrief JW, Popovich (eds) CAPD update Masson, New York, p 195–209
4. Potter DE, McDaid TK, McHenry K et al. (1981) Continuous ambulatory peritoneal dialysis in children. Trans Am Soc Artif Intern Organs 27:64–67
5. Salusky IB, Lucullo L, Nelson P, et al. (1982) Continuous ambulatory peritoneal dialysis in children. Pediatr Clin North Am 29:1005–1012
6. Baum M, Powell D, Calvin S, et al. (1982) Continuous ambulatory peritoneal dialysis in children. N Engl J Med 307:1537–1542
7. Salusky IB, Kopple JD, Fine RN (1983) Continuous ambulatory peritoneal dialysis in pediatric patients. A 20-month experience. Kidney Int 24 [Suppl 15]:101–105
8. Leichter HE, Salusky IB, Alliapoulos JC, et al. (1984) CAPD and CCPD in children: An experience of 3 1/2 years. Dial Transplant 13:382–388
9. Diaz-Buxo JA, Walker PJ, Farmer CD, et al. (1981) Continuous cyclic peritoneal dialysis. Kidney Int 19:145
10. Popovich RP, Moncrief JW, Decherd JB, et al. (1976) The definition of a novel portable/wearable equilibrium peritoneal dialysis technique (Abstract). Trans Am Soc Artif Intern Organs 5:64
11. Oreopoulos DG, Robson M, Izatt S, et al. (1978) A simple and safe technique for continuous ambulatory peritoneal dialysis (CAPD). Trans Am Soc Artif Intern Organs 24:484–489
12. Potter DE, McDaid TK, Ramirez JA (1981) Peritoneal dialysis in children. In: Atkins RC, Thomson NM, Farrell PC (eds) Peritoneal dialysis. Churchill Livingstone, Edinburgh, p 356–367
13. Alexander S (1982) CAPD in children. 2nd National conference on CAPD, Kansas City, MO, 15–17 Feb 1982
14. Balfe JW, Vigneux A, Willumsen J (1981) The use of CAPD in the treatment of children with end-stage renal disease. Perit Dial Bull 1:35–38
15. Fine RN, Salusky IB, Hall T, et al. (1983) Peritonitis in children undergoing continuous ambulatory peritoneal dialysis. Pediatrics 71:806–809
16. Keane WF, Comty CM, Verbrugh HA, et al. (1984) Opsonic deficiency of peritoneal dialysis effluent in continuous ambulatory peritoneal dialysis. Kidney Int 25:539–543
17. Rubin J, Rogers WA, Taylor HM, et al. (1980) Peritonitis during continuous ambulatory peritoneal dialysis. Ann Intern Med 92:7–13
18. Vas S (1981) Microbiological aspects of peritonitis. Perit Dial Bull 1[Suppl]:11
19. Rault R (1983) Candida peritonitis complicating uremic peritoneal dialysis: a report of five cases and review of the literature. Am J Kidney Dis 2:544–547
20. Krothapulli R, Duffy WB, Lacke C, et al. (1982) Pseudomonas peritonitis and continuous ambulatory peritoneal dialysis. Arch Intern Med 142:1862–1863

Pharmacokinetics of Various Antibiotics During CAPD

J. Rottembourg, P. Y. Cossette, B. Issad, and R. Mehamha

Introduction

The introduction of CAPD has renewed interest in peritoneal dialysis as a method for treating end-stage renal disease. The most frequent complication, peritonitis, is also the most frequent cause of failure of the technique. Peritonitis occurring during CAPD is clinically different from that following a surgical insult. Patients undergoing CAPD usually suffer some external contamination leading to infection. Dialysis therapy is used for treatment of infection. Effective antibiotic therapy must not only provide adequate serum and tissue levels, but must also be able to eradicate organisms that may persist in stagnant residual pools of dialysate within the peritoneal cavity. Thus, it would seem reasonable to attempt to obtain both adequate serum levels and dialysate concentrations.

The Kinetics of Antibiotics During Peritoneal Dialysis

During dialysis, solutes traverse the semipermeable membrane by diffusing along chemical concentration gradients and accompanying the bulk flow of water responding to hydrostatic or osmotic pressure gradients. The barrier consists of the peritoneal membrane, including the capillary endothelial cells, the mesothelial cells and their intercellular spaces, their basement membranes, and the interstitial spaces between them.

Factors which determine solute transport rate by ultrafiltration are the hydrostatic and osmotic pressure gradients, the membrane area, and the capillary filtration coefficient. Diffusion depends on the concentration gradient, membrane area and permeability, ionic charge, protein binding, and diffusivity, which is an inverse function of solution size. Because transport during peritoneal dialysis occurs predominantly by diffusion, both solute size and protein-binding are major determinants of the transport rate. Mass transport decreases as diffusion equilibrium is approached, and ultrafiltration by solvent drag removes solutes independently of molecular size until membrane sieving occurs.

With CAPD, transport of small solutes per unit time is slow because diffusion equilibrium is achieved or approached before the dialysate is replaced with fresh solution. The procedure is effective because it is continuous. However, larger solutes may continue to diffuse throughout the entire duration of the exchange. The maximal transport rate for any solute diffusing from plasma water when expressed as a

Table 1. Effect of peritoneal dialysis on drug kinetics [1]

Drug	Mol. weight	Percentage bound in plasma	Clearance ml/min		t½ life (h)	
			anuria	PD	anuria	PD
Gentamicin	543	0	2	4	50	20
Amykacin	586	4	1.5	6	60	20
Tobramycin	486	0	3	10	55	16
Cephaloridine	416	30	9	15	20	7
Cephalothin	396	70	15	15	12	6
Cefamandole	485	70	12	11	14	7
Carbenicillin	378	50	11	7	20	12
5-Fluorocytosine	129	5	5	15	100	25
Isoniazid	137	10		12	4	4
Ethambutol	204	20		9		

clearance is the flow rate of dialysis solution (usually 6–8.5 ml/min during long-dwell peritoneal dialysis). This can be sufficient to achieve steady-state plasma concentrations in a clinically acceptable range, but it has little or no impact on the concentration of most drugs in plasma because their natural clearances are considerably higher, even in uremic patients. Exceptions such as aminoglycosides and 5-fluorocytosine have been studied more carefully (Table 1). Because the clearance by continuous, long-dwell peritoneal dialysis approaches endogenous clearance in the anephric patient, the half-life of this restricted group of drugs should be significantly reduced by the procedure. Moreover, the removal rates of drug metabolites from the anephric patient may be considerably increased by CAPD procedure. Transport from the dialysate to the plasma can significantly increase the plasma concentration of many drugs, especially protein-bound drugs [1–3].

The efficiency of CAPD is often assessed by the measurement of equilibrium plasma concentrations. Although such concentrations are important in as much as they may reflect patient well-being, they are influenced by other factors, such as the solute input or production rate and elimination by residual renal function and extrarenal routes.

Factors Affecting the use of Antibiotics During CAPD

Method of Treatment During Peritonitis

Heparin is commonly added to the dialysate to prevent catheter pluging by proteinaceous deposits during treatment of peritonitis. Use of heparin has been felt to be important in preventing intraperitoneal adhesions and in maintaining the peritoneal membrane surface. Heparin has been shown to have an adverse effect on gentamicin activity and could be a potential problem for patients treated for peritonitis by means of intraperitoneal administration of antibiotics. A concentration of less than 3 U/ml of heparin should not adversely effect gentamicin therapy.

One of the major problems is that different protocols have been used by different investigators to study antibiotics: parenteral or local administration, automated or manual technique, volumes used per day ranging from 8 to 36 liters, variable timing of inflow intraperitoneal dwell and drainage of dialysate. Continuous lavage has also been a controversial question. Control studies show no significant advantage in using peritoneal lavage. Continuous lavage should be restricted to cases in which treatment is started late, in those with purulent dialysate, or for cases of fungal infections.

Method of Antibiotic Administration

The success of any dosage regimen depends upon the selection of an adequate loading dose and an appropriate maintenance dose.

Determination of Loading Dose

The loading dose can be determined from the volume of distribution (Vd) and the desired therapeutic blood level for those agents which follow first-order elimination kinetics. This is best illustrated by the aminoglycosides because the therapeutic blood levels of these substances are well-established. The loading dose can be calculated by the following equation:

Loading dose (mg/kg) = Vd (l/kg) × peak level (mg/l).

In addition, the Vd can also be used to determine the dose of drug required to achieve a therapeutic blood level after its removal by peritoneal dialysis. For example, if a preinjection blood level of tobramycin is 1.5 mg/l and one wishes to raise it to a peak blood level of 6 mg/l, the additional dose required can be calculated as follows:

Dose (mg) 15 l × 4.5 mg/l = 70 mg

where 15 l = Vd of tobramycin: 0.22 l/kg × 70 kg.

The difference between current dose and the desired peak blood level of 6 mg/l is 4.5 mg/l.

Because of intersubject variability, the prediction is more accurate if one uses the Vd for the individual patient rather than published values. The Vd for a given drug in a given patient depends on the metabolic status of the patient, including among other factors hydration and protein level. The Vd can be determined by administering an intravenous dose and measuring the concentration immediately thereafter. Assuming a one-compartmental model of elimination, Vd can be determined as follows:

Vd (l) = dose (mg)/blood level (mg/l).

Determination of Maintenance Dose

Many normograms are available for determining the maintenance dosage in renal patients with failure; however, it is unwise to rely on published data entirely. Judgment should be guided by the toxicity of the drug. Indeed, blood monitoring is essential with certain agents.

For the many drugs which possess a wide therapeutic margin, one can administer the drug according to the following method: The prescribed maintenance dose is one-half of the loading dose, and the dosage interval is equal to the individual half-life of the drug, as estimated from normograms or as reported. This principle, although oversimplified, is easy to remember and appropriate for patients on CAPD because clearance does not change with time.

Practical Methods of Antibiotic Administration (Tables 2 and 3)

For this review, only reports on CAPD were used. These studies investigated such factors as the extent of removal, the peritoneal and total body clearance, the Vd, and the dialysis half-life. Intraperitoneal administration was the method used, and many authors report the degree of absorption from the peritoneal cavity and the resultant blood levels observed. This gives an indication of the usefulness of the intraperitoneal route alone in achieving effective blood levels of antibiotics. Most of the reports have focussed on the disposition of the aminoglycosides and the cephalosporins in CAPD.

Aminoglycosides

Few aminoglycosides have been thoroughly studied during CAPD. The elimination characteristics have been described for both intravenous (I.V.) and intraperitoneal routes; it appears that transfer of these drugs is greater from the peritoneum to the blood than from the blood to peritoneum. In any case, administration of furosemide must be stopped during aminoglycoside administration.

Gentamicin: In patients on CAPD, the half-life following an intravenous dose is 36 hours. For those requiring gentamicin to combat systemic infection, a loading dose of 1.5–2 mg/kg of body weight is followed by a maintenance dose of 0.7–1 mg/kg per 36 h I.V. This regimen achieves a peak level of 6 mg/l and a trough level of 2 mg/l. If gentamicin is administered intraperitoneally (I.P.) at a dose of 1.5 mg/kg of body weight, a peak concentration of 3.2 mg/l is attained at the end of 6 hours. The half-life of the drug is 36 hours. A loading dose given I.P. or I.V. followed by an I.P. dose of 7.5–10 mg/l of dialysis solution will produce a steady-state concentration or 5–8 mg/l at 6 hours.

Tobramycin: The half-life in CAPD patients following an I.V. dose is 36 hours. A loading dose of 1.5–2 mg/kg of body weight followed by 0.75–1 mg/kg every 36 hours should maintain a peak level of 6 mg/l and a trough level of 2 mg/l. Following an I.P. dose of 1.5 mg/kg, a peak serum concentration of 2–4 mg/l is achieved

Table 2. Elimination of drugs during CAPD

Drug	t½ life (h) Normal	t½ life (h) ESRD	Vd (l/kg)	Total body clearance ml/min	Peritoneal dialysis clearance in ml/min	Percentage removed per time period (hours)	t½ life (h) CAPD
Gentamicin	2	49	0.23	NR	2.9±0.4	20 ±6.9/24	36 ± 9
Tobramycin	2	69	0.23	8.0±2.5	3.8±1.0	16.5±2.6/24	34 ±18
Cefazolin	1.5	36	0.10	5.7±0.6	0.9±0.3	NR	30 ± 9
Cefotaxim	1	2.5	0.40	NR	3.2	NR	NR
Cefoxitin	0.7	15	0.10	20 ± 4	1.4±0.6	NR	7.8±2.7
Cefamandole	1	20	0.2	20 ± 6	3.2±1.6	7.3±2.3/24	10 ± 7
Vancomycin	6	220	0.6	7 ±2	1.4±0.4	NR	90 ±25
Cotrimoxazole	12	36	1.5	1.3±0.3	NR	NR	NR

Table 3. Current use of drugs during CAPD

Drug		Dose	Dwell period (h)	Percentage absorbed	Serum levels (mg/l); Mean ± SD at h	
Gentamicin	LD	50 mg/l	6	50	3.5 ± 1.5	at 6 h
		1.5 mg/kg		80		
	MD	7.5 mg/l	6	–	3.7 ± 1.5	
Tobramycin	LD	50 mg/l	6	85	4.3 ± 0.6	at 6 h
		1.5 mg/kg	6	60	5 – 6	at 6 h
	MD	8 mg/l	6	50	5 – 6	steady state
Cefazolin	LD	500 mg/l	6	88	55 ± 6	at 6 h
	MD	250 mg/l	6	65	110 ± 20	steady state
Cefotaxine		100 mg/l	8	90	–	
Cefamandole	LD	500 mg/l	6	70	31 ± 5	
	MD	250 mg/l	6	–	–	
Vancomycin		10 mg/kg	4	60	6.3	
		500 mg/l	6	55	23.7	

LD, loading dose; MD, maintenance dose.

in 6 hours and after a maintenance I.P. dose of 7.5–10 mg given each 6 hours, a serum level of 3.5–7 mg/l is achieved. The degree of absorption is unknown.

Amikacin: the reported half-life is about 60 hours. After a loading dose of 250 mg/l in a 2-liter bag and a maintenance dose of 50 mg/l every 6 hours, a peak level of 30 mg/l is obtained, with a trough level of 15 mg/l.

Cephalosporins

Most cephalosporins are eliminated by renal mechanisms, and both glomerular and tubular secretion contribute to this elimination. Therefore, in the case of renal failure, the half-lives of most of these drugs will be prolonged to an extent which varies from 2- to 20-fold. The cephalosporins are characterized by a wide therapeutic margin. Toxicity is rare and appears only at serum concentrations several times greater than the minimum effective therapeutic concentration. In contrast to aminoglycosides, specific dosage recommendations for this group of drugs vary widely, in part because of the existence of a widely acceptable dosage range. In general, one can recommend that patients on CAPD receive the same dosage of cephalosporins as those with renal failure and that one can omit supplementary dosage to correct for peritoneal removal.

Five cephalosporin antibiotics have been studied after intraperitoneal administration in patients on CAPD. The drugs were absorbed efficiently (70%–90%) over the dwell period. During this period, bactericidal blood levels were achieved. For example, in the case of cefazolin, a loading dose of 500 mg/l given I.P. and a maintenance dose of 250 mg/l given every 6 hours will provide a peak level of 55 mg/l and a trough level of 110 mg/l. The total body clearance for cefazolin is 7–8 ml/min.

Miscellaneous Drugs

Cotrimoxazole: Following oral, I.P., or I.V. administration during CAPD, the half-life of the drug does not differ from that in patients with renal failure. I.P. administration leads to significant absorption, the degree of which appears to be enhanced by peritonitis. Half-life is 34 and 96 hours for trimethoprim (TMP) and sulfamethoxazole (SMZ), respectively. The loading dose should be 80 mg of TMP and 400 mg of SMZ, and the maintenance dose 50 mg/l of SMZ and 10 mg/l of TMP.

Vancomycin: on CAPD, the half-life of vancomycin is reduced to 60 hours, compared with the 200 hours obtained in renal failure patients. Vancomycin is rapidly absorbed through I.P. administration. During a 6-hour dwell period, 60% is absorbed. The half-life of elimination is similar during CAPD regardless of whether the drug is administrated I.P. or I.V. We recommend a loading dose of 1000 mg I.V. and a maintenance dose of 500 mg every 4 days. With the I.P. administration, a loading dose of 500 mg/l and a maintenance dose of 25 mg/l achieves good therapeutical levels.

Conclusion

The pharmacokinetics of antibiotics used in CAPD patients have to be carefully studied and should be compared with those obtained in renal failure patients. Residual renal function modifies the dosage regimen. To use tables available in the literature, one must be aware of the method of administration, the diffusion process, the dialysis regimen, the dwell time, the associated drugs, and the intensity of the inflammation process. Constant adjustment of dosage schedules is mandatory.

References

1. Maher JF (1981) Transport kinetics of drugs and peritoneal dialysis in advances in peritoneal dialysis. In: Gahl GM, Kessel M, Nolph KD (eds) Proceedings of the second international symposium on peritoneal dialysis. Excerpta Medica, Amsterdam, p 37–40
2. Rubin J (1981) Comments on dialysis solution composition, antibiotic transport, poisoning and novel uses of peritoneal dialysis. In: Nolph KD (ed) Peritoneal dialysis Martinus Nijhoff, The Hague, pp 240–274
3. Manuel MA, Paton TW, Cornish WR (1983) Drugs and peritoneal dialysis. Perit Dial Bull 3: 117–125

Prevention and Treatment of Peritonitis in Children on CAPD

E. P. Leumann and J. Nemeth

Problems Related to Peritonitis

Peritonitis remains one of the major complications of continuous ambulatory peritoneal dialysis (CAPD). The magnitude of the problem is illustrated in Fig. 1, which
summarizes our results obtained during the last 5 years in 11 pediatric patients (129
treatment months): All patients except patient no. 5 had at least one episode of peritonitis; the average length of hospitalization for peritonitis was 2 days per treatment
month. Outpatient treatment of peritonitis was started only in 1984. No patient
died, but CAPD had to be abandonded and hemodialysis initiated in patients no. 2
and 3.

Similar peritonitis rates have been reported in other pediatric series [1–3]. Thus
the incidence of peritonitis is still too high, even though the routes of bacterial in-
vasion of the peritoneum and appropriate preventive measures are well-known [4]
and the equipment presently available is adequate. Obviously, it is not the technique itself which is to blame, but rather human failure at several levels: not only at
the level of the patient and his family, but also at the level of the medical staff.

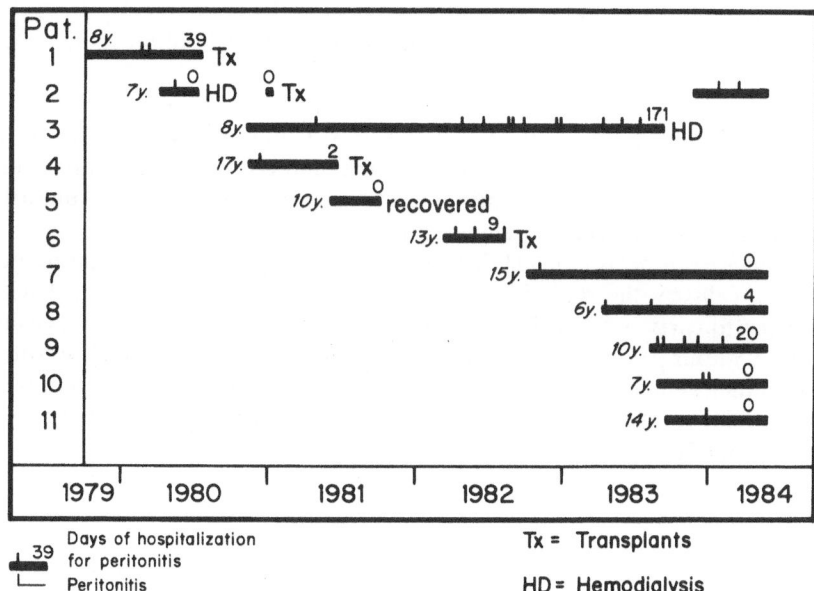

Fig. 1. Episodes of peritonitis (*vertical lines*) in 11 pediatric CAPD patients. Days of hospitalization for peritonitis are given for each patient. *Tx*, transplantation; *HD*, hemodialysis

Pediatric CAPD patients appear to have higher peritonitis rates than adult patients. However, these two groups of patients differ in two important respects: (a) the staff of adult programs is more experienced because of the greater number of patients, and (b) the pediatric patient, in contrast to the adult, does not usually perform the procedure. The burden of the procedure is primarily on the mother. The continuing stress often leads to parental fatigue, which we have observed in half of our patients. This is exemplified by patient no. 3, who did very well during the first year on CAPD despite an unfavorable social situation. However, repeated infections occurred subsequently which were clearly related to the mother's increasing exhaustion. On the other hand, the two patients who did *not* depend on their mothers because they performed the CAPD procedure themselves had the lowest infection rate of all our patients: Patient no. 7 had no peritonitis during 20 months of CAPD, and patient no. 11 had one episode during 9 months of CAPD.

Parental fatigue predisposes patients to episodes of peritonitis in three different ways: (a) CAPD is less carefully performed when the parent experiences fatigue, resulting in overt breaks in the antiseptic technique: (b) relatives without any CAPD training may be encouraged by the family to perform bag changes; and (c) minor problems such as an exit site infection or a disconnection are not immediately reported. The latter prevents the prompt initiation of simple preventive measures.

We were unable to determine how often improper handling occurred in our patients. However, we observed the latter two problems in four of the five families in whom parental fatigue was apparent. It should be a primary goal of any pediatric CAPD program to help these families in order to prevent or overcome parental fatigue [5].

Prevention of Peritonitis

The problems mentioned above clearly demonstrate where preventive measures are most likely to be effective:

Optimal instruction should be carried out by a single instructor, if possible, in order to keep all participants motivated. Instruction should also include training in uniform technique, regular follow-up visits, and continuing education, individually tailored to patient needs. Continuous supervision, a factor that is unfortunately often neglected, is essential to successful CAPD.

Family support is crucial [5]. This is best accomplished by regular home visits and phone calls by the dialysis nurse. Assistance of the mother by a backup person trained to carry out CAPD is extremely valuable. Our experience revealed that the fathers of our patients rarely performed bag changes (two of nine). Additional training rather should he provided for another person, e.g., the grandmother or some other relatives. Finally, patient selection is a delicate matter. CAPD is certainly not a good method for children whose parents are already experiencing depression before therapy is initiated. Continuous cycling peritoneal dialysis (CCPD) may be a valuable alternative to CAPD for patients whose families cannot tolerate the permanent burden of bag changes.

A *good CAPD technique* is essential, including optimal surgical insertion and fixation of the catheter. Unfortunately, stabilization of the catheter at the skin exit site is not always possible, especially in the hyperactive child. CAPD equipment and technique have to be impeccable. A decrease in the number of connections and disconnections might decrease the risk of infection. The windows of the room where CAPD is performed should always be closed during bag changes, and pets should not be allowed in the room. Betadine swabs are useful for clearing the exit site. However, we have observed a Betadine rash in three patients. Several procedures have been tried in an effort to prevent contamination during bag changes (antiseptics, sterilization, bacterial filters), but their value has yet to be proven [4, 6].

Finally, a few *additional measures* are important, e.g. good nutrition and proper personal hygiene. Routine home culturing of dialysate twice daily in infection-prone patients may help to detect bacterial infection before peritonitis becomes clinically manifest [7].

Treatment of Peritonitis

Therapy should be started as soon as possible. It should be effective and involve minimal discomfort to the patient. *Fig. 2* illustrates why it is important to start therapy immediately. The greater the delay (in hours) between the first symptoms and the start of therapy, the longer the time (in days) until the cloudy dialysate becomes clear. Patients should therefore come to the hospital as soon as cloudy dialysate is observed, and antibiotic therapy must be initiated immediately after one or two cycles of lavage. As an exception to this rule, diagnostic procedures and initiation of therapy may be done at home if the patient lives far away. Antibiotics should be ad-

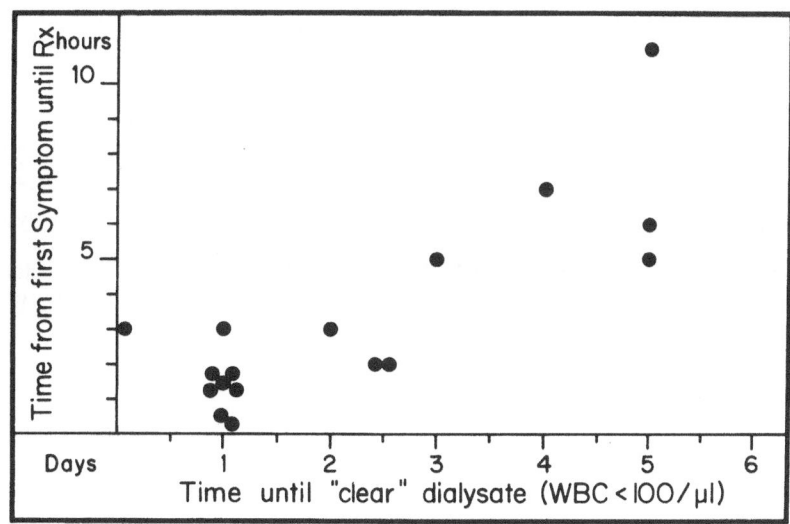

Fig. 2. Time elapsed between first symptom of peritonitis during CAPD and start of antibiotic therapy compared with time elapsed before dialysate is clear. Delays in beginning therapy (in hours, *vertical axis*) are associated with longer recovery times (in days, *horizontal axis*)

ded to the dialysate and continued according to the sensitivity of the organisms. In our series of 32 episodes of peritonitis observed in patients on CAPD, the majority of infections were caused by gram-positive organisms: 60% gram-positive, 9% gram-negative, 3% candida, and 28% unknown organisms. Nevertheless, we prefer to start therapy with both cefoxitin (150 mg/l) *and* gentamicin (first dose, 8 mg/l; thereafter, 6 mg/l) until the result of bacterial sensitivity is known. Depending on the results of sensitivity tests and on the clinical course, other antibiotics may be required [8]. Heparin (1000 µ/l) is added only as long as the dialysate is cloudy, and the usual schedule of bag changes is retained. Therapy is usually continued for 10 days. In cases of repeated infections or infection with candida, catheter removal is often necessary and should not be delayed [9].

Therapy should involve minimal discomfort to the patient. Initial lavage relieves pain. As we now carry out therapy on an outpatient basis, the patient's life is not significantly disrupted. It is hoped that preventive measures and improvement in the CAPD technique will ultimately reduce the incidence of peritonitis.

References

1. Baum M, Powell D, Calvin S, McDaid T, McHenry K, Mar H, Potter D (1982) Continuous ambulatory peritoneal dialysis in children. Comparison with hemodialysis. N Engl J Med 307:1537–1542
2. Eastham EJ, Kirpalani H, Francis D, Gokal R, Jackson RH (1982) Paediatric continuous ambulatory peritoneal dialysis. Arch Dis Child 57:677–680
3. Broyer M, Donckerwolcke RA, Brunner FP, et al. (1983) Combined report on regular dialysis and transplantation of children in Europe, XII, 1982. Proc Eur Dial Transplant Assoc 20:79–107
4. Oreopoulos DG, Vas SI, Khanna R (1983) Prevention of peritonitis during continuous ambulatory peritoneal dialysis. Perit Dial Bull [Suppl]3:18–20
5. Vigneux A, Hall Y, Willumsen J, Coughlin P, Balfe JW (1984) Pediatric CAPD – these families need help (Abstr). Perit Dial Bull [Suppl]4:S69
6. Parsons FM, Ahmed-Jushuf IH, Brownjohn AM, Coltman SJ, Gibson J, Young GA, Young JB (1983) Preventing CAPD peritonitis (letter). Lancet 2:907–908
7. Zaruba K, Oliveri M (1981) Prophylaxis of peritonitis in continuous ambulatory peritoneal dialysis (CAPD) by a simple microbiological patient self-check. Proc Eur Dial Transplant Assoc 18:275–279
8. Vas SI (1983) Microbiologic aspects of chronic ambulatory peritoneal dialysis. Kidney Int 23:83–92
9. Gray ED, Peters G, Verstegen M, Regelmann WE (1984) Effect of extracellular slime substance from staphylococcus epidermidis on the human cellular immune response. Lancet I:365–367

The Importance of the CAPD Nurse in Dealing with Patient/Family Burnout

T. L. Hall, M. Wilson, D. Davidson, and J. Foley

Introduction

Burnout or treatment fatigue has been loosely identified in both children and parents who undergo home peritoneal dialysis regimens. "Burnout" refers to a condition of stress within the child's family constellation which makes the CAPD/CCPD regimen intolerable. In our experience with 70 families, burnout has been an inevitability. The variables are: when will it occur? in what form will it be manifested and how long will it last?

Concepts and Goals of a Home Peritoneal Dialysis Management Program

Philosophic concepts essential to a pediatric CAPD/CCPD Program are:

1. Parents maintain the ultimate authority and responsibility for their child.
2. CAPD/CCPD is a successful maintenance treatment modality for children with end-stage renal disease.
3. Children undergoing CAPD/CCPD will have complications.

These three philosophical concepts, which are part of our program design, are useful to all members of the team in preparing for episodes of burnout. Firstly, it is important to remember that children belong to their parents and that parents hold the ultimate authority and responsibility for their children. Secondly, all team members must believe that CAPD/CCPD is a potentially successful treatment modality for children, and thirdly, every team member must acknowledge that children on home peritoneal dialysis regimens will have complications.

Critical to family education are the following concepts:

1. CAPD/CCPD procedures are simple, but the technique must be exact.
2. The child and his family are the first members of the team who cooperate and collaborate to provide CAPD/CCPD.
3. CAPD/CCPD is a family process.
4. Maintaining regular contact within the team is essential as well as advantageous.

The nursing staff begins to teach the four concepts listed above from the initial contact with each family. During training sessions, clinic visits, and any verbal consultations, one or more of these concepts are integrated into every interaction.

The goals of a home peritoneal dialysis management program can be summed up as follows:

1. To maintain each child in a well-dialyzed and biochemically stable state
2. To maintain each child on CAPD/CCPD in an infection-free state
3. To have each child's dialysis regimen require minimal changes in his/her family's lifestyle
4. To adjust the home peritoneal dialysis regimen so that each child can attend a school which is age-appropriate on a regular basis or otherwise fulfill developmentally appropriate tasks
5. To minimize hospitalization

Dealing with Patient/Family Burnout

These concepts and goals are then used to address manifestations of burnout. Previous end-stage renal disease (ESRD) treatment experiences of families will partially determine the initial response to CAPD/CCPD. The child and his family who are converting from hemodialysis usually experience a 3 to 6 month "honeymoon" period as described by Sorrels et al. [1] and usually do not develop symptoms of burnout until after that time. The child who begins CAPD after long-term conservative management during which careful preparation for CAPD/CCPD has been provided usually has a relatively smooth introductory period, provided the child is not severely ill.

Families who come to CAPD/CCPD following a failed transplant react with profound grief at the loss of the kidney and often have great difficulty in assimilating the training. Their early course of CAPD/CCPD can be quite stormy. The child who abruptly reaches ESRD requiring CAPD/CCPD has had little preparation for it. In addition, the families of these children experience grief over the loss of the child's health, and the parents have great difficulty making the initial adaptation to the therapeutic regimen. These last two groups frequently experience symptoms of burnout before CAPD/CCPD can even be started.

Early behavior patterns indicative of burnout are lateness to training appointments or clinic visits, failure to maintain accurate home records, and inappropriate responsibility shifts whithin the family. The latter include the parent who shifts responsibility for CAPD/CCPD to a child who is too young for that responsibility, or the older child who shifts responsibility for his own dialysis to a parent. Failure to take medication or perform exchanges, consistent unavailability by telephone, the inability to make decisions, and frequent episodes of infection are other behavior patterns indicative of treatment fatigue.

Nursing measures for dealing with burnout are varied. Regular telephone contact and home visits by the nursing staff provide support to families experiencing burnout. Referral to another family who has successfully coped with burnout is usually the most beneficial measure. Development of a referral list of families who are willing to be called on by other parents or children for support and/or ventilation is an important factor in planning to deal with burnout.

Table 1. CAPD/CCPD report card used as follow-up to regular clinic visits

Name _____	Your CAPD/CCPD Report Card		Date_____
Brought home records		Comments	
Brought food records			
Lab values	Normal value	Your value	Comments
Phosphorus	2.5 – 5.5		
Calcium	10 – 11.5		
Potassium	3.5 – 5.5		
Exit site	___ Yukky ___ OK ___ Beautiful	Comments	
Weight ___ OK ___ Need to gain ___ Too high	Comments	Blood Pressure ___ Normal ___ High ___ Low	Comments
Other things you need to know	Medication changes	Next clinic visit	

    The report card (Table 1) is used as a follow-up to regular clinic visits. In a technique similar to that used by school teachers for years, stickers can be attached to it as a reward or reminder that improvement is needed. The report cards are mailed to each child following each clinic visit. These report cards serve several functions: (a) They are rapid written reinforcement for any changes which must be made; (Written instructions are especially vital to families experiencing treatment fatigue); (b) They allow families to see the areas where they do not do as well in their own home without the scrutiny of staff; (c) They are a source of mail for the children. The response has been very favorable. The report card has been a major positive reinforcer.

    Implanting a Tenckhoff catheter in a doll or stuffed toy for performance of CAPD/CCPD allows the child an opportunity to practice the CAPD/CCPD technique and master the procedure. We frequently use these toys for initial training of both children and parents.

    The peritoneal dialysis cycler and conversion to CCPD has been a treatment method of major importance in dealing with CAPD burnout in families of very young children and in adolescents. With very young children, the parents' dialysis responsibilites are reduced to two times each day, and the daytime hours are free of dialysis exchanges. The teenager, who in our experience very frequently skips exchanges, also achieves free daytime hours. CCPD promotes dialytic compliance. It is very easy for the teenager to skip any or all CAPD exchanges without his parents' knowledge; however, it is very obvious if he or she does not connect to the cycler and dialyze each night.

Table 2. Incidence of peritonitis in family-performed dialysis at UCLA (August 1980 – March 1984)

Members trained per family	Training Sessions (n)	Experience (month)	Incidence of peritonitis	
			Episodes (n)	Rate (per patient – months)
One	20	339 (range, 2 – 40; mean, 17)	39	1/8.7
Two	15	209 (range, 2 – 26; mean, 14)	6	1/34.8
Total	35/70	548		

Summer camps for the children are another source of relief to fatigued parents and should not be overlooked.

Frequent episodes of peritonitis are thought to be indicative of burnout. Careful evaluation of peritonitis data can reveal areas which may require a change in methodology to reduce the infection rate. Table 2 shows such an example.

The information shown in Table 2 has led us vigorously to recommend training of two or more adults per family to carry out family-performed dialysis, as the data appear to indicate a reduction in the peritonitis rate when two adults are trained to perform the procedure.

The use of training sessions as a treatment for burnout should not be overlooked. Whenever possible, families whose child has suffered a failed transplant or arrived at ESRD unexpectedly should be given extended training. When parents or older children are taught in shorter sessions, which allows assimilation of information over 3 to 4 week periods, they have more time to deal with their grief and adapt more easily.

Retraining during burnout, especially when the sessions are presented as consultations, allows for ventilation as well as teaching. Use of primary nursing, i.e., one consistent nurse-teacher for all families is advantageous and is of particular importance for families experiencing burnout. The more diverse the life experiences and background of the professional team, especially the nursing staff, the more opportunities there are for successfully matching pairs of teachers and learners. The most successful CAPD/CCPD families make a strong identification with one staff member. In our experience, this staff member may be a nurse, physician, dietitian, or social worker. During episodes of burnout, changes in the dialysis regimen – whenever possible – should be initiated through this staff member, who can continuously set the family concrete goals and limits.

Finally, the initial distress call of a family experiencing burnout should be an indication to *bring them into the clinic,* of if this is not possible, to send them to a local physician for examination. Attempting to solve problems with families experiencing burnout does not work over the telephone. A distressed parent cannot make the assessments or decisions he or she can under normal conditions. Furthermore, such family members have difficulty following directions and need the opportunity to shift the responsibility, however briefly, to the professional staff.

In planning approaches for dealing with treatment fatigue, it is advisable for all team members to consider the following:

1. There are as many methods for dealing with burnout as the CAPD/CCPD team has the creativity to devise.
2. Adaptation to CAPD/CCPD should not be seen as having an end point; rather, it is a continuous process of accommodation.

Reference

1. Sorrels AJ, Mullins-Blackson C, Moncrief JW, et al. (1982) Getting back to reality: Psychosocial adjustments in CAPD ... continuous ambulatory peritoneal dialysis. Nephrology Nurse 4:22–23

Renal Transplantation in Children Treated by CAPD: A Report on a Cooperative Study

K. Schärer and R. N. Fine

Introduction

Successful renal transplantation (TP) is the ultimate treatment goal for almost all children with end-stage renal disease (ESRD). However, most children with ESRD require a prolonged period of dialysis treatment prior to TP. Since the advent of CAPD, an increasing number of pediatric patients have been managed by this technique, leading to a rising proportion of children on CAPD waiting for TP. Some pediatric nephrologists and transplant surgeons are hesitant to transplant children on CAPD because of the risk of peritonitis under immunosuppression, the presence of an unsuitable tissue bed for TP, or the fear of increased graft loss.

Only a few studies, primarily involving adult patients, have analyzed the effect of CAPD on the outcome of TP [1–6]. A single pediatric center has reported its experience with children who received grafts after being on CAPD for varying periods of time [7, 8].

Mechanical problems have rarely been encountered with TP for CAPD patients. Greater care on the part of the surgeons is apparently required to avoid puncturing the peritoneum in cases where the peritoneal cavity cannot be completely drained of all dialysate [2]. Usually, the graft is placed on the side opposite the catheter exit site to isolate the peritoneal catheter from the operative side.

Peritonitis, an obvious danger for pediatric patients, was first described in a 6-year-old girl who developed this complication immediately before TP and continued to have symptoms with positivie peritoneal fluid cultures in spite of antibiotic therapy. Following removal of the catheter at 4 weeks post-TP, the abdominal symptoms disappeared [2]. Pre-TP peritonitis poses an obvious danger in that it may create a nidus of infection in the peritoneal cavity which may become manifest after TP. Furthermore, a catheter left in situ might act as an irritating foreign body. It should be stressed, however, that comparative data on actuarial graft survival rates of patients undergoing TP following either CAPD or hemodialysis have not revealed a significant difference in outcome [2, 5, 7].

Because of the lack of data on the outcome of TP in pediatric patients on CAPD, a survey was performed among participants of the First International Symposium on CAPD in Children. This survey was accompanied by an inquiry on current policy in individual pediatric centers regarding suggested procedures for treating children by CAPD while awaiting TP.

Patients and Methods

A questionnaire was distributed among participants of the symposium asking for selected data on patients who were younger than 15.0 years at the start of CAPD and who subsequently underwent TP without hemodialysis immediately prior to TP. We asked for the patients' age, the number of episodes of peritonitis as defined by Pierratos [9], and other abdominal complications suffered while on CAPD both prior to and after TP. In addition, posttransplant data on the number of days on CAPD treatment, the number of hemodialysis sessions, the date of catheter removal, and the ultimate status of the patients were obtained. The participants were also asked to give their opinion on the present policy regarding TP in pediatric CAPD patients, especially with respect to the feasibility of TP in relation to episodes of peritonitis and on removal of the peritoneal catheter after TP.

Results

Reports for a total of 96 children were received: 52 reports from four American and 44 from 14 European pediatric centers. One child observed in a Japanese center and three children from a center in Israel were included in the group of European centers. Of the centers reporting, 11 contributed data on fewer than five children, but only two centers contributed more than ten patients. The patients reported on earlier by Balfe et al. [7, 8] are included in this study. Patients for whom the dates of the start of CAPD or of TP were unknown were excluded. The analysis of five patients who underwent a second transplant while being treated by CAPD was not included.

In Table 1, the *age* of the patients at initiation of CAPD is shown. The patients from the American centers were slightly but not significantly younger than those from the European centers. The mean time interval between the start of CAPD and the first TP was 11.6 months (Table 2). This interval was less than 12 months in 53% of all patients, between 1 and 2 years in 42%, and more than 2 years in 5% of the patients, with no significant difference between the American and the European patients.

Table 1. Age at start of CAPD treatment of 96 pediatric patients who subsequently received transplants

Age (years)	American centers (n, 52)	European centers (n, 44)	All centers (n, 96)
0 – 2	12	4	16
2 – 5	8	9	17
5 – 10	17	15	32
10 – 15	15	16	31
Mean age (years)	6.8	7.9	7.3

Table 2. Time elapsed between start of CAPD and first transplant

Interval (months)	American centers (n, 52)	European centers (n, 44)	All centers (n, 96)
0 – 3	5	3	8
3 – 6	10	8	18
6 – 9	7	10	17
9 – 12	4	4	8
12 – 15	11	4	15
15 – 18	8	4	12
18 – 24	3	10	13
24 – 36	2	1	3
> 36	2	–	2
Mean interval (months)	12.1	11.1	11.6

Before TP, a total of 180 episodes of *peritonitis* occurred in 70 patients during a period of 93.8 patient years on CAPD; which corresponded to one episode every 6.2 months for all 96 patients. Further abdominal complications observed before TP included: inguinal herniae, 10; tunnel infections, 4; cuff erosions, 3; pleural effusion, 2; umbilical herniae, 2; hernia at the site of pyelostomy, hernia at the site of the abdominal scar, ascites, scrotal swelling, or loss of ultrafiltration, one each, and other complications, 6.

Posttransplant peritonitis developed nine times in seven patients (two American, five European) from six centers. Details are given in Table 3. At the time of TP, these patients were younger than those without posttransplant peritonitis (mean age, 5.7 and 8.4 years, respectively (NS). The mean time period on CAPD before TP was 13.1 months for patients with posttransplant peritonitis as compared with 11.2 months for patients who were free of posttransplant peritonitis (NS). In five of the seven patients affected by posttransplant peritonitis, previous CAPD treatment had lasted for 12 months or more, compared with 64% in the grafted patients who did not develop this complication. In four patients with posttransplant peritonitis, one or more episodes of peritonitis occurred before TP. This corresponds to an overall incidence of one episode every 4.6 patient months, as compared with one episode every 6.4 patient months in patients without posttransplant peritonitis (NS). One 15-month-old child developed ascites and bowel perforation of unknown origin with subsequent peritonitis.

Three children with posttransplant peritonitis continued CAPD treatment after TP, apparently because of graft failure (Table 3), but none had hemodialysis after TP. The catheter was not removed from two of these patients until the last observation, 4 and 5 months after TP. In the third child (KD), the catheter was removed on day 38 due to peritonitis, and hemodialysis was initiated. The graft did not function in a fourth child (SW) in whom posttransplant peritonitis was diagnosed at day 7: *candida albicans* was cultured in a renal biopsy specimen and in the dialysate. Subsequently, the peritonitis resolved after removal of the Tenckhoff catheter, but the graft had to be removed, and 6 weeks later, CAPD was successfully resumed [7].

Table 3. Peritonitis in seven pediatric patients after transplantation (TP) following CAPD treatment

Initials of patients	Age at time of TP (years)	Pre-TP period on CAPD (months)	Episodes of pre-TP peritonitis while on CAPD	Diagnosis of post-TP peritonitis (days after TP)	Organism found in post-TP peritonitis	Other post-TP abdominal complications	Duration of post-TP CAPD	Time elapsed before catheter removal after TP (days)	Outcome at last post-TP observation
American patients:									
JB	1 3/12	15	1	5	E. coli Klebsiella	ascites with bowel perforation	0	14	F [9 months]
SW	1 11/12	2.5	0	7	Klebsiella Monilia		0	46	L→CAPD→ 2nd graft: F→died
European patients:									
ND	2 8/12	18	0	8 (asymptomatic)	Staphylococcus epidermidis	—	0	18	F [13 months]
DS	5 1/12	15	5	8		—	0	6 months	F [5 months]
KD	7 0/12	7	5	(2 episodes)		—	37 days	38	L→hemodialysis 2nd graft: F
JE	8 6/12	23	9	(2 episodes)		—	from day 3 (continuing)	not removed until month 4	L→CAPD [4 months]
JP	13 9/12	12	0 10 bouts of "allergic peritoneal reactions"		Bacterium anitratrum	—	5 months (continuing)	not removed until month 5	L→CAPD

F, funcioning graft; L, graft loss; in brackets: time post-TP at last observation.

Ascites was the most common abdominal complication after TP. It was noted mainly in three American centers, where it occurred in nine of 19, eight of 23, and three of five patients, respectively. Posttransplant ascites was reported in a single child from Europe. One patient developed a purulent abscess in the graft region which had to be drained surgically 6 weeks after TP, with good subsequent graft function. In addition, scrotal edema, abdominal hematoma, and sclerosing peritonitis were noted in one patient each.

The time of *catheter removal* varied greatly from center to center and from patient to patient. Dates on the exact time of catheter removal were available for 68 patients without posttransplant peritonitis (Table 4). In 19 patients, the catheters were removed at the time of TP; for the remaining patients, the time of removal ranged from 2 to 113 days after TP, with an average interval of 22 days. Although the mean time of catheter removal was the same in the American and European centers, a larger proportion of catheters in the United States and Canada were removed at the time of TP (14/43, compared with 5/25 in Europe). Only in 11 of the 68 cases did the time that the catheter was left in situ exceed 30 days. In nine of the 11 patients, some complication other than peritonitis occurred after TP: ascites (3 patients) graft abscess (1 patient) or insufficient graft function which required further CAPD (6 patients) or hemodialysis (3 patients).

In situations where *dialysis therapy* was needed after TP, CAPD was the method of choice for 17 patients and hemodialysis for seven patients, including three patients with posttransplant peritonitis. The *outcome of TP* at the last observation was assessed as follows: whereas 21 of 89 patients (24%) without posttransplant peritonitis lost their graft, graft loss occurred in four of seven patients who suffered this complication. A causal relationship between peritonitis and graft loss was, however, difficult to delineate from the data available. Nine of the 11 patients without posttransplant peritonitis whose peritoneal catheter was removed more than 30 days after TP had a functioning graft at the time of the last assessment. However, most of them required intercurrent dialysis therapy.

In all, 18 centers participated in the *inquiry on current policy for TP* in children treated by CAPD. All participants felt that children scheduled to receive grafts should be free of peritonitis or other abdominal complications before TP, but views on the duration of the peritonitis-free period differed (Table 5). As expected, most but not all centers indicated that the interval which must elapse after discontinuing antibiotic therapy before TP can be performed may be shorter. Four centers found that no antibiotic-free interval was needed prior to TP; only one center regarded a period longer than 2 weeks as necessary.

The critical question of whether the peritoneal *catheter* should be *removed* at time of TP and hemodialysis instituted if required subsequently received an affirmative reply from four centers and a negative one from 13 centers. The responses of the latter group regarding the appropriate time for catheter removal after TP were also far from being unanimous. Most centers who prefered to leave the catheter in place to allow for possible CAPD treatment after TP were of the opinion that (in cases where no further dialysis is required) the catheter should be removed between 7 and 14 days after TP (Table 6). However, four centers found that the catheter should be retained for a minimum of 90 days. This opinion differs somewhat from

Table 4. Time elapsed after TP when peritoneal catheter was removed in children previously treated by CAPD (without posttransplant peritonitis)

Days after TP	American centers (*n*, 43)	European centers (*n*, 25)	All centers (*n*, 68)
0	14	5	19
1– 7	6	–	6
8 – 14	7	4	11
15 – 30	9	12	21
31 – 90	5	3	8
> 90	2	1	3
Mean time (days)	22	22	22

Table 5. Criteria for transplantation in children on CAPD according to the inquiry conducted in 18 pediatric centers

Minimum number of days on CAPD required before transplantation	When patient is free of peritonitis and/or other abdominal complications[a]	When no antibiotic therapy is required[a]
0	–	4
2 – 3	2	–
4	1	2
7	2	6
10	2	1
14	6	4
20	1	–
28 – 30	4	1
> 30	–	–

[a] Figures indicate number of study participants giving affirmative response.

Table 6. Criteria for removal of peritoneal catheter in transplanted children previously treated by CAPD, according to the inquiry conducted at 18 patients centers

Time elapsed between TP and removal of peritoneal catheter (days)	Catheter removal when no further dialysis is required after TP[a]	Catheter removal after last post-TP CAPD treatment[a]
0 – 6	–	1
7 – 14	8	4
15 – 30	1	–
60 – 90	1	–
> 90	4	4
dependent on degree of renal function	–	2

[a] Figures indicate number of study participants giving affirmative response.

the actual figures reported by the same centers for previously observed patients (Table 4).

Finally, the question of whether, drugs may be administered through the peritoneal catheter after TP was answered affirmatively in six and negatively in nine instances.

The personal views expressed concerning problems of TP in CAPD children underscored fears that the catheter will end up being colonized if left in situ, but that delaying its removal is justified in cases where the graft does not function well immediately after TP or where ascites develops after TP.

Discussion

Since in the past many patients treated by CAPD, especially adults, were not regarded as suitable candidates for TP, problems arising in the CAPD patient prior to and following TP have been neglected. Only a few reports on adult patients treated by CAPD have dealt with this subject [1–6].

Posttransplant peritonitis in adult patients on CAPD has been described rarely. In two recent combined studies, none of 49 grafted adult patients had this complication [3, 5]. Our survey reveals a 7% incidence of posttransplant peritonitis in patients starting CAPD before the age of 15 years. This finding leads to the question of why children are more prone to posttransplant peritonitis than adult patients.

Three factors might be related to the development of posttransplant peritonitis in pediatric patients: (a) their youth, (b) repeated peritoneal infection during CAPD before TP, and (c) lack of immediate graft function. The extent to which these factors contribute to posttransplant peritonitis cannot be determined definitely at the present time. The slightly younger age of the risk group in our study might be explained by increased exposure to bacterial contamination or different immunologic reactivity as compared with older children. According to our data, it is not probable that repeated peritoneal infections prior to TP play a major role in causing posttransplant peritonitis. Although the time on CAPD treatment was slightly longer in the risk group, the incidence of pre-TP peritonitis per month on CAPD was not significantly different in children with and without post-TP peritonitis. Furthermore, three of the seven cases who developed post-TP peritonitis were peritonitis-free before TP.

It seems possible that insufficient immediate graft function requiring prolonged periods of peritoneal dialysis treatment and high doses of immunosuppressive agents are the primary factors responsible for transplant peritonitis in certain patients. In one adolescent patient reported to our survey but excluded from analysis because of the age limit, fungal peritonitis complicated graft failure and necessitated removal of the graft, followed by sepsis and death. In individual cases, it may be difficult to decide whether graft loss is the consequence of post-TP peritonitis or the primary event.

The second issue is the optimal time for posttransplant removal of the peritoneal catheter. In adult patients, it has been suggested that the peritoneal access be left in place for up to 90 days after TP [7]. According to our survey, long exposure is rare and, in fact, is believed to provoke peritonitis, although the data do not validate this concept. Continuing access to the peritoneal cavity in the period immediately following TP may be important for draining ascitic fluid [7].

Conclusions

From the experience reported, it is difficult to propose a uniform strategy for children on CAPD awaiting or undergoing TP. There is no contraindication for TP in these children, even when repeated periods of peritonitis have occurred before TP. It appears reasonable to require a *period of 1–2 weeks free of peritonitis* or other abdominal complications to elapse before considering a child as a candidate for grafting. Some centers feel, however, that this interval could be even shorter, especially if previous episodes of peritonitis were asymptomatic, while other centers extend this period up to 30 days. Most centers believe that the requirement of a 1- to 2-week period free of antibiotic therapy following peritonitis is desirable before TP.

Following TP, *CAPD may serve three purposes:* blood purification in case of graft loss, treatment of posttransplant peritonitis, and drainage of ascitic fluid. CAPD presents a suitable mode of treatment allowing efficient dialysis, even for prolonged periods of time, for the majority of children requiring blood purification. It appears that the prophylactic creation of an arteriovenous fistula in CAPD patients to allow hemodialysis in case of graft failure is generally not required.

Most participants in this survey indicated that the *catheter should be left in situ for 1–2 weeks after TP* even if no post-TP dialysis is required. Routine cultures of the peritoneal fluid are not recommended for cases without complications. Following the advice of participants, the external end of the catheter should be capped after TP. After initiation of good graft function, the catheter may be removed a few days after TP, especially if prospects for recovery are good (living donors, good immunologic matching, absence of severe uremic complications before TP). In favorable cases, some participants would suggest immediate removal of the catheter at the time of TP, especially if a vascular access is available. Where there have been frequent bouts of peritonitis before TP, it appears advantageous instead to pursue post-TP hemodialysis.

If any transient CAPD treatment becomes necessary after TP, some centers suggest that the catheter be removed about 1 week after the last day of CAPD. There are no contraindications for administering drugs by the intraperitoneal route after TP.

Difficulties in managing CAPD patients after TP may arise when fever caused either by peritonitis or by rejection develops. Frequent monitoring of the dialysis fluid for infectious agents is required in such cases.

Acknowledgements. We acknowledge with thanks the following colleagues, who have contributed to this survey with data from the following pediatric centers: S. R. Alexander (Portland, Orgeon), O. Amon and F. Bläker (Hamburg, FRG), H. J. Andersen (Odense, Denmark), J. W. Balfe (Toronto, Canada), K. E. Bonzel (Heidelberg, FRG), M. Broyer (Paris, France), A. Drukker (Jerusalem, Israel), R. J.

Hogg (Dallas, Texas), C. Holmberg (Helsinki, Finland), E. C. Kohaut (Birmingham, Alabama), E. Leumann (Zürich, Switzerland), R. H. K. Mak (London, UK), L. Monnens (Nijmegen, Netherlands), R. J. Postlethwaite (Manchester, UK), T. Sakai (Kanagawa, Japan), A. Tranaeus (Huddinge, Sweden), M. H. Winterborn (Birmingham, UK), and E. D. Wolff (Rotterdam, Netherlands).

References

1. Cardella CJ (1980) Renal transplantation in patients on peritoneal dialysis. Perit Dial Bull 1:12–14
2. Gokal R, Ramos JM, Veitch P et al. (1981) Renal transplantation in patients on continuous peritoneal dialysis. Proc Eur Dial Transplant Assoc 18:222–227
3. Ryckelynck JP, Verger C, Pierre D et al. (1984) Early posttransplantation infections in CAPD patients. Perit Dial Bull 4:40–41
4. Evans DH, Sorkin MI, Nolph KD et al (1981) Continuous ambulatory peritoneal dialysis and transplantation. Trans Am Soc Art Intern Organs 27:320–322
5. Shapira Z, Shmueli D, Yussim A et al (1984) Kidney transplantation in patients on continuous ambulatory peritoneal dialysis. Proc Eur Dial Transplant Assoc (in press)
6. Patel S, Rosenthal JT, Hakala TR (1983) Management of the peritoneal dialysis catheter after transplantation. Transplantation 36:589–590
7. Stefanidis CJ, Balfe JW, Arbus GS et al (1983) Renal transplantation in children treated with continuous ambulatory peritoneal dialysis. Perit Dial Bull 3:5–8
8. Balfe JW, Stefanidis CJ, Steele BT et al (1984) Continuous ambulatory peritoneal dialysis: clinical aspects. In: Fine RN, Gruskin AB (eds) End-stage renal disease in children. Saunders, Philadelphia, pp 135–148
9. Pierratos A (1984) Peritoneal dialysis glossary. Perit Dial Bull 4:2–3

Paediatric Nephrology

Proceedings of the Sixth International Symposium of
Paediatric Nephrology, Hannover, Federal Republic of
Germany, 29. August – 2. September 1983

Editors: **J. Brodehl, J. H. H. Ehrich**

1984. 74 figures, 89 tables. XXVII, 418 pages.
ISBN 3-540-13598-7

Contents: Plenary Lectures: Structure and Function of the
Renal Medulla. The Elucidation of Renal Transport Process:
A Multidisciplinary Approach. Immunopathogenesis of
Glomerular Diseases. Bacterial Virulence and Host Defence
in Acute and Recurrent Urinary Tract Infection. Philosophy
and Ethics of Multicenter International Controlled Clinical
Trials in Children. Paediatric Nephrology – Past Achieve-
ments and Future Goals. The Continued Care of Paediatric
Patients into Adult Life. – Symposia Presentations: Physiol-
ogy of Kidney Development. Clinical Aspects of the Developing Kidney. Nutrition in Paediatric Renal Disease. New
Techniques in Paediatric Dialysis Treatment. Acute Renal
Failure. Kidney Transplantation. Cystinosis. Psychosocial
Aspects in Children with Chronic Renal Disease. Immuno-
logically Mediated Tubulointerstitial Nephritis. Glomerulopathies in Systemic Diseases. Glomerular Diseases in
Special Populations. Immunology and Coagulation in Nephrotic Syndrome. Haemolytic Uraemic Syndromes. Recur-
rent Urinary Tract Infection. Vesico-ureteral Reflux and
Renal Scarring. The Neurogenic Bladder Dysfunktion.
Renal Dysplasias and Cystic Diseases. Diagnosis and Treatment. Vitamin D in Renal Diseases. Prostaglandins and
Inhibitors. – Subject Index.

The proceedings of the Sixth International Symposium of
Paediatric Nephrology, held in Hannover in the Fall of 1983,
document the state-of-the-art in the field. All of the papers
from the four plenary sessions and 95% of the symposia
presentations are included in this volume.
The wide range of topics chosen for discussion-scientific and
experimental research work, diagnostic procedures, therapeutic methods including dialysis and renal transplantation,
and metabolic and genetic aspects of children with renal
diseases – reflects the present status of paediatric nephrology worldwide.

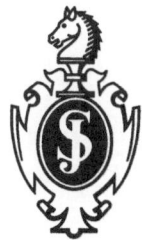

Springer-Verlag
Berlin
Heidelberg
New York
Tokyo